Innovations in Cancer and Palliative Care Education

Edited by

Lorna Foyle
Lecturer, Cancer and Palliative Care
University of Leeds

and

Janis Hostad
Lecturer/Education and Development Coordinator
Hull and East Yorkshire Hospitals Trust

Foreword by
Nigel Sykes
Medical Director
St Christopher's Hospice, London

Radcliffe Publishing
Oxford ● New York

Radcliffe Publishing Ltd
18 Marcham Road
Abingdon
Oxon OX14 1AA
United Kingdom

www.radcliffe-oxford.com
Electronic catalogue and worldwide online ordering facility.

_____

© 2007 Lorna Foyle and Janis Hostad

The authors have asserted their right under the Copyright, Designs and Patents Act 1998 to be identified as authors of this work.

All rights reserved. No part of this publication may be reproduced, stored in a retrieval system or transmitted, in any form or by any means, electronic, mechanical, photocopying, recording or otherwise, without the prior permission of the copyright owner.

British Library Cataloguing in Publication Data

A catalogue record for this book is available from the British Library.

ISBN-13: 978 1 84619 056 8

Typeset by Advance Typesetting Ltd, Oxford
Printed and bound by TJI Digital, Padstow, Cornwall

Contents

Foreword   v

Preface   vii

About the editors   ix

List of contributors   x

Acknowledgements   xii

1   High-fidelity clinical simulation in cancer and palliative care education   1
   Neil Pease

2   The use of competencies in palliative care education   13
   Robert Becker

3   Problem-based learning: not such a problem   24
   Jean Fisher

4   The conundrums of delivering chemotherapy care: tackling the
   educational challenges   37
   Krystina Koslowska

5   Leading the way: the role of education in achieving clinical standards
   in the haematological oncology setting   48
   Kirsten Midgley

6   Approaches to multi-professional radiotherapy education   62
   Kathryn Guyers

7   Taking the pain out of pain management teaching   70
   Sharon Wood

8   Teaching symptom management   85
   Sarah Callin and Fiona Hicks

9   Teaching ethics in cancer and palliative care   96
   Janet Holt

10   Information for service users: educational implications   107
   Sally-Ann Spencer Grey

11   Pre-registration nursing: cancer and palliative care education   125
   Julie MacDonald and Tracey McCready

12   Is nurse education in paediatric and adolescent oncology fit for
   purpose?   136
   Sue Fallon and Linda Sanderson

13   Educational strategies to improve palliative care for learning-disabled
   patients   148
   Jackie Saunders

14 Palliative care in nursing homes: an educational challenge   160
   Patricia Hirst and Anne Boyce

15 Family care: sensitive and dynamic approaches to teaching   169
   Pam Firth

16 Mapping the landscape: spirituality in cancer and palliative care
   education   185
   Elizabeth Foster

17 'Let's talk about it – we never do.' Sexual health in cancer and
   palliative care: an educational dilemma?   197
   Janis Hostad

18 Complementary therapies: progressing from knowledge to wisdom   220
   Ruth Sewell

19 Rehabilitation: imperatives in cancer and palliative care education   236
   Kim Platt-Johnson

20 Teaching approaches to survivorship issues in cancer care   251
   Candy Cooley

21 Health and social policy education: universally relevant, studiously
   avoided   260
   Lorna Foyle

Index   274

Foreword

This is the second book in the series *Dimensions in Cancer and Palliative Care Education*. The first book having placed cancer and palliative care education in its healthcare context, it is now time to look at some innovations in this field.

Palliative care is a specialty whose time has come. The NHS Cancer Plan published in 2000 had palliative care at its heart (or not too far from it, anyway) and in 2004 palliative care was dignified by its own guidance document from the National Institute for Clinical Excellence. In addition, although 'palliative care' and 'cancer' remain closely linked in the minds of many, the UK government imperative to make palliative care available to all who need it, regardless of disease label, has gathered pace. Having begun with the SNMAC/SMAC report of 1992 this drive has most recently found expression in a series of National Service Frameworks that have called for palliative care to be available to people with disorders such as neurodegenerative disease or heart failure. Outside the UK the WHO now regards palliative care as a fundamental component of Cancer Control Programmes, and there are signs that at last the pressing need for palliative care to have a similar status in HIV/AIDS programmes in sub-Saharan Africa and elsewhere is starting to be recognised by the agencies concerned.

British palliative care is unique among UK healthcare specialties in being provided to a considerable extent by providers outside the NHS. However, these voluntary providers for the most part receive a significant element of their funding from the NHS and so are not exempt from national priorities. This means that they also must answer to the agendas of equity and choice, as exemplified by the widening of access to palliative care for people with non-malignant conditions and to vulnerable and under-served groups. '

As a result there has never been a period when education in palliative care issues has been more topical or in demand, and some of the areas mentioned will be covered in the third book in this series (due to be published in 2008). Meanwhile, the present book gives us a three-dimensional view of how to respond to the demands on cancer and palliative care education today, set particularly in a British context but, of course, capable of extrapolation to other settings. These three dimensions of innovation can be summarised as: What do you teach? How do you teach it? To whom do you teach it? Innovation in all three aspects simultaneously may be difficult to achieve, but all who have a responsibility for education are faced with the challenges of making their teaching more effective (and demonstrating that they have done so), keeping abreast of advancing knowledge and clinical practice, and of reaching out to groups of learners who hitherto have been neglected.

Therefore this book contains chapters that might refresh those who teach a subject area regularly, and others that might help educators embark on handling a topic new to their teaching repertoire. On one hand the staples of cancer and palliative care teaching, such as pain and symptom control, chemotherapy and radiotherapy are covered, but with an aim of helping the reader freshen and reinvigorate their approach to the material. On the other hand there are descriptions of how to tackle less well-trodden topics such as sexuality, public communication and survivorship that both raise the profile of these important but overlooked subjects and provide encouraging pointers as to how to embark on helping others to learn about them.

As well as neglected subjects there are also considerations of how to reach neglected student groups such as nursing home staff and carers of people with learning disabilities. The increasing proportion of nursing home residents recognised to have palliative care needs, together with the under-access of people with learning difficulties to palliative care services, mean that these are vital pieces of educational outreach.

Throughout all this runs the need to assess the effectiveness of our teaching and the quality of the staff who participate in it. Both aspects of this requirement to assess are met by the use of competencies – what competencies do individuals have, and how have these been enhanced by the education in which they have participated? In attempting to give a multifaceted account of cancer and palliative care teaching as it is (or should be) today, this book also includes a consideration of the issues surrounding the use of competencies as a method of education outcome assessment.

The pressure for accountability in all kinds of service provision implies, among other things, an increasing professionalisation of healthcare education. Nursing and the Allied Health Professions have led the way and to a large extent it is from this background that this book and its forerunner have emerged. With the formation of the Academy of Medical Educators, doctors are catching up. But they will have to battle with the conundrum of how to balance the concentration on the role of educator with the maintenance of the role of clinician that alone can give clinical teaching life and credibility. This book will not solve that dilemma but it will be of significant help to anyone in this field whose concern is the delivery of effective and appropriate education.

Dr Nigel Sykes
Medical Director
St Christopher's Hospice, London
March 2007

Preface

The nature of education is multi-dimensional – hence the series title, *Dimensions in Cancer and Palliative Care Education*. The first book in this series, entitled *Delivering Cancer and Palliative Care Education*, looked at contextualising the role and relevance of cancer and palliative care education in current healthcare provision in a twenty-first-century culture of technological advancement. Inherent within this climate of scientific change, patients and healthcare professionals alike are seeking to connect and communicate at a deeper level when encountering each other during the healthcare experience of both patient and carer. Cancer and palliative care diagnoses often produce challenging and rhetorical questions for patients and lay carers as they struggle to achieve a more meaningful understanding of the nature of illness, life and existence itself. Clinicians today are probably challenged more by the esoteric components of care delivery than by the more practical and scientific elements. Both of these types of care are necessary, and a careful blend of these abilities is essential to ensure that a high standard of quality care is delivered and experienced. The education of clinicians to achieve these high standards is exacting and often requires some innovative approaches. With this in mind, we sought out those educators whom we had heard at conferences or who had been recommended to us because of their knowledge base and their command of their topic area. Invitations were issued, and the quantity and quality of the responses far exceeded the requirements for one book. Therefore there will be another volume in this series, which will cover aspects not addressed within this book (due to be published in 2008). The reader will not be disappointed by the contributions to the present book. Not only have the contributors shared their extensive knowledge base, but they have also divulged some very practical and original methods of teaching their topics.

As the chapters for this book were received, the title of the book – *Innovations in Cancer and Palliative Care Education* – became apparent without much deliberation as the composition and content of the chapters illustrated just how imaginative and innovative our contributors were in their educational role. Prepare to be as informed, intrigued and inspired as we were whilst editing the book.

This series was initiated in order to assist full-time educationalists in cancer and palliative care by extending their skills and knowledge in the delivery of these topics. Similarly, clinicians who have an educational responsibility and who are exploring different aspects of subject-specific topics and teaching methods will find a wealth of useful and practical information in this book. Educationalists in other fields of healthcare provision will also glean knowledge about different teaching styles and techniques with the possibility of enhancing their skills.

The authors' contributions provide the reader with a valuable resource with which to develop their knowledge of specific current themes in cancer and palliative care provision, while at the same time providing them with a diverse range of educational strategies.

Most of the chapters have been arranged in a specific order so as to maximise the learning experience. In a few chapters this format has not been adhered to, in order to accommodate the nuances and finer points of a particular topic. The quotes at the beginning of each chapter have been selected by the authors either to summarise the contents of the chapter or to stimulate the reader's thinking about the potential of the chapter. Each chapter includes an aim and learning outcomes in true educational tradition to guide the reader in achieving the appropriate learning from the chapter. The introduction and body of each chapter are intended to impart the information necessary to enable the reader to achieve the learning outcomes.

At the end of each chapter, in addition to the conclusion, key points summarise the pertinent issues and concerns that have been raised in the chapter, and a list of implications for the reader's own practice raises questions to challenge the reader's thinking and assist them in applying key concepts to clinical practice. Where appropriate, lists of further reading and useful resources have been supplied in order to assist the reader in their professional development.

This book has sought to demystify some of the educational processes, and it provides a kaleidoscope of teaching and learning theories and techniques for the subjects of cancer and palliative care. Some educational tools are provided for applying the theoretical aspects of palliative care and cancer education to the clinical care of those affected by a diagnosis of cancer and/or palliative care. It is hoped that this book not only inspires creative teaching but also, through this education, motivates clinicians to deliver total quality care in as many effective and innovative ways as possible.

> *If you have built castles in the air, your work need not be lost; that is where they should be. Now put the foundations under them.*
> *Henry David Thoreau (1817–1862)*

Lorna Foyle
Janis Hostad
March 2007

About the editors

Lorna Foyle MSc, BA Hons, Cert Ed, Dip HE Pall Care, NDN Cert, RGN Cert in Counselling, NLP Practitioner
Lecturer, Cancer and Palliative Care, University of Leeds

Janis Hostad MSc, BA Hons, Cert Ed, Dip HE Pall Care, NDN Cert, RGN Diploma in Counselling, NLP Practitioner
Lecturer/Education and Development Coordinator, Hull and East Yorkshire Hospitals Trust.

The two editors' combined experience in cancer and palliative care adds up to 40 years. The early part of their experience was firmly rooted in the clinical setting while in latter years their focus has switched to education and research.

List of contributors

Robert Becker
Lecturer
Shropshire and Mid Wales Hospice, Shrewsbury and University of Stafford

Anne Boyce
Palliative Care Clinical Nurse Specialist
Wheatfields Hospice

Sarah Callin
SR Pain Management Team
Leeds Teaching Hospitals, Leeds

Candy Cooley
Palliative Care Development Manager
South Worcestershire PCT

Sue Fallon
Lecturer
School of Healthcare, University of Leeds

Pam Firth
Head of Family Support
Isabel Hospice, Welwyn Garden City

Jean Fisher
Head of Education
St Michael's Hospice, Hereford

Elizabeth Foster
Macmillan Nurse, Specialist Palliative Care
North East Lincolnshire PCT

Kathryn Guyers
Lecturer
School of Healthcare, University of Leeds

Fiona Hicks
Consultant, Palliative Care Team
St James University Hospital, Leeds

Patricia Hirst
Macmillan Clinical Nurse Specialist in Palliative Care (Care Homes)
The Prince of Wales Hospice, Pontefract

Janet Holt
Senior Lecturer
School of Healthcare, University of Leeds

Krystina Koslowska
Macmillan Senior Chemotherapy Sister
Leeds Teaching Hospitals, Leeds

Julie MacDonald
Lecturer
Faculty of Health and Social Care, University of Hull

Tracey McCready
Lecturer
Faculty of Health and Social Care, University of Hull

Kirsten Midgley
Clinical Educator
Leeds Teaching Hospitals, Leeds

Neil Pease
Head of Education, Training and Development Centre
Bassetlaw Hospital, Worksop

Kim Platt-Johnson
Lecturer
School of Healthcare, University of Leeds

Linda Sanderson
Senior Lecturer
University of Central Lancashire

Jackie Saunders
Head of Education
St Nicholas Hospice, Bury St Edmunds

Ruth Sewell
Head of Special Projects
Penny Brohn Cancer Centre, Bristol

Sally-Ann Spencer Grey
Independent Lecturer and Consultant

Sharon Wood
Lecturer
School of Healthcare, University of Leeds

Acknowledgements

The production of this book has been supported by many people, and the following warrant a special mention.

Thank you to all the authors for your valuable contributions, and to Nigel Sykes for writing the Foreword.

To everyone at Radcliffe Publishing, thank you for your endless patience and support during the production of this book.

Dedications

To my parents Marie and Brian for teaching me all the important things in life, for always being there and believing in me.

To my daughter Crystal for making me so very proud, and for having the courage to be herself.

To Trevor, for completing my happiness.

Janis

To daughters Jenny and Elisa and sons-in-law Steve and Neil for their support, and for producing three wonderful grandsons.

To my grandsons Charlie, whose name means strength and who is my strength, Thomas, whose name means twin and who is twinned in my heart, and Toby, whose name means gift from God and who most certainly is a gift.

Finally, to Malcolm, whose unerring support and belief keep me inspired.

Lorna

Special dedication

Sadly, at the end of 2006 one of our chapter authors Tracey McCready died most untimely, at the age of only 43.

Tracey was a truly special person – genuine, gentle, warm and kind. She was a very dedicated, passionate and caring Nurse/Lecturer.

Unfortunately, her contributions to Cancer and Palliative Care, although great, had only just begun.

Her happy nature, enthusiasm, wicked sense of humour coupled with her great courage and capability, had a great impact on everyone she met.

Tracey always ensured she lived life to the full – a message to us all.

Chapter 1

High-fidelity clinical simulation in cancer and palliative care education

Neil Pease

> *I have been impressed with the urgency of doing. Knowing is not enough; we must apply. Being willing is not enough; we must do.*
>
> *Leonardo da Vinci (1452–1519, Italian draftsman, painter, sculptor, architect and engineer, whose genius epitomised the Renaissance humanist ideal)*

Aim

It is the aim of this chapter to introduce the reader to the concept of high-fidelity clinical simulation, and its possible applications in the field of cancer and palliative care education.

Learning outcomes

- Understand the perceived benefits and limitations of high-fidelity human patient simulation as a teaching tool.
- Examine high-fidelity clinical simulation as a strategy for educating both teams of staff and individuals in the management of rare or demanding clinical events in cancer and palliative care.
- Explore possible future uses of high-fidelity patient simulation in this field of care.

Introduction to patient simulation

Simulation has been described by Gabba (1996, p. 55) as 'a generic concept, which refers to the artificial replication of sufficient components of a real-world situation to achieve certain goals.' The aviation industry attempted to create the first rudimentary aircraft simulators in the 1920s, and by 1930 Edwin Link and his 'Link trainer' had become a standard instrument for flight training before the Second World War (Rolfe and Staple, 1986). Flight simulation has continued to develop over the decades, culminating in the current climate. Already qualified pilots are allowed to gain certification to fly different aircraft solely within a simulator, thus removing the need to pilot the specific aircraft in reality. This is due to the fidelity of the simulated experience, as a flight simulator can replicate a real aircraft with startling accuracy.

Healthcare has been profoundly hesitant to embrace the possible advantages of simulation for training staff in the management of rare or infrequently experienced events. The drive to create an accurate representation of the human form for teaching purposes has been predominantly driven by the anaesthetic community across the globe (Byrne *et al.*, 1994; Devitt *et al.*, 1995; Morgan and Cleave-Hogg, 2002). The first electromechanical *human patient simulator* was developed in 1968 in order to meet the needs of 'anasthesiologists' in the USA (Carter, 1969; Denson and Abrahamson, 1969). 'Sim One' was an extremely lifelike representation of the human form, and remains a credit to its creators in terms of morphological accuracy. The costs involved in the production of such a device (£270,000 by today's standards) and the reluctance of the medical community to embrace such a product ensured that 'Sim Two' was never produced. However, these early innovations in the area of human patient simulation did serve to stimulate the interest of the medical fraternity in the possible future uses of a simulated patient. Developments in computing impelled the advancement of the creation of a new breed of human patient simulators throughout the 1980s. At the time of writing, technology has progressed to a level where a high-fidelity patient simulator is readily available on the open market for multiple uses, not just within the anaesthetic arena.

What is a high-fidelity human patient simulator?

A human patient simulator is an engineered reproduction of a human being, driven by a blend of pneumatics, electronics and computer programming that is based upon mathematical modelling of human physiology. The product of such a process is a manikin that has palpable pulses, breathes spontaneously with functional lungs, has a patent airway and light-reactive pupils, and can be fully monitored both invasively and non-invasively. High-fidelity patient simulators also feature a drug recognition barcode-reader system which acknowledges the presence and dose of over 70 intravenous drugs, demonstrating the accurate physiological response of a 'real' patient exposed to pharmacological agents. The emergency care simulator (a portable version of the human patient simulator) also features bowel sounds and the ability to convulse. Both simulators can 'talk' by virtue of an 'actor' speaking into a microphone system to replicate the patient's voice. In addition, the manikin produces heart sounds, breath sounds and a recordable electrocardiogram, and can undergo urethral catheterisation.

Various mid-fidelity manikins possess some of these features, such as palpable pulses and breath sounds, but it is the physiological modelling that separates high-fidelity manikins from other forms of patient simulators. In high-fidelity simulators, the physiological modelling is interlinked as it is in a human being. In real terms, this means that if one variable, such as an increase in pulse rate, is altered, there will also be a reciprocal increase in other variables, such as cardiac output and systolic blood pressure. These changes are automatically instigated by the manikin and do not require manipulation by the operator (although this is a viable option for the person who is running the simulator).

In order to recreate the multiple pathogenic conditions that each simulator is capable of generating, there is a requirement for the operator to be able to 'speak' to the simulator in physiological language. For example, in order to lower the blood pressure of the 'patient', the operator may dramatically reduce the circulating blood volume. The risks posed to the simulated patient by taking this action are the same as would be experienced by a human patient. Furthermore, with the simulator running in real time, the simulated patient will become increasingly ill if the appropriate treatment regime is not instigated. In the case of the volume-depleted patient, the simulator may generate ischaemia on the electrocardiogram and ultimately suffer a hypovolaemic-related cardiac arrest. The more practical option for lowering the blood pressure would be to leave the circulating blood volume as standard, and to alter both myocardial contractility and the resistance factor of the peripheral vasculature, thereby avoiding the risk of complications resulting from a low circulating blood volume.

High-fidelity manikins are also available in paediatric and (more recently) infant versions. They are currently only produced by Medical Educational Technologies Incorporated (METI) in Sarasota, USA (www.meti.com). At the time of writing, only adult high-fidelity simulators have been used in the field of palliative and cancer education, although the use of paediatric manikins is a future possibility.

Advantages and disadvantages of high-fidelity human patient simulators

The main advantage of utilising human simulators is that the 'patient' cannot experience any harm at the hands of the learners, while repeated multiple pathogenic conditions can be recreated for educational purposes. Such conditions can be time scaled, and they provide the learner with the opportunity to experience rare events that are infrequently witnessed in clinical practice. The ability to recreate pathogenic conditions and the associated physiological manifestations demonstrates the advantage of simulators over medical actors – a common resource currently utilised in cancer and palliative care education (Heaven and Maguire, 1996). Problems with equipment, drugs or human interactions may also be integrated into the scenario. High-fidelity simulators are responsive to clinical intervention, and can therefore be cannulated, have intravenous fluids and drugs infused, and be defibrillated and intubated should the need arise. Although such invasive treatments are infrequently experienced in palliative care, the existence of a palpable pulse or audible breath sound supports the realism and credibility of the learning environment. Human actors do, of course, have an essential role to play in educational programmes such as 'breaking bad news' courses, but there is a limit to what a human actor can physically deliver as a 'sick' patient. Simulators can experience a cardiac arrest at the press of a button, or become increasingly ill as the scenario unfolds, accompanied by the associated physiological changes. This renders the situation more realistic and engaging than other forms of role play. The participants are subsequently required to make decisions in real time – an essential component of the educational experience, where decision making under stress could be a desired learning outcome of the scenario. Running high-fidelity simulators in real time requires participants to make clinical decisions at a pace that is dictated by the condition of the 'patient.' Flin *et al.* (2002) have provided a comprehensive overview of the themes and applications relating to decision making under stress.

Although the purported benefits of utilising simulation as an educational vehicle are many, there are some disadvantages of human patient simulation. The 'patient' can demonstrate a multitude of physiological manifestations, but facial expression, skin colour, skin turgor and pallor can never change. Invariably, this denies the student the opportunity to benefit from non-verbal forms of communication, an essential component of development within clinical practice. The actual simulators are extremely expensive, and therefore many health and educational institutions cannot afford them (in 2002, one adult and paediatric high-fidelity simulator cost over £200,000, including tax). As with any emerging technology, the reliability of such simulators can also be questionable. Although programmes can be pre-written to incorporate set pathogenic events, a high level of physiological understanding is required to operate the simulator. It is this understanding of human physiology that allows the simulator operator to manipulate bodily processes to meet the needs of the immediate situation.

High-fidelity clinical simulation centres

The use of high-fidelity simulators within the working environment, or as part of a teaching facility such as a college or university, has its limitations. Providing the operating requirements of the simulator in terms of piped medical gases (nitrogen, carbon dioxide, compressed air and nitrous oxide) limits their use to purpose-built clinical simulation centres. The number of such facilities is growing exponentially year upon year both in the UK and across the world (a list of current facilities can be accessed at www.bris.ac.uk/Depts/BMSC). The clinical simulation centre at Montagu Hospital, in Mexborough, South Yorkshire, opened in March 2003 and offers a simulation room which can replicate multiple clinical environments, a control room and a seminar room for debriefing purposes. This would be the standard room requirement for most facilities other than storage and office space. The majority of centres video-record scenarios for debriefing purposes and in order to consolidate the learning experience. At the Mexborough facility, digital cameras offer various angles from which to view and record events in the simulation room (*see* Figures 1.1, 1.2 and 1.3 opposite). One-way glass separates the control and seminar rooms from the simulation room. Pictures generated from the scenarios are linked live into the seminar room, giving delegates the opportunity to view events either on a large screen, or alternatively through the mirrored-glass dividing wall. Although the concept of students being videotaped is not a new one, at the Montagu facility it is emphasised that delegates are not being filmed as a mechanism for gauging their level of performance, but only to serve as a vehicle to stimulate debate as part of the debriefing process (Betzendoerfer, 1995; Raphael and Wilson, 2000). The process of group-mediated debriefing is a concept taken from the aviation industry (Dismukes and Smith, 2000), where facilitators adopt a supporting role as opposed to a lead teaching responsibility. The presence of clinical experts in the field of palliative and cancer care enhances learner support. Such experts are available to answer specific questions arising from the simulated practice, and facilitate students' personal development from the educational experience.

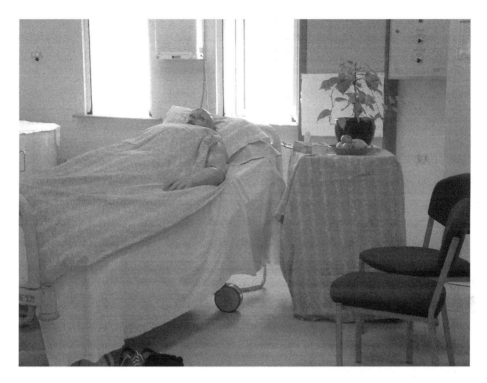

Figure 1.1

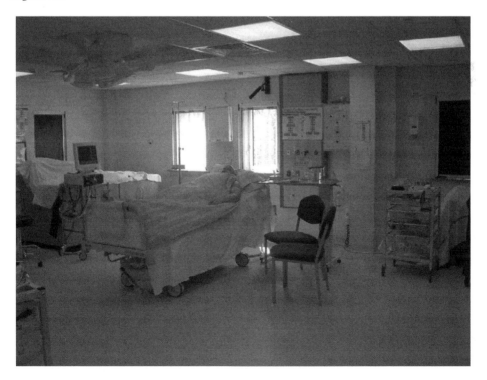

Figure 1.2

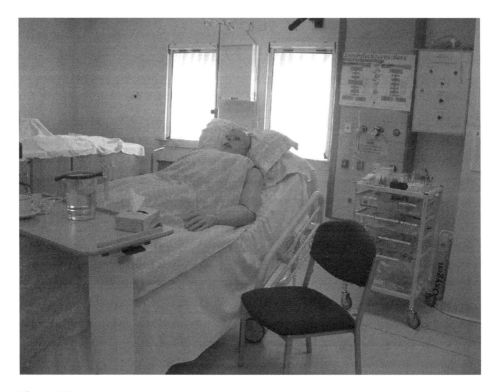

Figure 1.3

The evolution of high-fidelity simulation in cancer and palliative care education

As mentioned previously, high-fidelity simulation has its roots in anaesthetic and operating department practice. The question was posed as to whether the same technology could not be utilised to recreate simulated patients experiencing a palliative or cancer care emergency. After discussing the concept with staff at St John's Hospice in Doncaster, it became apparent that those working in this field were just as apprehensive about experiencing a palliative or cancer-based emergency as the anaesthetist was about dealing with such events in theatre or the intensive-care unit. Hospice, primary and secondary care staff all had their own infrequently experienced emergencies. These could not be recreated by a medical actor, and had previously only been deemed 'learnable' by experiencing them in real life.

Such events were categorised as follows:

- anaphylactic reaction to chemotherapy, a blood product or a pharmacological agent
- collapse of a relative or carer
- hypercalcaemia
- spinal cord compression

- major haemorrhage (both lower gastrointestinal and carotid 'blow out' have been simulated at the Montagu facility)
- end-of-life event
- finding an overdosed patient (due to euthanasia, accidental overdose, or the patient being in renal failure, leading to the accumulation of a pharmacological agent)
- relative wishing to reverse a 'Do Not Resuscitate' directive immediately post cardiac arrest.

Scenarios incorporating these events were jointly written by staff from St John's Hospice, Doncaster and Bassetlaw Hospitals NHS Foundation Trust and the Montagu Clinical Simulation Centre (also part of Doncaster and Bassetlaw Hospitals). Each scenario was trialled by other members of the group who were not actively involved in its writing. The pilot group included nursing, physiotherapy and medical staff from all levels. Scenarios were videoed for debriefing, and were gauged with regard to realism and accuracy of content, in addition to the quality of the projected learning outcomes. The question was debated as to whether this would be a credible vehicle for participants who wished to develop their knowledge of the management of such infrequent events. The production of nursing and medical notes, the acquisition of props and the use of actors in supporting roles, such as that of the patient's relative, all served to enhance the realism of each event. The patient simulator was programmed to recreate each condition, including end-of-life events, in which palliative care remains the only option offered by the facility where the patient dies. In line with all courses, a switchboard operator was positioned within the control room, allowing delegates to telephone for help or advice from within the simulation room. A member of the simulation centre staff also played various clinical roles within the simulated events, in order to help delegates to familiarise themselves with the environment. The scenarios ran in 'real time', and subsequently the simulator became increasingly ill at a rate comparable with a real emergency condition.

Multi-professional applications

Recruitment to the simulation centre courses in palliative and cancer care is by self-selection on the part of the learner, although the programme is now integrated into the palliative care modules of some universities, such as the palliative care course offered by Sheffield University. Courses generally operate with a mix of hospice, acute and primary care staff attending. The blend of delegates attending enriches the learning experience universally, and the dissemination of different ways of working, opinions and experiences enhances the perceived and expressed benefits of the day. All grades of staff from all professions are encouraged to attend, thus replicating the clinical environment. Although this supports the realism of the simulated event, operationally the palliative care scenarios are difficult to run from a functional perspective. When Accident and Emergency courses are being held, attention remains focused on the 'patient.' However, in cancer and palliative care courses the focus includes health and social care staff who are involved in the scenario, as well as the 'patient', relatives and friends. This leads to a very 'busy' simulation room, with the need to relay accurate information swiftly to those members of the simulation centre staff who are playing roles in the scenario. It is also necessary to change camera angles frequently, if the events are being recorded on film.

Why is high-fidelity clinical simulation important in palliative and cancer care?

Clinical simulation in palliative and cancer care has offered a new horizon of opportunities for educating staff in the management of infrequent events. Prior to the use of simulation in this format, the only way to learn about these events was through personal experience or the shared experience of another practitioner. Simulation offers a minimum of four scenarios conducted within a one-day course, with an average of three participants actively engaged in each recreated episode. For those not directly involved in the scenario, there is an opportunity to watch events as they unfold via the live visual feedback link, or by means of the observational wall. Post scenario, there is an opportunity to discuss the events that have transpired in a supportive, non-judgemental, confidential environment. Time is allocated within the programme to allow for such discussions – something that is infrequently experienced in the modern NHS. The human factors (Maurino *et al.*, 2001) and elements of *crisis avoidance* and *resource management* are also integrated into the debriefing (Flin and Moran, 2004).

Crisis avoidance and resource management principles focus broadly upon the following:

- situational awareness (being aware of the world around you, staying 'one step ahead of the game')
- the acknowledgment of human error and human performance; integrating the *Swiss cheese model* of error formation – an analogy to the barriers and holes that lead to the occurrence of errors (Reason, 2000, 2003)
- decision making
- teamworking and leadership
- resource management.

Other concepts that are integrated into the debriefing include sharing thought patterns (mental models), communication skills and the necessity for closing the communication loop. Discussions based around these prominent themes help delegates to better understand the effects that human factors have on the outcome of such situations.

Evidence of good educational practice

With all educational interventions, an evaluation of the learning experience is imperative as part of the quality control and governance mechanisms. In addition to a Likert scale questionnaire, which is circulated at the end of all courses, focus groups have been conducted to gain a deeper understanding of the effects of such interventions. By the end of 2006, approximately 150 staff will have completed the one-day palliative care course at the Montagu clinical simulation centre (this represents 12.5% of the centre's annual activity). A comprehensive qualitative review of all participants from the palliative care programme is still in its infancy, but themes emerging from focus groups of past delegates have included the following:

- increased confidence in the management of rare events
- a greater awareness of the need to plan for such events (one hospice in South Yorkshire rewrote its anaphylactic policy after taking part in the simulation centre course)
- consolidation of the participants' existing knowledge
- the opportunity to witness multiple rare events within a short space of time
- the time to communicate with colleagues away from the situational pressures of the work environment, including time to reflect upon the learning experience
- a high sense of personal achievement associated with completing a psychologically demanding educational event.

Specific comments from the focus groups have included the following:

> *I feel better about it [treating a case of anaphylaxis] having done that scenario. It's the next best thing towards a real-live event, and it does stick in your mind what you should do.*
>
> *General practitioner*

> *The beauty of that situation [simulated scenario] is that you respond to it and that it responds to you.*
>
> *Hospice registered nurse*

> *I probably got more belief in myself in what you're doing, rather than doubting something you are doing.*
>
> *Acute care registered nurse*

> *It would be good for people who want to do palliative care and are not quite sure.*
>
> *Hospice registered nurse*

> *It enhances your learning. Your accredited education is complemented by what you learned that day.*
>
> *Doctor working in palliative care*

Weller *et al.* (2003) offer an excellent insight into the perceived changes in practice in anaesthesia, after completion of a simulation-based course in crisis management.

Is this form of educational intervention needed in palliative and cancer care education?

From the wide range of courses available at the Montagu Clinical Simulation Centre, the palliative care one-day programme remains one of the most popular on offer. The course attracts staff from acute, primary and palliative care backgrounds. Scenarios are tailored to meet the skill level and needs of those taking part. Nevertheless, there are staff – not only within the palliative and cancer care arena, but also in all other avenues of healthcare – who remain critical of simulation as a credible means of learning. The principal criticism is that clinical simulation can never be the 'real thing', which of course it cannot. It is only by accepting simulation for what it is – an opportunity to participate in the recreation of a rare or demanding event – that the learner can truly benefit from partaking in the programme. The human form is infinitely more difficult to replicate than an aircraft cockpit, and consequently the level of realism that aviation simulation enjoys is not currently achievable in healthcare. But what are the available alternatives to help healthcare practitioners to prepare for these events? The existing options are limited, and consist of waiting for the manifestation of the event during practice. However, is this first experience of a possibly traumatic event the ideal time to be learning 'on the job'?

The credibility of the simulated experience relies upon the suspension of reality. The effort that goes into preparing the environment and the supporting props such as nursing notes and the physical appearance of the simulator pays dividends in convincing the learner that there is the necessary element of credibility for them to engage in the moment. In palliative and cancer care this credibility is sometimes stretched. The simulation room at the Montagu facility looks clinically orientated, making it less believable as, for example, a client's home. However, feedback from participants identifies how delegates look beyond the immediate environment and are engaged with the realism of the situation.

Future developments

The mobile version of the human patient simulator has recently been trialled in a hospice environment for the first time. Although operating away from the simulation centre has disadvantages, such as the loss of a live video link to the scenario, there are also multiple benefits with regard to capturing the reality of the true working environment. The hospice pilot featured a patient who had attempted suicide by taking an overdose of an opiate-based drug, and the collapse and cardiac arrest of a hospice visitor. The first one-day course conducted solely within a hospice is now planned for the very near future, when the operating of a full programme can actually be tested in the workplace.

Other developments include the theoretical use of the paediatric simulator to recreate emergencies or challenging ethical scenarios in paediatric oncology and palliative care. The sensitivity of these programmes would require much fore-thought and cognitive support for participants if a course was to be offered on this theme. Such is the level of realism offered by courses within the simulation centre that it is not uncommon for delegates to find the experience emotionally unsettling. Courses in paediatric oncology and palliative care may be challenging the boundaries of what is acceptable under the umbrella of learning, for staff other than those working in the specialiy of a children's hospice or other area of expertise

---

Key points

- The first human patient simulator was developed in 1968 in the USA.
- Clinical simulation has its roots in anaesthesia and operating department practice.
- A patient simulator is a recreation of the human form, with the high-fidelity versions demonstrating mathematically modelled interwoven human physiology.

- By using high-fidelity patient simulators, a plethora of medical and ethical situations can be recreated which run in 'real time.'
- Effort must be devoted to the suspension of reality if the learner is to engage with the process.
- The drawbacks of simulation include morphological limitations of the manikin, operating requirements and financial cost.

Conclusion

High-fidelity clinical simulation in palliative and cancer care education is a new concept. This modality of educational intervention offers the learner the chance to experience rare clinical or emotionally challenging events, without any risk to a real patient or any other consequence of action. More importantly, simulation provides the opportunity to practise such events before one has to deal with the situation in actual clinical practice. High-fidelity simulation has limitations, specifically in relation to the morphological appearance of the manikin. Some of these drawbacks are alleviated by the interlinked physiological modelling of the simulator, providing palpable pulses, heart sounds and other physiological markers that are not present in other forms of simulation. The use of props such as medical notes and pre-prepared case histories helps to create a realistic learning environment for those taking part.

The future for clinical simulation in the field of palliative and cancer care is full of opportunity. The portable Emergency Care Simulator has the potential to offer such educational experience in the workplace, where the question of realistic surroundings pales into insignificance. There is also the possibility of using paediatric simulators in oncology and palliative care, although careful deliberation and action planning would be required for such a programme to be successful.

Implications for the reader's own practice

1 What are your personal views with regard to high-fidelity simulation in palliative and cancer care education? Specifically, would you want to use simulation to either learn by, or to provide education to others?
2 What are the other benefits and drawbacks of simulation that have not been mentioned in this chapter?
3 Does the cost of purchasing such equipment equate to the perceived benefits of learning in this way?
4 'You can only learn this type of thing by doing it for real.' What are your opinions of such a statement?

References

Betzendoerfer D. TOMS: team-oriented medical simulation: briefing, simulation, debriefing. *Proceedings of The Anesthesia Simulator as an Educational Tool.* 1995. pp. 51–5.

Byrne AJ, Hilton PJ, Lunn JN. Basic simulations for anaesthetists. A pilot study of the ACCESS system. *Anaesthesia.* 1994; **49:** 376–81.

Carter DF. Man-made man: anesthesiological medical human simulator. *J Assoc Adv Med Instrument.* 1969; **3**: 80–86.

Denson JS, Abrahamson S. A computer-controlled patient simulator. *JAMA.* 1969; **208**: 504–8.

Devitt JH, Kurrek M, Fish KJ. Anaesthesia simulators. *Can J Anaesth.* 1995; **42**: 952.

Dismukes R, Smith G. *Facilitation and Debriefing in Aviation Training and Operations.* Aldershot: Ashgate Publishing; 2000.

Flin R, Moran N. Identifying and training non-technical skills for teams in acute medicine. *J Qual Safety Health.* 2004; **13**: 80–84.

Flin R, Salas E, Strub M *et al. Decision Making Under Stress.* Aldershot: Ashgate Publishing; 2002.

Gabba D. Simulators in anesthesiology. In: *Advances in Anesthesia. Volume 14.* St Louis: Mosby Year Book Inc.; 1996.

Heaven C, Maguire P. Training hospice nurses to elicit patient concerns. *J Adv Nurs.* 1996; **23**: 280–86.

Maurino D, Reason J, Johnston N *et al. Beyond Aviation: human factors.* Aldershot: Ashgate Publishing; 2001.

Morgan PJ, Cleave-Hogg D. A worldwide survey of the use of simulation in anaesthesia. *Can J Anaesth.* 2002; **49**: 659–62.

Raphael B, Wilson J. *Psychological Debriefing: theory, practice and evidence.* Cambridge: Cambridge University Press; 2000.

Reason J. Human error: models and management. *BMJ.* 2000; **320**: 768–70.

Reason J. *Human Error.* Cambridge: Cambridge University Press; 2003.

Rolfe JM, Staple KJ. *Flight Simulation.* Cambridge: Cambridge University Press; 1986.

Weller J, Wilson L, Robinson B. Survey of change in practice following simulation-based training in crisis management. *Anaesthesia.* 2003; **58**: 471–3.

Further reading

- Maurino D, Reason J, Johnston N. *Beyond Aviation: human factors.* Aldershot: Ashgate Publishing; 2001.

- Montagu Clinical Simulation Centre; www.montagusimulation.co.uk

- Raphael B, Wilson J. *Psychological Debriefing: theory, practice and evidence.* Cambridge: Cambridge University Press; 2000.

- Reason J. Human error: models and management. *BMJ.* 2000; **320**: 768–70.

- Weller J, Wilson L, Robinson B. Survey of change in practice following simulation-based training in crisis management. *Anaesthesia.* 2003; **58**: 471–3.

Chapter 2

The use of competencies in palliative care education

Robert Becker

Eighty per cent of success in life is related to attitude rather than competency.

Anon.

Aim

The aim of this chapter is to review the development of competency-based education in cancer and palliative care over the last decade and to discuss the issues and implications for current and future curriculum development.

Learning outcomes

- Understand the notion of competence and its place in professional practice.
- Recognise the principal issues that underpin developments surrounding competency assessment in cancer and palliative care education.
- Appreciate the need for a more balanced, holistic approach to the assessment of cancer and palliative care education that is both achievable for practitioners and reliable for assessors.

Introduction

Measuring the effectiveness of cancer and palliative care education is fraught with difficulty. The use of the word 'effective' in itself implies that there is an end point and outcome that is objective and achievable, but the reality is somewhat different. It is by no means clear as to what education in cancer and palliative care is trying to achieve competence in, and the means of doing this are at best overly complex (Becker, 2000) and at worst reductionist of the whole concept of holistic care (Koffman, 2001). As the opening quote suggests, competence is about more than attaining a given level of skills, knowledge and experience. It is also concerned with the attitudes and behaviours exhibited during the utilisation of these attributes. This central issue could be evaded in cancer and palliative care education simply by concentrating on the concrete science involved. Assessment of competency would then be much more factually based and could provide benchmark standards for all. However, this fails to do justice to the dynamic relationships that exist between patients and carers, the social, cultural and ethical influences that shape these interactions, and the development of complex interpersonal and intrapersonal skills that run concurrent with such care. This is the true essence of cancer and palliative care, and therefore the real challenge is to develop education that can capture this and foster learning that is useful to the practitioner, sound in its knowledge base and internalised in such a way that correct attitudinal and behavioural traits are demonstrated in professional practice. Competency assessment is most certainly not a universal panacea for finding this Holy Grail of education, but where it is sensibly applied, rigorously piloted and evaluated and fit for purpose, it can make a valuable contribution. This chapter will attempt to examine the developing paradigm of competency assessment, its strengths and inherent limitations, the missed opportunities and the potential way forward in our evidence-based health-care culture.

How has competency assessment evolved?

Competency assessment in an educational context has evolved primarily from the work of Benner (1984), with influences from the learning taxonomy devised by Bloom (1984). The model takes into account increments in the performance of a given skill based on experience as well as education. It also provides a basis for clinical knowledge development and potentially for career progression in clinical nursing.

The driving force towards developing competency assessment in cancer and palliative care over the last decade has been the publication of a number of key documents. *The NHS Cancer Plan* (Department of Health, 2000) determined the strategic direction for the development of a national, high-quality, uniform and equitable cancer service. Following on from this came the *Core Competency Framework* (Royal College of Nursing, 2003), which attempted to pull together a uniform framework of standards for cancer nursing across four levels of practitioner and a wide range of skills. The Royal College of Nursing published its own *National Core Competency Framework* for nurses working in specialist palliative care (Royal College of Nursing, 2002). Both of these documents have as their baseline premise the notion that competencies can best be assessed by the medium of observable behaviour in practice, backed up by a plethora of both written and verbal evidence. However, higher education institutions (HEIs) find themselves, in the UK at least, with a proliferation of accredited courses for qualified staff at all levels that may be qualitatively excellent in the academic sense, but which tend to concentrate on competency assessment via demonstrable critical thinking ability – and therein lies the paradox. How can the professions develop an acceptable model of competency assessment that embodies the best of both approaches?

Why is it important?

It is important because we are now at a juncture in cancer and palliative care education that demands much more integrated and creative thinking from educationalists if the needs of the cancer patient and their family at all stages of the disease process are to be met. Education at all levels must reflect the dynamic nature of an ever changing clinical environment and the evolving roles of those caring for these patients in whatever setting. That education should be both academically and clinically rigorous in the widest sense and where possible measurable in terms of clearly defined outcomes. It is with regard to this latter point that the development of competency assessment fits best and can help the professions to come closer to defining their expertise and credentialling competent and confident practitioners.

What is competency?

Educators have been attempting to accurately define the notion of competence for several decades, and have yet to reach an informed consensus in this debate (Lillyman 1998). Although competency standards for pre-registration education have been agreed for some time now (United Kingdom Central Council for Nursing, Midwifery and Health Visiting, 1999), attempts to define and assess specialist and advanced levels of practice in cancer and palliative care still continue (Royal College of Nursing 2002, 2003). Generally speaking, competence in a given set of skills can be defined as 'The skills, knowledge, experience, attributes and behaviours required by an individual in order to perform the job effectively' (Royal College of Nursing, 2002). In order to work it therefore relies on the formulation of agreed competency statements which are then identified at different levels of practice.

At pre-registration level it is well established that it is the role of clinical staff to conduct practice-based assessments, as they are seen as more credible and up to date with regard to practice-related issues. The issue of grading competency to practise in pre-registration programmes is straightforward. In the majority of cases the assessor is simply required to make a judgement which indicates 'yes' or 'no' against a given competency statement. For the protection of the public, absolutes such as this are necessary and form an essential part of good ethical and professional standards, yet the objectivity of such judgements is as much open to question as any other system. Those involved in delivering cancer and palliative care education may well have a more detailed knowledge base, but few are in the position to consider themselves clinically active in any substantial way and therefore as clinically qualified to assess skills competence.

Clearly with qualified and experienced staff a different approach is needed. Authors such as Benner (1984), who saw nurses moving from 'novice to expert' along a continuum, have provided us with a much clearer idea of the ways in which adults learn in the 'real world' of practice, and their work relates closely to the four patterns of knowing which Carper (1978) suggests should be present in each act, namely empirical knowledge, aesthetic knowledge, personal knowledge and ethical knowledge. Carper's work has stood the test of time, and elements of these four patterns can be observed in current codes of conduct (Nursing and Midwifery Council, 2004).

At post-qualification level the assessment of clinical skills is more complex and is predominantly based on self-judgement validated by educators and only occasionally by practitioners. This assessment usually involves the following:

- reflective essays, diaries and journals – linked to competencies

- portfolio development, sometimes incorporating competencies
- critical incident analysis.

This kind of reflective-process-centred assessment is indeed one way out of a difficult dilemma, and it is popular with HEIs because it makes it much easier and more acceptable to validate and assess the work produced against clearly defined academic criteria. However, it is suggested that the ability to think and write effectively at a given academic standard about clinical issues does not necessarily translate into competence in clinical skills, no matter how articulate, insightful and academically sound the material that is produced. To this day, higher education remains unsure about validating modes of assessment that put the judgement of competency in the hands of practitioners in a work environment. At present, no form of clinical assessment involving competencies can be said to be wholly objective. Indeed, this may never be fully achievable because of the holistic nature of care delivery and the multiple, extraneous variables that can influence such assessment at any one time. The evidence does suggest that an assessor's influence on how a nurse learns when caring for the dying is severely restricted by such factors (Degner *et al.*, 1991). Therefore universities perhaps have a valid point.

There are a number of ways to describe the domains inherent in both learning and competence, but for the sake of simplicity an adapted version of Bloom's (1984) taxonomy which emphasises individuals moving from a lower level of knowledge to a higher level of evaluation can be used in conjunction with a variation of Benner's (1984) 'novice to expert' thesis, which acknowledges critical thinking ability combined with technical skills. The work of Schon (1987) must also be considered, principally because she recognised that it was the 'artistry' of practice which helped to differentiate between competent and expert practitioners.

Domains of competence

- *Knowledge competence* is the retained (baseline and advanced) knowledge of a given subject which is needed for the execution of both technical and inter-personal skills.
- *Technical competence* consists of the learned psychomotor skills and techniques necessary to perform specific tasks.
- *Cognitive/analytical competence* involves the development of intellectual skills and revolves around accumulated knowledge and the ability to use high-level thinking skills to resolve problems effectively.
- *Ethical/personal behavioural competence* is characterised by the possession of appropriate personal and professional values and behaviours and the ability to make sound judgements when confronted with ethical dilemmas.
- *Affective competence* can be described as emotional intelligence (Goleman, 1996), and refers to our ability to deal with emotions and develop appropriate attitudes.

It is self-evident that all of these areas overlap and contribute to the collective expertise and wisdom of a competent practitioner, but could there perhaps be a further area which is not so clearly defined, but which has been acknowledged by a number of authors as significant in the repertoire of skills needed for successful practice in palliative care (Heslin and Bramwell, 1989; Davies and Oberle, 1990; Degner *et al.*, 1991; Taylor *et al.*, 1997) This refers to the artistry discussed by Schon

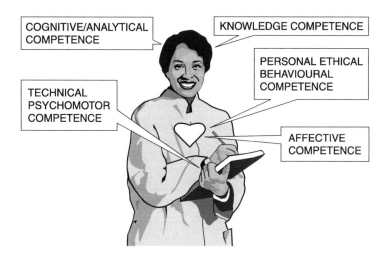

Figure 2.1 Professional competence in a palliative care context.

(1987) and the personal and professional maturity to address the challenging intrapersonal issues intrinsic in caring for dying people and their families. It involves the ability both to maintain self-esteem and self-worth by acknowledging and questioning personal behaviours and feelings as an integral part of effective functioning, and to discuss and reflect periodically on the meaning and significance of life and death events in relation to work by drawing on insights and spiritual awareness. It also involves being able to recognise and attempt to understand personal reactions and feelings that are generated from time to time as a natural consequence of working with the dying and bereaved, and to reflect on how this affects the care that is given in sensitive situations.

It would be arrogant to assume that such virtues are unique to palliative care, but they do play a significant part in the long-term personal and professional growth of those people who choose to work in this field. Education developments that either ignore or only superficially acknowledge this complex element fail to address the reality of competence to practise in the long term. A good example of the success of this approach comes from the work of a group of Norwegian educators who integrated group supervision over a two-year period as an integral part of the follow-up to a postgraduate palliative care programme that was competency focused (Landmark *et al.*, 2004). The students reported the expected increases in both knowledge and skills, but also improved abilities in self-reflection and self-awareness, which gave deeper meaning to their work.

Applications to cancer and palliative care education

The sheer complexity of many clinical skills today demands that professions move beyond the 'see one, do one, show one' approach of old, and the fields of cancer and palliative care are good examples of the intricacy and blend of qualities and skills that are needed. What competencies can do, therefore, is to make clear and explicit the precise knowledge and skills that are needed in order to provide care, and their popularity reflects the perceived imbalance in nursing in recent years towards valuing academic qualifications over clinical practice (Crouch, 2005). This has been recognised by both educators and managers of services who are beginning to use competencies to develop educational programmes (Wilkie *et al.*, 2001). In America, the Robert Wood Johnson Foundation has supported the development of educational competencies for end-of-life care that can be integrated into mainstream undergraduate nursing curricula, in recognition of the dearth of palliative care-related teaching that was prevalent throughout the country (Ferrell *et al.*, 1999).

Undergraduate medical education is now beginning to recognise the need for palliative care skills, acknowledging that the palliative approach needs to be integrated into the training of all doctors in the UK (Association for Palliative Medicine, 1992). Subsequently, the average number of hours devoted to such education has increased significantly, and some of the strategies used are competency based (Field and Wee, 2002). By contrast, however, the formal teaching of such skills in UK nursing faculties remains ad hoc at best (Lloyd Williams and Field, 2002), and no such national imperative yet exists (Cooley, 2004), despite government recognition of the need for it (Department of Health, 2004).

There is a real and urgent need for baseline competencies in both palliative and cancer care to be clearly spelt out and actively integrated into the undergraduate curricula of all healthcare professions. Achieving this goal is much more difficult, as governments worldwide are inclined towards giving guidance rather than directives, and are reluctant to engage in the politics of university education and professional governing bodies. However, it is abundantly clear that one of the best ways to successfully influence and shape the attitudes and skills of healthcare professionals in the palliative care approach is to begin from day one in their professional education with a coherent competency development strategy that is assessed in theory and practice and validated at source.

The European Association of Palliative Care (EAPC) has recently produced a report and key recommendations for the advancement of nurse education in Europe (De Vleiger *et al.*, 2004). This offers a set of useful criteria against which education programmes can be developed in those countries where palliative care is in its infancy, and it successfully draws together the threads of a holistic, multimodal approach based on skills development.

Small-scale initiatives involving educational competencies for specific skills, such as delivering cytotoxic therapy and setting up syringe drivers, are already well thought out in healthcare trusts and hospices, and reflect local initiatives to improve care. These are often linked to modules of study accredited by local universities on specialist degree pathways, and they give practitioners the opportunity to obtain qualifications that are recognised by professional bodies alongside HEIs (United Kingdom Central Council for Nursing, Midwifery and Health Visiting, 2001). Now growing apace following the introduction of the National Institute for Clinical Excellence (2004) guidelines for improving palliative care for people with cancer are educational initiatives and service development linked to the key recommendations of this important document. Areas such as psychological support, spiritual care and bereavement services are currently being looked at from a competency perspective (Gordon and Mitchell, 2004).

One of the most potentially influential developments linking job competencies to pay scales and professional development is the Knowledge and Skills Framework (Department of Health, 2004) of the *Agenda for Change* (Department of Health, 2005). This extensive and complex initiative is currently being rolled out across the

UK in the mainstream NHS sector of care, and is designed to support career progression and personal development of staff across many disciplines. The idea is that managers will be able to identify the knowledge and specific skills that an individual needs to use in their job and, when these are achieved, to provide a basis for career and pay progression. It is anticipated that the framework will able to use and link with current and emerging competence frameworks.

It is directly relevant to palliative care practitioners in a variety of disciplines, as many are employed by the NHS, and a considerable number of those who are employed by hospices have their pay directly linked to NHS rates, conditions of service and therefore job descriptions. The core components that will be reviewed and graded on a 4-point scale to establish competency and pay progression embrace a broad and generic range of skills applicable to many disciplines in a vast array of jobs. The real challenge will be to devise descriptors and competencies that reflect the true nature and unique characteristics of the palliative care approach, to enable a fair and equitable assessment of the individual's performance in their job. It is suggested that the content and structure of future education initiatives in both the cancer and palliative care field via HEIs in particular will therefore need to reflect the competency levels and statements that are intrinsic to this framework, if they are to be of relevance to the staff concerned and supported by hard-pressed service managers.

Conclusion

The assessment of competence in human interactions is an esoteric, abstract and subjective pursuit, and therefore by definition it is unachievable in any quantifiable way. The unique dynamics of human interactions at a time of major life crisis are just that – unique. However, it is possible to identify the common characteristics of a given situation and to devise verbal, psychomotor and behavioural responses that are culturally and ethically acceptable as good practice, and from this to develop competency statements. Unfortunately, this exercise will always be inherently flawed, because it ignores the variables that can influence practice. It is unrealistic to hypothesise that a given situation can be exactly replicated in practice to allow the opportunity for self- and peer assessment of performance against the given competency benchmarks. The paradox is clear – context is everything. Practitioners are being asked to make reliable judgements of observable practice that may contain elements of spontaneous, emotion-laden, compassionate and sometimes intuitive actions of a professional carer towards a patient and their family.

The skills that are being assessed may be demonstrated in an acute medical ward, an Accident and Emergency department, a quiet room in a local community hospital, a crowded outpatients department or a patient's home. The environmental, social and relationship variables that can influence the context and outcome of this conversation are limitless. What should not be forgotten, of course, is the potential influence of the assessor as either passive observer or active participant, and lastly, but most importantly, the perceived competence and confidence of the person who is being assessed on that given day. When all of these factors are taken together, one begins to get some idea of just how difficult the true notion of competency assessment really is. Much more work is needed in the development of realistic, jargon-free, achievable and reliable competency assessment tools that can be used by both educators and clinicians.

The professions involved in palliative care and educationalists alike must be wary of falling into the trap created by much of western industrialised society, which considers that any given human action and interaction can be broken down into its constituent parts and the outcomes accurately predicted. Although this approach undoubtedly has its merits and helps us to understand patterns of behaviour, conversely it can create a defensive, litigation-obsessed and reductionist approach to healthcare.

The way forward

Used wisely, competence-based assessment of professional development can help to provide HEIs, hospice educators and Workforce Development Directorates with useful information to inform the following:

- education and training commissioning with local providers
- identification of appropriate modes of delivery of education
- facilitation of competency acquisition in the workplace
- provide a uniform, clinically relevant and standardised content for cancer and palliative care education programmes.

It can also help individual practitioners to:

- plan and develop their career pathway
- identify their own training and education/skill requirements
- access appropriate education initiatives
- self-assess their performance in relation to Individual Performance Review (IPR) and the development of a Personal Development Plans (PDP).

It has the potential to provide managers with a robust system for:

- assessing ongoing competency as part of the IPR and PDP process
- informing future roles and responsibilities, job description and person specification development (Department of Health, 2005)
- measuring competency within a team to inform skill mix review and staffing establishment
- identifying workforce training needs
- monitoring progress towards achieving national targets and standards.

Key points

- There is a real and urgent need for baseline competencies in both palliative and cancer care to be clearly spelt out and actively integrated into the undergraduate curricula of all healthcare professions.
- Competency-based education initiatives need to face up to the challenge of integrating and supporting the development of intrapersonal integrity as a key component of the curriculum.

- Assessment tools should be written in readable, jargon-free language, and should be sufficiently focused to be relevant to everyday practice in a given area.
- Competency assessment is not a universal panacea for successful education, but where it is sensibly applied, rigorously piloted and evaluated and fit for purpose, it can make a valuable contribution.

Further study

If you have access to the Internet, log on to www.cancernursing.org, where you can register free, and then follow the links to the Introduction to Palliative Care Nursing course (Becker, 2005). This free-to-access course has an integral competency development tool that is geared towards the non-specialist, can be used in multiple work environments and will challenge you to examine your own perceived competence in using the palliative approach to care. It has been extensively evaluated in practice, peer reviewed, published and developed over several years, and it has the added advantage of clarifying and validating for you what you perceive you are already competent at, where this is evident. This is important to our professional development, as it can sometimes be difficult to acknowledge and articulate what we know we are good at in our job when the culture of caring is so often centred around identifying the problems rather than the achievements. The evidence base presented by this competency tool is but one small step in this direction, and is offered to you as an opportunity to engage in such work.

Implications for the reader's own practice

1 Does your job description accurately reflect the full range of skills that you regularly use in a palliative care context? If not, can you do something about this?
2 How do you rate your own competence in caring for the dying and bereaved?
3 Getting support for yourself in an ongoing professional relationship with a trusted confidant is a key part of successful practice when working regularly with the dying and bereaved. How do you achieve this?
4 What is the provision for palliative care education in your local area? Find out and challenge the educators to provide evidence of links to practice-based competency.
5 Can you be proactive and engage with the challenge of self- and peer assessment of your competency? You will find this difficult, but also empowering.

References

Association for Palliative Medicine. *Palliative Medicine Curriculum for Medical Students, General Professional Training and Specialist Training.* Southampton: Association for Palliative Medicine; 1992.

Becker R. Competency assessment in palliative nursing. *Eur J Palliat Care.* 2000; 7: 88–91.

Becker R. *An Introduction to Palliative Care Nursing*; www.cancernursing.org

Benner P. *From Novice to Expert: excellence and power in clinical nursing practice*. Menlo Park, CA: Addison Wesley, 1984.

Bloom BS. *Taxonomy of Educational Objectives*. Boston, MA: Allyn & Bacon; 1984.

Carper B. Fundamental patterns of knowing in nursing. *Adv Nurs Sci*. 1978; **1**: 13–23.

Cooley C. Core skills: nursing cancer. *Int Cancer Nurs News*. 2004; **16**: 45.

Crouch D. Proving your competency. *Nurs Times*. 2005; **101**: 22–4.

Davies B, Oberle K. Dimensions of the supportive role of the nurse in palliative care. *Oncol Nurs Forum*. 1990; **17**: 87–94.

Degner LF, Gow CM, Thompson LA. Critical nursing behaviours in care for the dying. *Cancer Nurs*. 1991; **14**: 246–53.

Department of Health. *The NHS Cancer Plan: a plan for investment, a plan for reform*. London: Department of Health; 2000.

Department of Health. *The NHS Knowledge and Skills Framework and the Development Review Process*. London: Department of Health; 2004.

Department of Health. *Agenda for Change*. London: Department of Health; 2005.

De Vleiger M, Gorchs N, Larkin PJ *et al*. *A Guide to the Development of Palliative Nurse Education in Europe. Palliative nurse education: Report of the EAPC Task Force*. Milan: European Association of Palliative Care; 2004.

Ferrell BR, Grant M, Virini R. Strengthening nursing education to improve end-of-life care. *Nurs Outlook*. 1999; **47**: 252–6.

Field D, Wee B. Preparation for palliative care: teaching about death, dying and bereavement in UK medical schools 2000–2001. *Med Educ*. 2002; **36**: 561–7.

Goleman D. *Emotional Intelligence: why it can matter more than IQ*. London: Bloomsbury; 1996.

Gordon T, Mitchell D. A competency model for the assessment and delivery of spiritual care. *Palliat Med*. 2004; **18**: 646–51.

Heslin K, Bramwell L. The supportive role of the staff nurse in the hospital palliative care situation. *J Palliat Care*. 1989; **5(3)**: 20–6.

Koffman J. Multi-professional palliative care education: past challenges, future issues. *J Palliat Care*. 2001; **17**: 86–93.

Landmark B, Wahl J, Bohler A. Group supervision to support competency development in palliative care in Norway. *Int J Palliat Nurs*, 2004; **10**: 542–8.

Lillyman S. Assessing competence. In: Castledine G, McGee P, editors. *Advanced and Specialist Nursing Practice*. Oxford: Blackwell Science; 1998.

Lloyd Williams M, Field D. Are undergraduate nurses taught palliative care during their training? *Nurse Educ Today*, 2002; **22**: 589–92.

National Institute for Clinical Excellence. *Improving Supportive and Palliative Care for People with Cancer*. London: National Institute for Clinical Excellence; 2004.

Nursing and Midwifery Council. *Code of Professional Conduct: standards for conduct performance and ethics*. London: Nursing and Midwifery Council; 2004.

Royal College of Nursing. *A Framework for Nurses Working in Specialist Palliative Care: competencies project*. London: RCN Publications; 2002.

Royal College of Nursing. *Core Competency Framework for Cancer Nursing: delivering effective patient care*. London: RCN Publications; 2003.

Schon D. *Educating the Reflective Practitioner*. San Francisco, CA: Jossey Bass; 1987.

Taylor B, Glass N, McFarlane J *et al*. Palliative nurses' perceptions of the nature and effects of their work. *Int J Palliat Nurs*. 1997; **3**: 253–8.

United Kingdom Central Council for Nursing, Midwifery and Health Visiting (UKCC). *Fitness for Practice Summary*. London: UKCC; 1999.

United Kingdom Central Council for Nursing, Midwifery and Health Visiting (UKCC). *Standards for Specialist Education and Practice*. London: UKCC; 2001.

Wilkie D, Kay M, Judge *et al*. Excellence in teaching end-of-life care. *Nurs Health Care Perspect*. 2001; **22:** 226–31.

Chapter 3

Problem-based learning: not such a problem

Jean Fisher

We only think when we are confronted by a problem.

John Dewey

Aim

The aim of this chapter is to provide an overview of the process of *problem-based learning (PBL)*, highlighting the importance of the role of facilitation as part of this process. Exploration of the development of a PBL package for palliative care education will be followed by discussion of the part that PBL can play in both uni-disciplinary and multi-disciplinary education in palliative care.

Learning outcomes

- Understand the principles underpinning PBL.
- Compare and contrast the roles of facilitator and teacher within the context of cancer and palliative care education.
- Discuss the rationale for using PBL as a tool for providing relevant and effective palliative care education.

Introduction

What is PBL?

PBL has been utilised in medical education for many years (Boud, 1998). It is an active learning process, based on adult learning theory (Knowles, 1989; Rogers and Freiberg, 1994). PBL is a method whereby 'problems' or 'cases' are used by a group to generate their own set of learning needs. Having identified topics and subject areas where knowledge gaps exist, individual group members, or subgroups, take responsibility for undertaking review of relevant literature, or exploration of a research base, and then giving feedback to the group as a whole.

PBL differs from both *action learning* and *case-based learning*. In action learning a group of individuals come together to work on a problem experienced by one of the group members, in order to clarify issues and explore alternatives (McGill and

Brockbank, 2004). In traditional 'case-based' teaching, the case is used either to identify knowledge gaps which the lecturer/teacher then attempts to fill, in a pedagogical manner, or to reinforce aspects of learning that have already been covered (Woods, 1994). In PBL, however, the group makes the decisions about the areas that need more knowledge or understanding, and then assumes ownership of the explorations necessary for the learning to be shared. It is therefore andragogical in its approach (Knowles, 1989), with the group leader taking on a facilitating rather than a teaching role. There are four key components necessary for PBL, namely the problem, the facilitator, the group and the time frame.

The problem

The problems, or cases, used in PBL are carefully constructed to cover a range of practical and non-practical issues that can arise in practice. Each case is designed to accurately reflect healthcare contexts and situations. A case evolves page by page, with each new statement or series of statements, leading to group discussion and the generation of potential learning issues. Each group working with a case will create their own list of learning issues, congruent with their experience and expertise (Downey and O'Brien, 1999). From experience it has been seen that a group can work with the same problem more than once, since their learning issues will change over time as they develop as practitioners.

The facilitator

For PBL to work successfully, the tutor/group leader must adopt not a teaching mode, but a facilitative one. The role of the facilitator is pivotal. The first and, arguably, most fundamental element in this role is the creation of the appropriate environment for PBL – an atmosphere of safety for group members is essential. The key functions of the facilitator are to initiate and organise the process and to ensure that the group maintains focus and clarifies their learning issues. The facilitator must resist the urge to become 'the teacher', even when he or she has a body of knowledge/skill in the area. Instead, the group leader needs to encourage the group members to share together the knowledge acquired. Azila *et al.* (2001) noted that PBL requires a significant shift in stance and approach among students and teachers. In our experience this has certainly been true.

   Much has been written about whether or not it is preferable for the facilitator to have a thorough subject knowledge base. Eagle *et al.* (1992), in a trial using 10 groups and 35 PBL cases, found that the 'expert' tutors (i.e. those with a good level of subject knowledge of the field being studied) enabled the generation of twice as many learning issues as the 'non-expert' tutors. The learning issues were all appropriate to the case. Hay and Katsikitis (2001) conducted a randomised trial of PBL groups facilitated by 'expert' and 'non-expert' facilitators, and found that the 'expert' group achieved higher scores in a post-course test. However, Bochner *et al.* (2002) found that first-, second- and third-year dental students felt that the facilitator's familiarity with PBL was as important as their level of subject knowledge. In our own experience we have found that facilitation skills are of paramount importance, and sometimes group members can be frustrated by a facilitator who seems 'determined to teach' because he or she has significant expertise in the subject area.

In an evaluative study, Dolmans *et al.* (1994) found that three factors were important in facilitators/tutors of PBL, namely guiding the students through the learning process, commitment to the learning, and having relevant subject knowledge. In subsequent work, Dolmans *et al.* (2001) have highlighted the value of the facilitator's group dynamics skills. This skill set was described by students as particularly valuable in ensuring that all group members 'pull their weight' in addressing the learning issues. Dolmans *et al.* (2002) highlighted the fact that the subject expert tutor is more likely to direct discussion using their own knowledge than is the facilitator who has no great knowledge of the subject matter, who is more likely to use process facilitation. Dolmans *et al.* (2002) go on to suggest that this finding means it is essential for the facilitator to be a reflective practitioner and educator, so that they do not over-direct the group's discussion and activities. On one of the courses run by this author, a facilitator took responsibility for researching a learning issue (alongside the participants) because it concerned a specific practice issue that was little known to her. This worked well, as the course participants perceived this to be active involvement in developing the learning for all.

There may be occasions when the provision of a subject 'clinical expert' within the feedback session is of benefit, but this is not essential. Where this has been done, it has proved helpful to set specific parameters for the involvement of the 'clinical expert' in advance, in order to ensure that they fully understand the PBL process and their own role in it. These limits may be that they will contribute on a particular aspect or learning issue, or that they may be asked to provide 'added-value' comments or insights after each learning issue has been fed back to the group as a whole by the participant with responsibility for that learning issue. When this approach is adopted, it is crucial to ensure that the group members' contributions are still perceived as key to the overall learning experience, with the expert input being regarded as a 'bonus.'

The group

PBL is ideally suited to the types of small groups that are often encountered in palliative care education, as noted by Forbes (1994), who also discussed the need for context-led use of PBL. Woods (1994) suggests that PBL can successfully be utilised with groups of 30 to 300, citing the McMaster University chemical engineering programme as an example. It is claimed by Woods (1994) that groups can facilitate their own learning, without the requirement for huge numbers of tutors to be involved. However, the nature of palliative care education is such that large group teaching of any type requires enormous skill in order to tackle the delicate and often personal and painful issues in a meaningful but safe way. From experience it has been seen that, although groups may be able to use PBL effectively for some elements, even small groups may 'shy away' from really complex non-clinical issues, unless a true sense of safety has been established. This is more difficult to achieve without facilitators.

The group members need to fully understand PBL and be willing and indeed expect to participate fully in the identification of need and the shared learning process – in other words, to be a team within the activity. Willingness to take risks and make mistakes is an important prerequisite for PBL to be successful. Recognition of the case as an opportunity to develop knowledge, skills and confidence by testing out ideas and theories and sharing knowledge and learning is crucial for group members. The notions of honesty and sensitivity within the group are fundamental and need to be fostered, so that the other elements necessary for PBL can occur. All of these elements can be put in place when a skilled facilitator is available to aid the group development phases described by Adair (1986) as being a prerequisite for achieving good group performance.

The process of PBL

In order to utilise PBL, two sessions of around one to two hours, one to two weeks apart, work well. In the author's experience, longer gaps between sessions one and two can lead to a degree of process disengagement among group members.

Session 1

In the first session the case will be discussed and learning issues identified. Group members may each have a copy of the pages of the case, or the case may be read out loud, or PowerPoint/overhead projectors may be used to display the information page by page. Each group will need a scribe, who makes brief notes on a flipchart of group discussion under the following subheadings:

- facts – what the group knows
- ideas and thoughts
- learning issues – areas that the group identifies as knowledge/skills gaps.

The group members will also decide who will explore which learning issues prior to the second session.

Session 2

The follow-up session provides an opportunity for group members to share their learning through mini-presentations, discussion, debate, reflection and even role play. Written information, reference lists and the evidence base for material delivered are all useful. Members of groups that are used to PBL develop these as a matter of course, to help themselves and each other.

PBL and palliative care education

The overall aim of any palliative care education programme must be to develop, change and enhance practice, thereby improving the palliative and supportive care that is offered to both patients and families (Kenny, 2001). PBL can be used when considering clinical, interpersonal, managerial, organisational, ethical and attitudinal aspects of any case that is developed (Downey and O'Brien, 1999). It is this very flexibility that makes PBL ideal for palliative care education, as we have such complex concepts, knowledge and ideas to explore, in ways that are meaningful to students of all types and disciplines. Sensitive and subtle educational approaches are required to enable practitioners to grasp both the principles and the nuances of practice that are fundamental to providing excellent palliative care.

Reflection and reflective practice are at the heart of palliative care (Duke and Copp, 1994). Reflection is also fundamental to PBL, as group participants consider their own knowledge, skills and understanding gaps in order to come up with a set of learning issues. In addition, reflection will help practitioners to identify the gaps in their confidence and comfort zones. This is essential if we are to provide holistic care in the context of life-threatening illness, dying, death and loss.

Within Western culture and healthcare, death remains relatively unacceptable – we have not yet moved too far from Gorer's (1965) description of a death-denying society. Within nursing literature, death anxiety has been researched and discussed (Beck, 1997; Georges and Grypdonck, 2002). These issues have been explored in detail by Farley (2004) in the first book of this series. Wong *et al.* (2001) have successfully utilised PBL as a technique for tackling some of the attitudinal issues surrounding death and dying for student nurses, who often experience death anxiety when caring for dying patients. The technique enabled individuals to perceive that much of their experience was shared by their colleagues, and they thereby gained support from each other. Although the need for nurses to have close personal contact with palliative patients in order to develop a therapeutic relationship with them has been highlighted, it has been shown from experience that the same concerns with regard to death anxiety and the building of close relationships are just as pertinent for all disciplines within the team. PBL can also serve as an excellent medium for the multi-disciplinary team to explore these issues, as a case can be constructed in such a way as to encourage discussion. For example:

> *Jenny, the third-year student nurse undertaking community practice placement, seems reluctant to accompany team members on home visits to Joe, and confides to Paul, the GP trainee, that she is finding it difficult to care for Joe and to talk to his wife.*

Developing the PBL palliative care package

St Michael's Hospice, Hereford has been providing formal and informal education for a number of years. As part of that process the hospice has been involved with the local Vocational Training Scheme (VTS) for general practitioners (GPs), providing visits, placements and taught sessions on hospice and palliative care. The local GP trainers had already developed PBL packages for use on this scheme and in other areas of primary care. They approached the hospice to explore whether a collaborative venture to produce a PBL package with a series of palliative care cases would be possible. Following initial observations of these two GP trainers utilising PBL within their VTS course, this author was encouraged by the potential breadth and depth of topics that could be developed from one case, and the energy and enthusiasm that were generated in each session that they witnessed. Reviewing the literature confirmed that this was one of the advantages of PBL as a learning strategy (*see* section on strengths of PBL on p. 30). Over 50 potential learning issues were identified that were thought to be valid and pertinent. These ranged from sperm banking to aspects of symptom control, and assisted suicide. Slowly, and in collaboration with our GP colleagues, a series of eight cases was developed and refined. Throughout this process the principles of case design, as discussed by Dolmans *et al.* (1997) and outlined below, were utilised. A process that was initially predicted to be easy turned out to be quite complex, in order to complete cases that were realistic, but without extraneous or superfluous detail. Colleagues helped to curb an instinctive desire to create paradigms of excellence, and instead to build evolving scenarios designed to promote discussion, debate and learning opportunities.

Developing PBL cases: principles for effective case creation

Cases should meet overall course learning objectives.
Case content should reflect appropriately the professions and levels of prior knowledge of group members.
Presentation of basic science should be in the context of the clinical situation to encourage the integration of learning.
A number of cues should be contained in each case to promote discussion.
Cases should be relevant to current or future practice.
A case should be open enough to sustain discussion and facilitate exploration of alternatives and options.
Self-directed learning using a variety of learning resources and modalities should be generated by the case.

(Adapted from Dolmans *et al.*, 1997)

Application and evaluation in practice

Since the pack was first developed and launched, it has been used with single-discipline groups, primarily doctors, but also in a limited way with nurses. Many doctors are already familiar with the approach and idea of PBL and so can readily begin to work on a case. A number of qualified nurses have not encountered such student-centred strategies before, having been trained at a time when more traditional, didactic approaches were used. This represents a significant disadvantage in the sense that there is often insufficient time to introduce the concept in a short programme of learning, and to obtain adequate levels of understanding and engagement with the process, and participant confidence. Student nurses are now encouraged to take greater responsibility for their own learning, and this is likely to mean that PBL will be more readily used in palliative care nurse education in the future.

Hughes and Lucas (1997) reported significant successes with the use of PBL with multi-disciplinary groups. PBL cases have been used by the author with multi-disciplinary teams, particularly in primary healthcare. One of the observed outcomes of this has been changes in team dynamics. Some team members seem to have been surprised by the levels of knowledge among colleagues, and by the nursing team members' capacity to search out the evidence base for aspects of practice. Although this is purely anecdotal evidence, informal discussion with teams indicates that relationships have improved and developed as a consequence. This is in addition to the intended outcomes of enhanced knowledge and confidence in dealing with palliative care situations. As good palliative care relies upon collaboration and multi-professional teamworking, these improved relationships will hopefully be of direct benefit to patient care and patient and family support.

Formal evaluation of the package has so far been limited to participant feedback and comment. From the data, it appears that most of those who have experienced the pack have found it beneficial and stimulating, as outlined below:

> What a lot of issues in one situation! It was interesting to look at the less practical aspects as well as the obvious symptom control. (Participant 10, Group A)
>
> I didn't expect to do a role play in the case, but it proved very useful and promoted lots of discussion. (Participant 3, Group B)
>
> I had not realised how much knowledge we already had amongst the team. That was a real surprise to me. (Participant 4, Group B)
>
> I wonder if we wasted time on long, complex discussions. (Participant 6, Group A)
>
> It was good to learn together and from each other. (Participant 5, Group A)
>
> I think we have learnt a lot about each other as well as about palliative care. (Participant 1, Group A)
>
> I thought at the start I would feel really stupid – I think I was surprised by how much I did know but never trusted myself with before. (Participant 2, Group B)
>
> The thing that concerns me is did we pick the right learning issues, or did we miss important things out? (Participant 8, Group B).

Strengths of PBL as a learning strategy

As with any approach, PBL has both critics and proponents. Prior to involving the hospice in the project, it was important to review the evidence in order to elicit the advantages and limitations of PBL. Much of the work that was located was related to medical education, but it was encouraging to discover that internationally PBL has been used for a range of health disciplines, including chiropractic practitioners (Bovee and Gran, 2000). There is a small amount of literature and research on palliative care in particular. The following brief literature review is an attempt to answer some crucial questions about the value and efficacy of PBL.

Do students enjoy PBL?

One of the fundamental beliefs of hospice education departments is that participants should enjoy their learning opportunities, and are more likely to benefit from learning opportunities that they can reflect on positively. Albanese and Mitchell (1993) undertook a review of the literature and meta-analyses, and found that students perceived PBL to be both nurturing and enjoyable. Antepohl and Herzig (1999) undertook a randomised controlled trial of PBL versus lecture-based learning. The PBL group (consisting of 63 students) derived benefit from the interdisciplinary learning elements of the programme, the teamwork and the fun of PBL. This was in the context of a course on basic pharmacology, which might not be anticipated to generate comments about 'fun.' The results of a study by Abacioglu *et al.* (2004) on the use of PBL on a clinical cancer management course were encouraging, with positive feedback from participants about the use of the approach. Bligh *et al.* (2000) explored student perception of PBL as a teaching methodology, and found that PBL students had a higher level of satisfaction with the course than did their traditionally educated colleagues.

The criticism has been raised that although PBL may be interesting and fun for some, not all students find it so (Farrow 1995). In a thoughtful and well-balanced review, Albanese (2000) suggested that even if knowledge acquisition and clinical skills are no more greatly enhanced by the use of PBL than by traditional programmes, the enhanced working environment for both students and teaching staff that has consistently been found in studies undertaken means that PBL is an appropriate learning tool. Student feedback has shown that PBL is perceived positively with regard to creating a positive environment for active learning.

Several studies have explored student concerns with regard to PBL. Azila *et al.* (2001) found that students were worried that they might not select the right learning issues. In this author's first experience of using PBL, she felt some concern that the group were 'missing' some important issues. GP colleagues suggest that the group's selected issues are the right issues for that particular group at that particular time. There may be some justification for the notion that a higher number of learning issues might serve to overwhelm the group and thus to demotivate them from learning. The work of Birkholz *et al.* (2004) focused on the learning needs of student nurses with regard to death and dying. The needs identified by the students linked very closely with competencies for the provision of high-quality end-of-life care devised by the American Association of Colleges of Nursing. This would suggest that those students, at least, could identify appropriate things to learn about. Individuals who have been using group-generated learning agendas over time will recognise most of the topics that come up – there is homogeneity therein. (This then raises the question of why it is so difficult to come up with clear national frameworks for what should be included in medical and nursing curricula!)

Does PBL work?

Do students learn? What about academic achievement? Is learning sustained? And does practice develop as a consequence?

There have been various suggestions with regard to the theory of how PBL works. Albanese (2000) postulated that in fact contextual learning is not the basis of PBL, but that information-processing theory, cooperative learning theory, self-determination theory and control theory are all involved. The experiential learning theory proposed by Rogers and Freiberg (1994) includes the following principles.

- Learning occurs when the subject matter is directly relevant to the participants.
- Learning is facilitated best when threats to the participants are minimised.
- Learning lasts longest and is deepest when self-initiated.

This author suggests, from her experience of using PBL, that it is in fact experiential theory that is most closely relevant to PBL.

Albanese and Mitchell (1993) found that although students did equally well in clinical examinations and faculty evaluation, there were potential deficits in their cognitive knowledge. In a Canadian review, Chang *et al.* (1995) suggested that learning may in fact be no greater than that achieved using traditional teaching techniques and methods. Hughes-Caplow *et al.* (1997) found that retention of knowledge was improved, and also that use of PBL encouraged deeper thinking about material within a case, rather than merely factual recall. This is obviously particularly pertinent with regard to the ethical and psychosocial aspects of cancer and palliative care cases. Depth of thinking has been evidenced by the range of learning issues raised by groups on our courses, including euthanasia, talking with children about a parent's impending death, and the rights of same-sex partners. These examples demonstrate that a case can generate much more than obvious clinical and symptom control issues.

Alexander *et al.* (2002) evaluated a three-year undergraduate nursing programme and found that their PBL students exceeded the educational outcomes. Similarly, Antepohl and Herzig (1999) found that PBL students scored slightly higher in their end-of-course exams. Bovee and Gran (2000) also found that, in a multiple-choice-test situation, the PBL students obtained the same scores as their traditionally educated colleagues.

With regard to eliciting practice development, a number of studies have explored the role of PBL in changing clinical activity. Borduas *et al.* (1998) utilised a PBL approach when introducing clinical practice guidelines for the management of congestive heart failure. A total of 1,698 practitioners undertook this programme, and the 3- and 6-month post-course test results, together with chart evaluation, indicated sustained use of the guidance initiated with the PBL scheme. This might appear to be a vast and inevitably expensive programme, but if the practitioners have all now embedded the guidance into their practice, the time and money will have been well spent. There is little evidence that cancer pain guidelines have been successfully disseminated and utilised across the UK. In fact, most areas have spent time and money preparing local guidance, despite the logic of having clear national guidance distributed.

Davis *et al.* (2004) ran a PBL teleconferencing course with 20 primary healthcare physicians and found that their prescribing patterns for the management of paediatric asthma changed following the course. Practice changes were maintained over a 12-month period. These are particularly encouraging findings, as we all know that it is entirely possible for individuals to attend educational events without any practice-based development occurring as a consequence! Informal 3-month post-event follow-up with students suggests that there have been changes to clinical practice, as indicated below:

I do think more about the anti-emetics I prescribe now, having considered more options in the case we reviewed. (Participant 1, Group A)

We do discuss our palliative patients more as a team now than we used to. I find that really helpful. (Participant 4, Group A)

I feel as if my point of view is valued now, and we are certainly involved by the team much more and earlier. (Participant 7, Group A)

A number of studies, including one by Antepohl and Herzig (1999), have highlighted the development of collaborative working and teamworking that PBL fosters. Dean *et al.* (2003) utilised a self-reporting methodology with 76 students and found that they felt more prepared with regard to interpersonal skills, collaborative working and holistic care. Course organisers endorsed the students' perceptions. As these aspects are core to the business of palliative care, this seems to be a solid endorsement of PBL as an appropriate educational tool. Antepohl *et al.* (2003) conducted a follow-up questionnaire study of 446 graduates of a PBL curriculum, and obtained a 77% response rate. The majority of the participants felt well prepared, particularly with regard to communication, collaboration with other professionals and critical thinking. From the PBL palliative care workshops undertaken to date, participant evaluation suggests that teamwork and collaboration have improved and there is enhanced awareness of one another's professional roles and strengths. Broomfield and Humphris (2001), in a study designed to identify the cancer education needs of GPs, found that the most commonly occurring themes concerned addressing psychological issues, knowledge and information, and teamwork and communication. The GPs in the study were keen to be involved in their learning and to avoid the use of didactic methodology.

Another benefit of PBL is that it does engender motivation, individual responsibility for learning and the whole notion of self-directed learning. Bahrain medical students involved in a PBL programme were found to develop high levels of self-directed learning skills (Al Haddad and Jayawickramarajah, 1991). Bligh *et al.* (2000) and Biley and Smith (1998) also found that students were well motivated and took personal responsibility for their own learning and actions. Thomas (1997) noted these elements as two of four key achievement areas resulting from the use of PBL in medical education, the others being the development of clinical reasoning and the structuring of knowledge within a clinical context. All of these are relevant in all areas of healthcare education, but are arguably extremely pertinent to palliative care, where all elements of knowledge – scientific, intuitive, personal and ethical, according to Carper (1978) – may be required if appropriate, individualised care is to be offered.

In today's climate of lifelong learning and the ever increasing pace of change in healthcare, it is crucial that all learning programmes foster these fundamental principles. School education in the UK has been criticised for creating dependency among students, who expect that the teacher will provide a rigid framework concerning what to learn and how to produce 'the right answer' (Claxton, 2002). This leaves young people ill equipped for the problem-solving and learning in action that are required in most working contexts. The General Medical Council (1993, p. 23) has stated the need to promote 'learning through curiosity and critical evaluation.' It is clearly important for all educationists to continue to encourage and support this aim, and PBL is an excellent medium by which to achieve it.

PBL and changing technology

PBL has primarily been used as a face-to-face learning activity. However, some teams and universities are already adopting Web-based approaches. Sydney University developed a 72-case Web-based programme, used for years one and two of the medical curriculum (Carlile *et al.*, 1998). Davis *et al.* (2004) have successfully utilised teleconferencing as a medium for PBL. The idea of palliative care PBL on the Web is certainly a possibility, but great care would need to be taken to develop the required kind of group dynamics, particularly if sensitive issues are likely to arise – and from experience it has been seen that in palliative care they usually do!

The use of information technology, teleconferencing and Web-based learning is still really in its infancy in the UK, but is very well established elsewhere. We have much to learn from the experience of practitioners and educators in other countries. As economic and time constraints increasingly restrict the ability of healthcare practitioners to attend courses, we shall need to rely more and more upon other learning opportunities. The difficulty in the case of palliative care education is that although the technical and scientific knowledge can, theoretically, be relatively easily imparted and learned, the most difficult elements relate to attitudinal stances, communication skills and the kind of personal 'stuff' that often emerges in a supported, face-to-face learning context, but may never do so in front of a computer screen. Issues relating to modern technology and learning opportunities have been discussed in detail by Kwa Kwa (2004) in the first book of this series.

Key points

- PBL is distinct from and different to both case-based and action learning.
- The success of PBL depends on the facilitation skills of the group leader/tutor.
- PBL can be used for both uni-disciplinary and multi-disciplinary education, and to consider a range of issues – both concrete and more abstract in nature.
- PBL has been shown to enable deep and sustained learning that can have a significant impact on clinical practice.
- Although PBL is ideally suited to a face-to-face approach, in a changing health economy other modalities need to be utilised and evaluated.

Conclusion

This chapter has explored the definition and mechanics of PBL and has considered a framework for its use. The author has attempted to give a balanced overview of both the benefits and the drawbacks of PBL, despite herself being an advocate of this approach to learning. The process of developing a PBL package specifically for palliative care education has been described, and its implementation in a rural county in the UK has been explored. Finally, challenges have been issued to colleagues to explore how education practice can be developed, to keep in step with modern technology and the constraints imposed by the current organisational and economic climate, yet still to 'get to the heart' of palliative care practice.

Implications for the reader's own practice

1 How involved are your students in deciding what they need to learn?
2 What educational needs do you and your colleagues need to address in order to adopt a more facilitative role?

3 How much evaluative work do you do in order to ascertain how the education that you undertake influences practice change?

4 In what ways could you incorporate a PBL approach into some of your teaching? What hurdles would you need to consider?

References

Abacioglu U, Sarikaya O, Iskit S *et al.* Integration of a PBL multi-disciplinary clinical cancer management course into undergraduate education. *J Cancer Educ.* 2004; **19:** 144–8.

Adair J. *Effective Teambuilding.* London: Gower; 1986.

Albanese M. PBL: why curricula are likely to show little effect on knowledge and clinical skills. *Med Educ.* 2000; **34:** 729–39.

Albanese M, Mitchell S. Problem-based learning: a review of the literature on its outcomes and implementation issues. *Acad Med.* 1993; **68:** 52–81.

Alexander JG *et al.* Promoting, applying and evaluating problem-based learning in the undergraduate nursing curriculum. *Nurs Educ Perspect.* 2002; **23:** 248–53.

Al Haddad MK, Jayawickramarajah PT. Problem-based curriculum: outcome evaluation. *Med Teacher.* 1991; **13:** 273–9.

Antepohl W, Herzig S. PBL versus lecture-based learning in a course of basic pharmacology: a controlled randomised study. *Med Educ.* 1999; **33:** 106–13.

Antepohl W *et al.* A follow-up of medical graduates of a problem-based learning curriculum. *Med Educ.* 2003; **37:** 155–62.

Azila NM *et al.* Encouraging learning how to fish: an uphill but worthwhile battle. *Ann Acad Med.* 2001; **30:** 375–8.

Beck CT. Nursing students' experiences of caring for the dying patient. *J Nurs Educ.* 1997; **36:** 408–15.

Biley FC, Smith K. 'The buck stops here': accepting responsibility for learning and actions after graduation from a Problem-Based Learning nursing education curriculum. *J Adv Nurs.* 1998; **27:** 1021–9.

Birkholz CG *et al.* Students' self-identified learning needs: a case study of baccalaureate students designing their own death and dying course curriculum. *J Nurs Educ.* 2004; **43:** 36–9.

Bligh J, Lloyd-Jones G, Smith G. Early effects of a new problem-oriented curriculum on students' perceptions of teaching. *Med Educ.* 2000; **34:** 487–9.

Bochner G *et al.* Tutoring in a problem-based curriculum: expert versus non-expert. *J Dent Educ.* 2002; **66:** 1246–51.

Borduas F *et al.* An interactive workshop: an effective means of integrating the Canadian Cardiovascular Society clinical practice guidelines on congestive heart failure into Canadian family physicians' practice. *Can J Cardiol.* 1998; **14:** 911–16.

Bovee M, Gran DF. Comparison of two teaching methods in a chiropractic clinical science course. *J Allied Health.* 2000; **29:** 157–60.

Boud D, Feletti G. *The Challenge of Problem Based Learning.* London: Kogan Page; 1998.

Broomfield D, Humphris G. Using the Delphi technique to identify the cancer education requirements of GPs. *Med Educ.* 2001; **35:** 928–37.

Carlile S *et al.* Medical problem-based learning supported by intranet technology: a natural student-centred approach. *Int J Health Informatics.* 1998; **50:** 225–33.

Carper B. Fundamental patterns of knowing in nursing. *Adv Nurs Sci.* 1978; **1:** 13–23.

Chang G *et al.* Problem-based learning: its role in undergraduate surgical education. *Can J Surg.* 1995; **38:** 13–21.

Claxton G. *Building Learning Power.* Bristol: TLO; 2002.

Davis RS *et al.* Changing physicians' prescribing patterns through problem-based learning: an interactive, teleconference case-based education programme and review of problem-based learning. *Ann Allergy Asthma Immunol.* 2004; **93**: 237–42.

Dean SJ *et al.* Preparedness for hospital practice among graduates of a problem-based, graduate-entry medical programme. *Med J Aust.* 2003; **178**: 163–6.

Dolmans D *et al.* A rating scale for tutor evaluation in a problem-based curriculum: validity and reliability. *Med Educ.* 1994; **28**: 550–58.

Dolmans D *et al.* Seven principles of effective case design for a problem-based curriculum. *Med Teacher.* 1997; **19**: 185–9.

Dolmans D *et al.* Relationship of tutors' group dynamics skills to their performance ratings in problem-based learning. *Acad Med.* 2001; **76**: 473–6.

Dolmans D *et al.* Trends in research on the tutor in problem-based learning: conclusions and implications for education practice and research. *Med Teacher.* 2002; **24**: 173–80.

Downey P, O'Brien D. *Hereford PBL Pack.* Hereford: Hereford PBL; 1999.

Duke S, Copp G. Reflection in palliative care. In: Palmer C, Burns D, Bulman C, editors. *Reflective Practice in Nursing.* Oxford: Blackwell; 1994.

Eagle CJ, Harasym P, Mandi H. Effects of tutors with case expertise on PBL issues. *Acad Med.* 1992; **67**: 465–9.

Farley G. Death anxiety and death education: a brief analysis of the key issues. In: Foyle L, Hostad J, editors. *Delivering Cancer and Palliative Care Education.* Oxford: Radcliffe Publishing; 2004.

Farrow R. Problem-based learning at medical school. 'Some think it thrilling but not all do.' *BMJ.* 1995; **311**: 1643.

Forbes JF. Towards an optimal teaching programme for supportive care. *Support Care Cancer.* 1994; **2**: 7–15.

General Medical Council. *Tomorrow's Doctors: Report of the Education Committee.* London: General Medical Council; 1993.

Georges J, Grypdonck M. Moral problems experienced by nurses when caring for terminally ill persons: a literature review. *Nurs Ethics.* 2002; **9**: 155–78.

Gorer G. *Death, Grief and Mourning in Contemporary Britain.* London: Cresset Press; 1965.

Hay PJ, Katsikitis M. The 'expert' in problem-based and case-based learning: necessary or not? *Med Educ.* 2001; **35**: 22–6.

Hughes L, Lucas T. An evaluation of problem based learning in the multi professional education curriculum for the health professions. *J Interprof Care.* 1997; **11**: 77–88.

Hughes-Caplow J *et al.* Learning in a problem-based medical curriculum: students' perceptions. *Med Educ.* 1997; **31**: 440–47.

Kenny L. An evaluation-based model for palliative care education: making a difference. *Int J Palliat Nurs.* 2001; **5**: 189–93.

Knowles M. *Andragogy in Action.* London: Chapman and Hall; 1989.

Kwa Kwa J. Clinical governance in 'face-to-face' and 'online space' palliative care education. In: Foyle L, Hostad J, editors. *Delivering Cancer and Palliative Care Education.* Oxford: Radcliffe Publishing; 2004.

McGill I, Brockbank A. *The Action Learning Handbook: powerful techniques for education, professional development and training.* London: Routledge; 2004.

Rogers C, Freiberg HJ. *Freedom to Learn.* 3rd ed. Basingstoke: Macmillan; 1994.

Thomas R. Problem-based learning: measurable outcomes. *Med Educ.* 1997; **31**: 320–29.

Wong FMY, Lee WM, Mok E. Educating nurses to care for the dying in Hong Kong: a problem-based approach. *Cancer Nurs.* 2001; **24**: 112–21.

Woods DR. *Problem-Based Learning: how to gain the most from PBL.* Hamilton: Waterdown; 1994.

Chapter 4

The conundrums of delivering chemotherapy care: tackling the educational challenges

Krystina Koslowska

> *In all affairs it's a healthy thing now and then to hang a question mark on the things you have long taken for granted.*
>
> *Albert Einstein (1879–1955)*

Aim

How did you achieve competence in chemotherapy administration? How were you trained and educated? What framework did you follow? Was it accredited?

These are questions that nurses who have been delivering chemotherapy for a number of years find difficult to answer. The responses are a little murky, not clear cut.

For many, their emergence as a chemotherapy nurse has been rather ad hoc. They certainly *feel* that they have always been competent, but they are not entirely sure either how it happened or whether they could prove it on paper. It used to be common practice to learn on the job from someone else who had learned on the job, and to follow a competency framework developed by a mentor or hospital in the absence of any guidance from professional bodies. There were few recognised chemotherapy education programmes. Accreditation was reserved for university and college courses, and most nurses didn't go to university or college to learn about chemotherapy.

Thankfully, the climate has now changed and there are standards and guidance that recognise the importance of training and education in this specialty. Demonstrating and maintaining competence is a key topic. Experienced chemotherapy nurses now find themselves teaching what they were never taught, and thinking of doing it in ways that they would never have imagined. This chapter explores the emerging climate with regard to achieving competence in chemotherapy nursing and managing the educational needs of staff. It also looks at the realities of the chemotherapy environment and asks how education can be best provided to meet the needs of the cancer workforce.

Learning outcomes

- Identify the main drivers that have influenced and are influencing the development of chemotherapy education.
- Recognise the importance of accessing education and achieving competence when caring for patients who are receiving chemotherapy.
- Reflect on your own clinical areas and identify barriers to learning and achieving competence.
- Analyse how barriers to learning can be overcome in relation to achieving competence in chemotherapy administration.

Introduction

What has influenced the need for competence in chemotherapy?

Chemotherapy nursing education is central to providing excellent patient care. Chemotherapy nurses know that it has been a long time coming. In 1998, the Royal College of Nursing (RCN) published its clinical practice guidelines for the administration of cytotoxic chemotherapy. These guidelines recommended that chemotherapy should be given by professionally qualified practitioners who were able to demonstrate competence. Practitioners were to have regularly updated continuing education and were to be educated by academically and clinically qualified staff. This guidance was welcomed as a step towards recognising that the education of chemotherapy staff should be formalised, but it gave no indication as to what that education should look like, other than mentioning the topics that should be covered. Further clarity was provided by the *Manual of Cancer Services Standards* (Department of Health, 2000a), which had drawn from the Calman–Hine Report, *A Policy Framework for Commissioning Cancer Services* (Calman and Hine 1995), and which was used as the basis for cancer chemotherapy inspections in the form of peer review. This document created a stir, as it defined the need for chemotherapy education at a specific level. It stated the need for oncology staff administering chemotherapy to have taken either the now obsolete English National Board (ENB) N59 course or an in-house training course equivalent to it. The difficulty was that the ENB course was not easily accessible nationally. How were NHS trusts to ensure that staff accessed these courses? Alternatively, how were they to evidence their own courses, many of which had been put together without any educational input from a recognised body? The standards further complicated matters by suggesting that staff should not administer chemotherapy unless they were undertaking or had undertaken such a course. The reality at that point was that many nurses who were already giving chemotherapy had not had access to the required education. There was a lot to be done in a short time, and as a result NHS trusts throughout the country entered into negotiation with academic establishments to provide a route for delivering this education.

The revisiting of these standards and the publication of the current quality measures in the *Manual of Cancer Services* (Department of Health, 2004) set down very clearly the revised government expectations. The new measures require experienced named chemotherapy nurses for each chemotherapy service qualified to level III in cancer-related studies with at least one module in chemotherapy.

These nurses are to have responsibility for training in chemotherapy administration and for the review of chemotherapy competency. They have to ensure that training for all chemotherapy nurses is delivered according to the local Cancer Network agreed programme and that competence is assessed annually. In addition, staff who are not authorised to administer chemotherapy are unable to practise, and unsupervised and medical staff are subject to training and competence review, with those delivering chemotherapy having to provide evidence that they are fit to practise.

The implications of these standards mean the reorganisation and rethinking of chemotherapy services as trusts are addressing and have addressed the less than ideal practices that were common prior to peer review. This has involved:

- analysing the route of chemotherapy education and ensuring access to provision of level III and Network agreed learning
- looking to the local Cancer Network for guidance on the content of chemotherapy programmes
- agreeing who within their organisation has the responsibility for chemotherapy training and competency assessment
- developing ways to capture training and competence records
- ensuring that medical and nursing staff attend training and are assessed as competent prior to administering chemotherapy unsupervised
- ensuring that chemotherapy is delivered at all times by suitably qualified staff.

These changes have not been easy to manage, as difficulties in the reality of the working world have made seemingly sensible measures awkward to implement. Senior chemotherapy nurses have struggled with the idea of accessing education in order to tick the box that says they need to have it, when in reality many of them have been and are involved in creating and teaching on the very learning packages that they are expected to access. For less senior nurses working in increasingly busy environments, there is a real challenge to arranging to be released to attend educational programmes. Clinical environments struggle to support traditional education methods in a climate that finds nurses working under conditions of increasing workload and complexity, where staff regularly work longer than their contracted hours and staffing levels are minimal. These issues partly explain the current situation in chemotherapy nursing. There are simply not enough nurses who have undertaken cancer specialist training (Department of Health, 2000b). The whole ethos of training has changed. Trust- and Network-wide coordinated approaches are replacing training developed and delivered within individual workplaces, with nurses needing to collaborate across the service in new ways to make this happen. It has also impacted on the realities of staffing. As some chemotherapy regimens are impossible to deliver within a day-case setting, provision must be made around the clock for authorised chemotherapy nurses to be available to practise, so that treatment provision can continue. This is difficult in environments where medical staff may have been called upon to provide this service out of hours. Suggesting that medical staff no longer take part in this process will result in improved patient care, as competent nurses who deliver chemotherapy on a regular basis are the most suitable practitioners to manage the complications of cytotoxic drug delivery. However, this further highlights the urgent need to ensure that nurses are trained swiftly and have available the support necessary to manage the complexities of the patients who require this treatment.

Why is there a need for a coordinated approach to achieving competency?

In many clinical areas, nurses have developed into skilled practitioners with excellent capabilities, while in others the acquisition of skills has been less rigorous. Nurses joining the specialty often have little or no skill in chemotherapy delivery, and their development is largely dependent upon the standards set in the environment in which they work (Kelly and Crowe, 2004). Yet chemotherapy administration is a complicated process that requires a constantly changing body of knowledge and presents a high risk to the patient (Kanaskie and Arnold, 1999). Cytotoxic agents are often highly toxic, as they are rarely, if ever, selective solely for cancer cells (Neal and Hoskin, 1994). At worst, incorrectly administered chemotherapy can prove fatal, and there is a need for a nursing workforce that is able to respond to the increasingly complex nature of treatment administration in this field. Nursing has progressed rapidly and is at the forefront in ensuring that patients receive their treatment safely. This can only be achieved through the acquisition of specialist knowledge and skills and the development of competence. As the specialty develops, it is becoming more common to find nurse-led chemotherapy services. Increasingly, nurses are taking responsibility for the assessment of patient toxicities, organisation and management of the patient pathway, and the patient care needed for chemotherapy complications through the manning of 24-hour telephone advice lines.

Nurses are also almost entirely responsible for the delivery of these cytotoxic agents, which requires advanced expertise in cannulation, the management of venous complications and the care and management of central venous catheters. Many environments have developed nurse-led insertion of these catheters, particularly peripherally inserted central venous catheters, yet administration of chemotherapy with its inevitable toxicity is fraught with risk. Nearly all cytotoxic drugs could theoretically produce a hypersensitivity reaction, many are capable of causing chemical phlebitis and venous irritation, and practitioners must be capable of preventing, detecting and managing extravasation when vesicant drugs are used (Allwood et al., 2002). It should also be remembered that exposure to cytotoxic drugs is potentially hazardous, as they are known to be mutagenic, teratogenic and carcinogenic. Personnel must be protected from the effects of these drugs through the acquisition of skills in safe handling, which can only be attained by adequate training.

How does this impact on the wider picture for cancer and palliative care education?

The number of patients receiving chemotherapy is increasing, and the ways in which chemotherapy is delivered are changing. As the demand for overnight beds has increased and medical knowledge and experience have grown, the percentage of patients receiving chemotherapy within the inpatient setting has shifted. Changes to chemotherapy regimens and greater confidence in managing complications now mean that the majority of patients can receive chemotherapy as outpatients, and the proportion of patients who do so will continue to grow in the future. In some circumstances patients receive chemotherapy at home, in the form of ambulatory intravenous infusions delivered via a central venous catheter (usually initiated in the acute setting), intravenous chemotherapy delivered by a trained nurse, subcutaneous injections or, increasingly, oral cytotoxic drugs. In an age where 80% of cancer patients are being cared for in the community and patients want to stay at home for longer (Royal College of Nursing, 2003), it is inappropriate to consider a need for nursing chemotherapy education only in the acute setting. People who are receiving this treatment can have contact with health professionals in any healthcare setting, and it is important that all nurses involved in the pathway – not just those specialising in cancer care – have the knowledge and skills necessary to ensure that they are sufficiently competent and confident to deal with the issues of the chemotherapy patient (Department of Health, 2000b). For example, district nurses are frequently requested to become involved in the monitoring and care of chemotherapy patients at home, and many of them have little experience of this specialty. They are called upon to make assessments of patient toxicities and to manage central venous catheter care, and consequently need to obtain knowledge from the acute nursing services to help them to manage the situations that they encounter. When nurses are asked to perform beyond their knowledge base and they endeavour to manage complications with which they are unfamiliar, patients are at risk of inappropriate referral back to the acute setting and are exposed to potentially unsafe practice. A move to introduce education and training and increase competence in working with this patient group would be welcomed.

There is a growing understanding that palliative care should be available throughout the course of the disease process and not just in the terminal stages (Royal College of Nursing, 1996). The majority of chemotherapy is given with a palliative aim, and as patients are actively supported at home, community palliative care nurses must not be excluded from any educational provisions that are made. In addition, as the decision to discontinue chemotherapy is not always clear cut, it is not uncommon for patients to present to hospices with the need for nurses to have some level of chemotherapy knowledge. All of these professional groups must be considered in the evolving picture of what chemotherapy education should be about.

How can chemotherapy education be adapted for all nursing groups?

The national agenda is thus to ensure that nurses within acute settings who are delivering chemotherapy are educated to a minimum level. Looking at the provision of chemotherapy care in the community and a typical patient pathway, patient safety must be maximised by encouraging intervention from professionals in the acute and community services who adopt a collaborative approach to patient care. To be able to do this efficiently, community nurses need to have access to chemotherapy educational provision. Primary care is changing as community staff are called upon to increase their efficiency and apply their skills to a variety of specialty settings. They should have access to clinical supervision, professional advice, continuing professional development, reliable IT support and the knowledge and skills that they need to provide high-quality care (Department of Health,

2002). So who should lead the development of this education across the community and acute sectors? What should it consist of? How should it be delivered? And what will different professional groups need to learn?

Cancer Networks have been advised to agree upon what chemotherapy education should be provided across their acute trusts (Department of Health, 2004). No such guidance exists for primary care, although it has been suggested that community service providers should ensure that programmes of education are available for nurses caring for cancer patients in the community (Royal College of Nursing, 1999). The cancer nurses who are recognised as having the greatest expertise in a particular specialty are nurse specialists. These specialists are generally located in the acute trusts. As such, this is a good opportunity for Cancer Networks to lead work with acute trusts and chemotherapy specialists to develop programmes that guide nurses within the specialist chemotherapy and community settings with regard to learning to be achieved and competence to be attained.

There is a strong case for nationally driven educational guidance. However, the existing competency frameworks may serve to indicate what the content of an educational package should contain. One Cancer Network, in embarking upon this work, reviewed the competency frameworks that were available at the time. Recognised work that had been undertaken regionally included that of the Cancer Care Alliance (2000). They eventually based their work on that undertaken by the National Board for Scotland (2001). Since then, a competency framework for training in the administration of chemotherapy to children has also been published (Royal College of Nursing, 2005), and Skills for Health has produced chemotherapy-related National Workforce Competencies (details of which can be found at www.skillsforhealth.org.uk) mapped to the Knowledge and Skills Framework.

In deciding how to proceed, the Cancer Network in question addressed the issue of competence levels in nursing practitioners. Clearly, the staff groups across the various healthcare settings had different needs. Identifying appropriate levels was a complex matter, and the Network considered the following:

- Level 1 – non-qualified staff, and qualified staff with minimal involvement in chemotherapy assessment and administration
- Level 2 – supervised registered practitioner
- Level 3 – registered practitioner
- Level 4 – expert practitioner.

As education at Level III and above was available from the local academic institution, development of a Network competency and educational framework was concentrated at Levels I and II. This served to reinforce the complexities of chemotherapy care, and key discussion points included debate on issues such as the following.

- Where nurses are regularly administering only one type of chemotherapy, is it necessary for them to achieve Level III education, even if they practise unsupervised?
- Where community nurses are caring for patients who are receiving chemotherapy that is home based, but they are not actively involved in its delivery, should the required competence be Level I or II?
- Should community nurses overall be expected to access Level I or II education?
- What is meant by 'supervised' practice?

- In reality, less experienced nurses across the healthcare settings attend to patients independently. Is there a better way to distinguish between the competence required in Levels I and II?

It was clear throughout the process that there was difficulty in articulating the different depth of knowledge and skills required in competencies that spanned the two levels. Organisations undertaking similar work, regardless of how that work is approached, must be mindful of the need to produce competencies that reflect working practices without expecting generalist nurses to undertake a level of education and training which is inappropriate for their needs. In addition, it is equally important to ensure that competencies reflect a minimum standard of safe practice and understanding. Achieving this balance is a key challenge in managing this educational provision.

Subsequent development of an educational framework included a scoping exercise to identify the type of educational provision that Cancer Network services felt was most useful, and their preferred method of delivery. Trusts and primary care settings were unanimous in preferring to provide their own educational input, with guidance on content to be provided by the Network. Ensuring that all healthcare establishments provided nurses with the same knowledge and education was seen as important, but all preferred to use the traditional in-house study-day approach to deliver a programme.

How should chemotherapy education be delivered?

Traditional taught study days are the mainstay of chemotherapy education, but have associated difficulties in today's climate. With new responsibilities attached to senior chemotherapy staff and the anticipated increase in training, establishments will be hard pressed to support all in-house programmes. Staff at the forefront of patient care can experience difficulty in taking time out to access programmes on the particular days when they are offered (Jenkins, 2005). In addition, according to current thinking the lecture format of teaching involves passive learning, where learners are not required to be actively involved and information is made available through recall. As fewer cognitive skills are used, lower-level learning is often the outcome (Philips, 2005). Conversely, a rapidly emerging mode of teaching is through the use of e-learning, which if developed carefully should employ active learning strategies. Active learning engages the student in higher-order thinking which allows the assimilation, application and retention of learning. Chemotherapy education, with its practical nature, is well suited to this model, and it is felt that once they are experienced, most learners prefer an active learning approach (Philips, 2005). Associated advantages of e-learning include the release of educators, which enables them to spend time with learners as coaches and facilitators in the acquisition of practical skills. Importantly, staff have the opportunity to access learning at a time when it is most convenient for them to do so, and organisational boundaries are minimised, allowing acute and community staff to access programmes. With appropriate organisational and financial support, it is also possible for e-learning to be linked to a technological infrastructure that allows student management and tracking, presentation of materials and student testing, through the use of a learning management system. Thus the capturing and recording of evidence of learning can be made easier.

Interactive learning is being used to educate many healthcare providers in a variety of settings (Caldwell, 2005). Consideration should be given to employing e-learning as a strategy for providing this type of education and overcoming the organisational restrictions that create barriers to learning.

What are the difficulties in adopting a new approach to learning?

Development of an appropriate e-learning package is a time-consuming occupation, requiring collaborative working between identified subject matter experts, e-learning companies and organisational IT experts. Finances must be identified to fund the project, and proper design of the format is imperative (Jeffries, 2005). Where there is little expertise in developing packages, care must be taken to ensure that subject matter experts provide as much detail as possible to enable e-learning companies to produce worthwhile products. e-Learning companies are not chemotherapy experts, and therefore information may be interpreted wrongly. Including an interactive element in the product is essential in order to engage the student in a way that ensures they will learn from the experience. The package must be easy to navigate and should record modules as they are completed, so that the learner can pick up and drop the learning as necessary. Modules should be tested so that competence in theory can be assessed. The Cancer Network described above is actively pursuing the development of such a package to meet the needs of its nursing staff.

Using e-learning as a teaching approach can be more daunting for those nurses who feel less computer literate than their colleagues. Inevitably, the adoption of e-learning assumes both that nurses are IT literate and that they have access to IT facilities (Hegge *et al.*, 2002). Therefore, in circumstances where these criteria may not be fulfilled, it is important to explore the possibility of e-learning being used alongside traditional teaching methods, with students given the option of choosing between the two. Undoubtedly, e-learning technology requires a commitment from the organisation to ensure that staff have the skills necessary to access this type of learning and the opportunity to do so. For example, healthcare settings that have only one terminal available in a clinical area for all staff do not facilitate the e-learning development of staff, and this is why this type of education sometimes has its limitations.

What is the future for chemotherapy education?

The use of e-learning as a tool for chemotherapy education has yet to be evaluated. However, as technology continues to develop, there is a real opportunity for knowledge in this field to be acquired through interactive e-learning packages. Encouraging a flexible approach is paramount in order to maximise the opportunities for learning. Nurses need encouragement to address their electronic learning needs and to develop using this method of learning so that they can maximise the potential educational advantages available to them.

Key points

- Excellent care of the chemotherapy patient is only possible through appropriate education and competency assessment of the individuals who provide that care.
- Programmes of chemotherapy learning for acute trusts should be Network driven.
- Nurses who are involved in chemotherapy delivery or care of the chemotherapy patient in the community have different educational and competency requirements to nurses who are delivering chemotherapy in the acute setting.
- Realistic chemotherapy competency assessments that reflect their practice roles are required of community nurses.
- Networks should consider the needs of and ensure provision of education for community nurses who are involved in the chemotherapy patient pathway.
- Traditional routes of education have associated barriers to learning in the chemotherapy climate.
- Alternative routes of education should be considered alongside traditional routes. e-Learning can provide a novel way of accessing educational programmes, and may be more appropriate for some chemotherapy practitioners and settings.

Conclusion

Nurses who are caring for chemotherapy patients within acute trusts and community settings require education in the care of this patient group. Government measures dictate the need for trusts and Cancer Networks to formalise the approach that they use in ensuring education and resulting competence are achieved. Community staff should not be forgotten in the provision of these frameworks, to ensure the best possible care for patients and the continuation of safe standards of practice. Designing a framework is a complex matter, due to the differing needs of staff. However, every effort should be made to ensure that education is provided in a form that is accessible to all, with input from specialist practitioners during its development. Consideration should be given to embracing technological advances when planning how education should be delivered. e-Learning provides a real opportunity for nurses to undertake programmes that overcome some barriers to learning, and should be developed in future to take more of a leading role in chemotherapy nursing education.

Implications for the reader's own practice

1 Who are the nursing professionals involved in the care of chemotherapy patients in your work environment?
2 Where are the gaps in chemotherapy knowledge and skills across these staff groups?
3 What is the current chemotherapy education provision available to you and to other staff in the patient pathway?
4 How appropriate is the educational provision in relation to the roles that staff perform?
5 What would be the benefits of a collaborative approach to this education?
6 What are the barriers to chemotherapy education in your work environment?
7 How could these barriers be overcome?
8 What would be the benefits and costs of introducing e-learning as a method of education?

References

Allwood M, Stanley A, Wright P. *The Cytotoxics Handbook*. 4th ed. Oxford: Radcliffe Medical Press; 2002.

Caldwell R. Community health nursing in a virtual setting. *J Nurs Educ.* 2005; **44:** 147–9.

Calman K, Hine D. *A Policy Framework for Commissioning Cancer Services.*

Report by the Advisory Group on Cancer. London: Department of Health; 1995.

Cancer Care Alliance. *Cancer Care Alliance Chemotherapy Competency Framework.* Middlesborough: Cancer Care Alliance; 2000.

Department of Health. *Manual of Cancer Services Standards.* London: Department of Health; 2000a.

Department of Health. *The Nursing Contribution to Cancer Care.* London: Department of Health; 2000b.

Department of Health. *Liberating the Talents.* London: Department of Health; 2002.

Department of Health. *Manual of Cancer Services.* London: Department of Health; 2004.

Hegge M, Powers P, Hendricks L *et al.* Competence, continuing education and computers. *J Continuing Educ Nurs.* 2002; **33:** 24–33.

Jeffries P. Technology trends in nursing education: next steps. *J Nurs Educ.* 2005; **44:** 3–4.

Jenkins A. On the fast track. *Nurs Standard.* 2005; **19:** 77–9.

Kanaskie K, Arnold E. New ways to evaluate chemotherapy competencies. *Nurs Manage.* 1999; **30:** 41–4.

Kelly C, Crowe M. *Chemotherapy Nursing Briefing Paper.* National Chemotherapy Advisory Group; 2004.

National Board for Scotland. *The Core Curriculum for the Administration and Safe Handling of Cytotoxic Chemotherapy.* Edinburgh: National Board for Scotland; 2001.

Neal A, Hoskin P. *Clinical Oncology: a textbook for students.* London: Edward Arnold; 1994.

Philips JM. Strategies for active learning in online continuing education. *J Continuing Educ Nurs.* 2005; **36:** 77–84.

Royal College of Nursing. *A Structure for Cancer Nursing Services.* London: RCN Cancer Nursing Society; 1996.

Royal College of Nursing. *Clinical Practice Guidelines. The administration of cytotoxic chemotherapy.* London: Royal College of Nursing; 1998.

Royal College of Nursing. *The Administration of Cytotoxic Chemotherapy. Technical Report.* London: Royal College of Nursing; 1999.

Royal College of Nursing. *A Framework for Adult Cancer Nursing.* London: Royal College of Nursing; 2003.

Royal College of Nursing. *Competencies: an integrated competency framework for training programmes in the safe administration of chemotherapy to children and young people.* London: Royal College of Nursing; 2005.

Further reading

- Ali N, Hodson-Carlton K, Ryan M. Web-based professional education for advanced practice nursing: a consumer guide for program selection. *J Continuing Educ Nurs.* 2002; **33:** 33–9.
- Quinn F. *Principles and Practice of Nurse Education.* 4th ed. Gloucester: Stanley Thornes Ltd; 2000.
- Thede L. *Computers in Nursing.* Philadelphia, PA: Lippincott; 1999.

Chapter 5

Leading the way: the role of education in achieving clinical standards in the haematological oncology setting

Kirsten Midgley

> *Education is the great engine of personal development. It is through education that the daughter of a peasant can become a doctor, that the son of a mineworker can become head of the mine, that a child of farm workers can become the president of a great nation.*
>
> *Nelson Mandela (1994)*

Aim

The aim of this chapter is explore quality issues in healthcare and how they impact on the specialty of haematological oncology care. The impact of gaining accreditation in the haematological oncology setting will be explored, as well as the role of the clinical educator in ensuring that quality of care is delivered. A variety of clinical models and learning styles will be explored.

Learning outcomes

- Consider the role of clinical education when developing a cancer, palliative or haematological oncology-specific care learning programme.
- Gain knowledge of a variety of clinical education models and how they may be applied in post-registration cancer education and continuing professional development.
- Examine the implications of learning styles for developing a specialist educational and training programme in haematological oncology.

Introduction

Quality in healthcare is not new, and in the literature it can be traced back to the time of Florence Nightingale. Quality has been a prominent component of healthcare policy for the last 10 years. JACIE is an acronym for *Joint Accreditation Committee of ISCT and EBMT*. Its origins are in the work of the International Society for Cellular Therapy (ISCT), the North American Foundation for the Accreditation of Cellular Therapy (FACT) and European Blood and Marrow Transplantation (EBMT), but its essence is in quality, a quality bone-marrow transplantation (BMT) programme. The JACIE vision is that all European BMT centres will follow and meet this quality programme. BMT is a relatively new medical discipline. In the 1960s, it was undertaken experimentally as a last resort. However, today BMT is recognised as a proven treatment for many haematological malignancies, and the medical and nursing fields of BMT continue to evolve. Education is pivotal to the success of any policy initiative, and JACIE accreditation is no exception. Nurse education and training are an essential standard for any centre that is seeking JACIE accreditation. This chapter will explore the concept of clinical education during 'in-house' post-registration education and training and continued professional development. The term 'in-house' refers to locally delivered education and training courses. Thus the education and training are not formally led by an academic institution, nor do they usually have academic rigour.

Background

JACIE standards were originally drawn up in 1996, to provide minimum guidelines for centres that perform haematopoietic cell transplantation and therapy or that provide support services for such procedures. The JACIE standards are based on the standards developed in America by FACT, which in turn resulted from the merger of laboratory standards developed by the ISCT and the clinical and training guidelines produced by FACT. Standards were developed by agreement from the medical literature and contributions of experts in the field of transplantation to provide regulation of BMT. The primary objective of the JACIE standards is the promotion of robust quality-driven medical and laboratory practice in haematopoietic progenitor cell transplantation. Success in terms of these measures leads to the acquisition of full accreditation by qualified peer inspection.

Quality is now of paramount importance in healthcare, particularly as society demands a more effective and accountable health service. Quality refers to fitness for use. However, for quality to be successful within any institution or business – large or small – all members of the organisation need to take part. *Total quality management (TQM)* is a culture that aims to continually improve the performance of all functions and departments of a company or institution (Holmes, 2002). For any institution or company that wishes to adopt a TQM approach, a robust educational policy is therefore crucial for ensuring the cooperation, commitment and involvement of all of its members.

Nurse education and training are an essential component of the JACIE standards.

> *B3.710 Programmes must have nurses and nurse supervisors*
> *formally trained and experienced in the management of*
> *patients receiving haematopoietic progenitor cell*
> *transplants*
> *B3.730 Training must include haematology/oncology patient*
> *care: administration of high-dose therapy, growth*
> *factors and immunosuppressive medications;*
> *management of infectious complications associated*
> *with compromised host defence mechanisms;*

> *administration of blood products; and an appropriate*
> *degree of intensive nursing care*
>
> *(JACIE Accreditation Manual, 2005)*

It would be short-sighted and impractical to consider 'formal' education as just that which is academically driven. Guidance from the JACIE document acknowledges that, within their definition, formal training may include in-service education and training such as review classes, course, conferences, or on-the-job training that addresses specific topics. Importantly, evidence of training and education in these core competencies must be documented. Such standards clearly demonstrate recognition of the important role that nurse education and training play in a quality programme and service, in which clinical education must have a crucial part.

Pre-registration education and training should prepare the learner for practice at the point of registration, whilst continuing professional development must be geared to the post-registration renewal process and the standards of professional practice that the nursing profession requires.

A key facet of any type of education is unquestionably the aim of helping and encouraging each learner to reach their full potential or, from a humanistic viewpoint, the achievement of self-actualisation and maximum potential for personal growth (McKenna, 1995). Yes, there are certainly others, but for any educator – whatever their area of practice – seeing a learner achieve important milestones is immensely rewarding. Nursing has embraced the importance of education through its commitment to lifelong learning. It is important to realise that nurse education and training may vary in approach. The conventional approach involves formal education and training, which is academically driven, usually with the attainment of a qualification as a measure of success, and it is necessary for professional practice. However, a significant but less often acknowledged approach is work-based training and education, which does not often result in any formal qualification being obtained, is usually run 'in-house', and is motivated by the achievement of competency in a specific skill, with a record of attendance kept.

Defining clinical education

Clinical education has been defined as follows:

> *A teaching and learning process which is student focused and may be student led, which occurs in the context of client care. It involves the translation of theory into the development of clinical knowledge and practical skills, with the incorporation of the affective domain needed for sensitive and ethical client care. Clinical education occurs in an environment supportive of the development of clinical reasoning skills, professional socialisation and lifelong learning.*
>
> *(McAllister, 2001, p. 3)*

This description encompasses the attainment of knowledge, skills and attributes that are required in order to become both a competent professional and a proficient practitioner. Clinical education is a fundamental and irreplaceable aspect of preparing students for the reality of their future professional role (Grahn, 1989; Williams and Webb, 1994). Indeed, if we subscribe to the notion that nursing is an 'action profession' that nurses learn by doing it (Neary, 2000), the role of clinical education in pre-registration training is crucial. However, when a nurse qualifies and becomes a registered practitioner, then in reality the educational and training journey is just beginning, not ending. In today's healthcare climate the emphasis is on an accountable and responsible service that is responsive, safe, efficient and effective, and thus the role of continuing education and development is crucial. Historically, the role of clinical educators was traditionally ensconced in pre-registration nurse training, but no more. During the last 10 to 15 years there has been a growing emphasis on the role of clinical education for qualified (post-registration) nursing staff and for nursing teams as a whole, with the emergence of clinical educator roles, particularly in specialist fields of nursing.

These roles are usually funded by hospital trusts rather than by academic institutions.

Clinical education is concerned with the real world of professional practice, based on holistic learning that involves the reassignment, reorganisation, application, synthesis and appraisal of previously attained knowledge, along with the acquisition of new knowledge and skills (*see* Box 5.1). These goals are particularly pertinent to education in the haematological setting, as they facilitate and enable both the educator and the learner to address and explore the complexity of haematological oncology care.

Box 5.1   Goals of clinical education for healthcare professionals (adapted from Higgs *et al.*, 1991, cited in McAllister, 2001)

- An understanding of health, disease and the healthcare structure.
- An awareness of one's own attitudes, beliefs and values with regard to health and illness.
- An understanding of the roles within the multi-disciplinary healthcare team.
- Clinical competencies and skills relevant to the learner's field, including interpersonal, communication, clinical, reasoning and psychomotor skills and competencies.
- Evidence-based interactions and actions.
- Patient/client education.
- Time and workload management.
- Development of coping skills.
- Computer and technology skills.
- Critical analysis and personal development.
- Quality clinical practice.
- Professional accountability and responsibility to patients, employers and self.
- Commitment to develop and maintain professional competence and skills.
- Skills needed to ensure lifelong learning.
- Ability to respond to the challenges and changes in healthcare needs.

Unsurprisingly, it is argued that the clinical setting best promotes the integration of theory and practice, particularly the problem-solving and clinical decision-making skills that are essential in real-life patient care (McAllister, 2001). This is clearly true in pre-registration nurse training and education, but what about the scenario of clinical education for qualified nursing staff? Theoretically, it is easy to argue that the situation and practice should be the same. However, the reality is a little different. During pre-registration training the learner has protected clinical time in which to learn and develop, largely due to their supernumerary status. However, once they have qualified, this protected learning changes. Clinical demands, time pressures and simply getting the job done will result in a change of emphasis for the practitioner.

Pre-registration training encourages the learner to become a reflective practitioner and a knowledgeable doer, and promotes self-directed learning. Post registration the impetus changes. The practitioner no longer has academic pressures, and requirements to encourage and stimulate active clinical learning no longer prevail. The emphasis and drive for learning have changed. Often there is no longer a measurable educational goal to achieve, and learning is truly more self-directed. The desire for team acceptance, usefulness, role fulfilment and ultimately the need for career progression become the driving force. Without the academic drive and distinct measurable outcome, do practitioners always continue the clinical learning that was so actively encouraged throughout their pre-registration training? For clinical educators this is a fundamental question that needs to be considered and addressed, although it is unclear whether there is any answer that will apply to all.

Post registration, each practitioner will have different desires and motives to learn and develop. Some will be eager to continue to learn and develop, while others will need direction and guidance, so is this so different from other areas of teaching and learning? Without a formal structured process, many healthcare professionals will struggle to continue the learning that is essential for professional and individual growth and development. Today, however, with the introduction of the *Agenda for Change* and the *Knowledge and Skills Framework (KSF)*, this attitude may change, with the emphasis on the application of knowledge and skills essential for professional success and development. It is through mechanisms such as the KSF that individuals may be challenged to acknowledge and hopefully even embrace the importance of continuing clinical education both for their own personal development and to ensure the continued delivery of high-quality nursing care. A significant approach may be to map the required haematological competencies needed for JACIE and other measures – for example, Cancer Standards (Department of Health, 2004b) – back to the KSF, thereby providing the learner with a clear view of the required professional development journey.

Another key difference between pre- and post-registration nurse learners is that in the post-registration setting the learner is utilising clinical knowledge and practical skills that have already been learned. During pre-registration nurse training the learner develops skills of critical thinking, enabling them to recognise the ever changing nature of knowledge, and they learn to seen human experience from more than one perspective (Pickering and McAllister, 2001). As with other areas of adult learning, in the post-registration setting, each learner will bring different skills and knowledge and different educational and training experiences to bear. The clinical educator has a crucial role in helping to bring together this prior learning, so that all of the learners can learn and develop both independently and from each other. To employ the terminology of Benner (1984), they facilitate the learner's journey from 'novice to expert.' A fundamental skill that is required on this journey is reflection.

Learning from experience is probably one of the most important life skills. It can often be taken for granted or carried out intuitively without conscious awareness (Honey and Mumford, 2000a). Nursing is an action profession, and consequently a large amount of learning is achieved through clinical experience. It is crucial that this learning is conscious learning, so that we learn from our experiences. Key to this conscious learning is reflection. Dewey (1933) argued that there could be no true growth as a result of learning solely from experience, but only by *reflecting upon experience*. Schön (1983) suggests that, through reflective practice, learners develop an analytical understanding of the recurring experiences of a specialised field, and can make new sense of uncertain or unique situations that they encounter. Reflective practice undoubtedly helps learners to make sense of their experiences and become competent practitioners. Thus it is crucial that those facilitating clinical education take reflective practice seriously (Lincoln *et al.*, 2001) and utilise it effectively.

Within post-registration clinical education there is an expectation that each learner is responsible for their future learning and development. It is important that clinical educators engage with their learners to help to develop appropriate learning plans and packages. By engaging with the learner you give them some ownership of the learning process. This can be done through a training needs analysis (TNA), which is the first and essential step in the training and educational strategy of an organisation, and is necessary to meet the educational and training needs of both healthcare professionals and service demands (Gould *et al.*, 2004). If possible, a TNA should involve all potential stakeholders (i.e. employees, service users, education providers and commissioners). It is important that the training and education needs of the organisation are clearly acknowledged and reflected in the TNA (Gould *et al.*, 2004). There is the risk of conflict between organisational needs and individual staff needs. However, if sensitively addressed, a TNA will give individual staff members some ownership, particularly if they can see that the TNA and their responses have been translated into a training programme. Within BMT, the JACIE standards provided the framework for both the TNA and the educational and training pro-gramme, but by encouraging staff to identify learning areas within this framework it gave them some tenure in this process. A TNA is a valuable starting point for any clinical educator. TNA methods will vary according to what is suitable for the clinical area, and they should be rigorous yet practical. Suggested methods include face-to-face interviews, focus groups, questionnaires, observation and telephone questionnaire, or a combination of methods (Gould *et al.*, 2004). When the training and educational needs have been identified, it is important to determine how these will translate into a clinical education programme.

Models of clinical education

> *Theory without practice is vacuous, but practice without theory is like someone going to sea without a map in a ship without a rudder.*
> Clark (1982), cited by Jackson (1986)

> *...it is important that the map you choose gets you where you want to be taken.*
> Jackson (1986), cited by Johns (1994)

Models are not a new concept to nursing, as they provide direction. A knowledge and understanding of the various models of clinical education that are available allows educators to work and teach in a way that best suits their needs and those of their learners and the service as a whole (McLeod *et al.*, 2001). Within cancer and palliative care education, the use of models encourages the educator to make sense of, order, improve, articulate and teach the process that is being experienced (Pickering, 1987). It is vital that the learner understands and appreciates the model that the educator has chosen, so that they have an awareness of the design and the expectations of them as learners and what they can hope to gain from the process. The models of clinical education have developed from the diverse disciplines involved in clinical education. Consequently, when choosing a model, the clinical educator must take into account not only the philosophies that underlie the relationship between the educator, the learner and the patient, but also the way in which adult learning is perceived and valued, the attitudes and preferences of the various professions and professionals, and the practicalities of time, money and space (McLeod *et al.*, 2001).

Six different types of model will now be described, and possible examples from the cancer and/or palliative care setting will be given. Although it is beyond the scope of this chapter to explore these models in more detail, these introductions should provide the clinical educator with a range of options to examine further in order to determine what would be most appropriate for their clinical practice. In many cases this may be a combination of models.

Descriptive models

There are a number of clinical education models that take a broad view and describe the various elements of the process. One such model is the *trigonal model of clinical education* proposed by Farmer and Farmer (1989), which identified that clinical education has three interrelated components:

1 *constituents* – the people involved in the process (e.g. students, patients, families, clinical educator and other clinicians)
2 *concepts* – the knowledge and theories of clinical education
3 *context* – the setting in which the education occurs (e.g. classroom, hospital, community).

An example of this methodology is described by the Royal College of Nursing (2003) in *A Framework for Adult Cancer Nursing*, in the Fife Primary Cancer Care Education Strategy. In this approach the patient and his or her family are placed at the centre of the care learning experience. Many courses are offered, including clinical skills-based, clinical needs-led or generic cancer care specialties in various settings. Specific competencies are accompanied by transferable skills from clinical (acute, palliative and community), educational and research environments. A database notifies staff of the availability of courses and when they need updates.

Integration models

These models are subsets of the descriptive clinical education models. Integration models provide a framework for the coordination of academic and clinical elements –that is, they aim to address the theory–practice gap. This is perhaps one of the most popular approaches within nursing. Greatorex *et al.* (2002) describe the development of a short course cancer education programme for qualified and non-qualified nursing staff, the main aims being to reduce the theory–practice gap and help attendees to improve their patient care. The short course enhances the learner's knowledge so as to enable them to critically examine their particular field of practice. Similarly, Barker *et al.* (2004) developed a palliative care education programme for community-based nurses. This was a network-wide, skills-based course in palliative care, founded around a theoretical framework. A key aim was that the learner would acquire transferable skills of good assessment that could be applied in any palliative care setting (National Council for Hospice and Specialist Palliative Care Services, 1998).

Developmental models

Developmental models assume that learners progress through hierarchical steps and that development occurs through the interaction between the learner and their environment (Sprinthall and Thies-Sprinthall, 1983). These models are concerned with how learners make sense of the experience as well as the actual outcome of the clinical education (Wittman and Schwartz, 1991). The *Knowledge and Skills Framework (KSF)* (Department of Health, 2004a) is a good example of this approach, as clinical areas everywhere will be deciding how to apply this approach with their teams. Wetherall (2004) describes the application of the core competency framework within the cancer care setting, which pre-dates the publication of the KSF. The framework aimed to provide a consensus for assessing and developing nurses' clinical competencies, with the ultimate aim of improving the quality of care for cancer patients and their families wherever care is provided.

Interactive process models

These models describe the actual interactive process of clinical education – that is, what really occurs during the everyday exchange between the clinical educator and the learner (McLeod *et al.*, 2001). This type of methodology mirrors the clinical supervision process.

Collaborative models

Collaborative models have emerged more recently, reflecting an increasing interest in collaborative learning, and the value of learning among peers and multi-disciplinary learning. Johnson and Johnson (1990) developed a conceptual style to collaborative learning. They identified five basic components of a collaborative learning situation, namely positive interdependence, face-to-face interaction, individual accountability, cooperative skills and group processing. The RCN Cancer Nursing Society (1996) recommended that consideration should be given to whether some elements of education and training should be uni-disciplinary or multi-disciplinary. Johnson *et al.* (2004) have described the development and establishment of a clinical rotation programme in cancer and palliative care nursing. This programme involved acute care provision and hospice and community palliative care.

Teacher–manager model

This is a relatively new model that has not been widely examined in the literature. The teacher–manager model was developed by Romanini and Higgs (1991). Unlike the previous models, it does not fit into one category but rather it embraces aspects of all five categories. Within this model the clinical educator is seen as a proactive facilitator of the whole learning programme and a manager of the clinical learning programme (McLeod *et al.*, 2001). The teacher–manager model was developed as a tool to aid the design, implementation and evaluation of learning programmes in an array of educational settings (Romanini and Higgs, 1991), particularly nursing. This approach may be particularly useful in clinical areas that have a dedicated clinical educator who can take sole responsibility for the development and implementation of the programme.

Learning styles

Having identified an appropriate model of clinical education that is suitable for the clinical setting, it is also important to consider how people learn. Learning is such an elementary process that it often gets taken for granted, the convenient assumption being that in adulthood we have learned how to learn and need no further help. Trainers may often assume that learners are 'empty buckets waiting to be filled by whatever training method the trainer favours. The fact that the buckets are different shapes and sizes is conveniently overlooked' (Honey and Mumford, 2000b). It is clear that people vary not just in their learning skills but also in their learning styles, as do the educators.

Learning style refers to the attitudes and behaviours that determine a learner's preferred way of learning (Honey and Mumford, 2000a). It is important that the clinical educator is aware of their own learning style as well as how their learners learn, as this will probably influence the way in which they teach. Knowledge of the learners' preferred learning style can help to direct the educator to activities that suit their learners' learning style. This may seem more useful in one-to-one teaching sessions than in group sessions, although knowledge of the preferred learning styles of a group of learners could be used to split the group into smaller defined groups, who could then be taught according to their particular learning style. The educator may decide to use his or her knowledge of different learning styles to ensure that each teaching session engages attributes from each learning style. Similarly, a clinical educator can choose to use the knowledge of his or her learners' preferred learning style, knowing how those individuals learn in clinical practice.

In busy haematological oncology care settings, both professionally and personally, education can often take a back seat. However, if the learner can see the value of learning, they are more likely to engage readily in the process. Importantly, those with an educational role in the haematological oncology setting need to teach others to appreciate individual learning styles. This not only encourages increased learning, but can also ultimately improve patient care.

Challenges

Healthcare is facing many challenges in the twenty-first century, and cancer and palliative care is no exception. The concept of and drive for quality are embedded in the culture and philosophy of the NHS. A programme such as the JACIE standards for BMT is one such example of a quality programme. Quality is everyone's concern, although ensuring that everyone realises they have a part to play can often be problematic. It is here at the beginning of a quality programme, as well as in the ongoing process of the programme, that education has a significant role to play.

> *Reassuring patients is a hard thing to do – a knowledgeable nurse is welcoming, knows who you are and why you are there, stands out when you are feeling insecure, anxious, uncertain and afraid.*
>
> *(Royal College of Nursing, 2002)*

Service users have ever increasing demands and expectations of healthcare and the professionals who provide the service. Education is pivotal in meeting those needs and expectations, and in both personal and professional development – never more so than in a busy haematological oncology setting where art and science need to be finely balanced.

If education is to become embedded in the ethos of healthcare, it needs resources. Although financial implications are associated with delivering clinical education and training programmes, it would appear that the most important resource is time. Time is often a rare resource in healthcare for the following reasons.

- The role of work-based learning is essential for nursing development, but learners also need time away from the clinical setting in order to learn.
- Clinical educators often face the competing demands of clinical requirements and educational needs. Perhaps, as a profession, nursing needs to consider incorporating personal growth and learning into the working week.
- During pre-registration training the learner has dedicated study time and opportunities for learning and development. However, competing demands mean that haematological oncology is often only fleetingly considered or may be omitted altogether.

Another significant challenge for clinical educators in post-registration oncology education and training is the diversity of experience of their learners, ranging from the newly qualified to those with significant experience in the clinical field – sometimes with more experience than that of the clinical educator. Ultimately, the motivation to learn will vary from one learner to another, so the challenge for the clinical educator is to engage all of their learners in a variety of settings. It is important to consider new and varied ways of working, such as the use of a variety of teaching styles (e.g. lectures, focus groups, seminars, work-based learning, e-learning) and settings. The clinical educator's own motivation and willingness to try to meet the varied needs of their learners will in itself encourage learning.

Personal reflection

As a clinical educator for haematology and medical oncology, this author has had sole responsibility for the implementation of the training and education programme for JACIE within her Unit, and as such has encountered many of the problems described above. This author has utilised many elements of the 'teacher–manager model' of clinical education as the preferred model for developing the clinical education and training programme in BMT, and whilst being the facilitator and manager of the whole learning programme, learner participation was ensured through TNA and ongoing evaluation. Learner involvement does encourage some degree of ownership. To date, questionnaires have been utilised as the main method of data collection, as this is probably the least threatening method, while at the same time giving useful results. The questionnaires have always allowed space for the respondent to express their opinions. The response rates have varied, but have always exceeded 50%. The biggest problem that was encountered was time – that is, dedicated time for learners away from the clinical area. This time was necessary for the delivery of the training and education programme, and it was essential in order to meet and engage the different needs of my adult learners. The staff were divided into learning groups according to grade/band, in an attempt to have staff of similar experience together where possible. A framework gives a training programme structure, so the key areas identified in the JACIE standards were used. A varied programme was developed that used a variety of learning strategies, including lectures, group work, videos, learning packages, etc., to engage the learners. In addition, all staff within the BMT programme received a training and education folder in which to collate handouts, learning packages, etc. from the taught sessions, to utilise as a record of training and education and to facilitate personal development.

It was clear that despite the support of senior staff it would not be possible for all staff to be released to attend every training session. Consequently, all staff were given the same written information. The JACIE education and training requirements are quite broad and diverse, making it impossible for one person to deliver the whole programme, so clinical experts help to support the programme as appropriate. It is important that the training and education programme is flexible enough to address not only clinical changes and the requirements for accreditation, but also the changes and challenges in nursing (e.g. the KSF). In addition, one should always consider new ways of delivering information and reaching the intended audience.

Key points

- The role of haematological oncology care education in a quality programme is essential.
- The role of clinical education in the post-registration oncology setting has an important contribution to make.
- New ways of providing specific cancer and palliative clinical education should be a priority for development.
- Meeting the different learning needs and styles of learners in an oncology setting should always be a consideration.

Conclusion

Informal approaches to clinical education in the post-registration education setting have much to offer. In the current climate, clinical educators must be mindful of the competing demands, and need to consider new ways of approaching clinical education. Training and education are essential for a quality haematological oncology service, and also have a role to play in maintaining staff morale and staff retainment. A significant change in healthcare which should help the clinical educator in their drive to embed clinical education in the organisational philosophy is the KSF, introduced as part of the *Agenda for Change*. The KSF defines and describes the knowledge and skills that NHS staff need to apply in their work in order to deliver quality services. Its aim is to provide a single, consistent, comprehensive and explicit framework on which to base review and development for all staff (Department of Health, 2004a). The KSF represents a significant opportunity which, so long as more than lip service is paid to it, will promote clinical education, training and development. The clinical educator has a vital role in engaging the 'hearts and minds' of their learners in the post-registration arena to ensure that this opportunity for nursing growth and development is not missed. As the NHS strives to meet the challenges of healthcare in the twenty-first century, clinical education and the role of the clinical educator have never been more important, particularly in the advancing and highly technological setting of haematological oncology.

Implications for the reader's own practice

1 What is your role in delivering quality in an oncology setting?
2 How could you implement a model of clinical education in your clinical area?
3 How could you assess and meet the needs of the different learning styles of your learners?
4 How would you evaluate the effect of a clinical education programme in the oncological post-registration setting?
5 How do you know that your clinical haematological oncology education is successful?

References

Barker S, Gibbs G, Hill A *et al.* Palliative care education for community-based nurses. *Cancer Nurs Pract.* 2004; **3**: 29–33.

Benner P. *From Novice to Expert: excellence and power in clinical nursing practice.* Menlo Park, CA: Addison-Wesley; 1984.

Department of Health. *The NHS Knowledge and Skills Framework (NHS KSF) and the Development Review Process.* London: Department of Health; 2004a.

Department of Health. *Manual of Cancer Services.* London: Department of Health; 2004b.

Dewey J. *How We Whink.* Boston, MA: DC Heath; 1933.

Farmer S, Farmer J. *Supervision in Communication Disorders.* Columbus, OH: Merrill Publishing; 1989.

Gould D, Kelly D, White I. Training needs analysis: an evaluation framework. *Nurs Standard.* 2004; **18**: 33–6.

Grahn G. Educational situations in clinical settings. *Radiography Today.* 1989; **55**: 26–7.

Greatorex T, Cresswell A, Hirst P *et al.* Developments in education. *Cancer Nurs Pract.* 2002; **1**: 26–30.

Holmes K. Total quality management. In: *ACCA Study Text Paper 3.5. Strategic business planning and development.* London: BPP Publishing Ltd; 2002.

Honey P, Mumford A. *The Learning Styles Questionnaire: 80-item version.* Maidenhead: Peter Honey; 2000a.

Honey P, Mumford A. *The Learning Styles Helper's Guide.* Maidenhead: Peter Honey; 2000b.

Jackson M. On maps and models. *Senior Nurse.* 1986; **5**(4): 24–6.

Johns C, editor. *BDNU Model: caring in practice.* London: Blackwell Science; 1994.

Johnson DW, Johnson RT. *Learning Together and Alone: cooperative, competitive and individualistic learning.* Boston, MA: Alyn & Bacon; 1990.

Johnson M, Mennon A, Richardson A. Establishing clinical rotation programmes in cancer and palliative care nursing. *Cancer Nurs Pract.* 2004; **3**: 29–34.

Joint Accreditation Committee of ISCT and EBMT. *JACIE Accreditation Manual.* 2nd ed. Barcelona: JACIE; 2005.

Lincoln M, Stockhausen L, Maloney D. Learning processes in clinical education. In: McAllister L, Lincoln M, McLeod S *et al.*, editors. *Facilitating Learning in Clinical Settings.* Cheltenham: Nelson Thornes Ltd; 2001.

McAllister L. An adult learning framework for clinical education. In: McAllister L, Lincoln M, McLeod S *et al.*, editors. *Facilitating Learning in Clinical Settings.* Cheltenham: Nelson Thornes Ltd; 2001.

McKenna G. Learning theories made easy: humanism. *Nurs Standard.* 1995; **9**: 29–31.

McLeod S, Romanini J, Cohn E *et al.* Models and roles in clinical education. In: McAllister L, Lincoln M, McLeod S *et al.*, editors. *Facilitating Learning in Clinical Settings.* Cheltenham: Nelson Thornes Ltd; 2001.

Mandela N. *Long Walk to Freedom.* London: Little Brown & Co.; 1994.

National Council for Hospice and Specialist Palliative Care Services (NCHSPCS). *Reaching Out: specialist palliative care for adults with non-malignant diagnoses.* Occasional Paper No. 8. London: NCHSPCS; 1998.

Neary M. Responsive assessment: assessing student nurses' clinical competence. *Nurse Educ Today.* 2000; **21**: 3–17.

Pickering M. Supervision: a person-focused process. In: Crago M, Pickering M, editors. *Supervision in Human Communication Disorders: perspectives on a process.* San Diego, CA: College Hill Press; 1987.

Pickering M, McAllister L. Clinical education and the future: an emerging mosaic of change, challenge and creativity. In: McAllister L, Lincoln M, McLeod S *et al.*, editors. *Facilitating Learning in Clinical Settings.* Cheltenham: Nelson Thornes Ltd; 2001.

Romanini J, Higgs J. The teacher as manager in continuing professional education. *Stud Continuing Educ.* 1991; **13**: 41–52.

Royal College of Nursing. *Quality Education for Quality Care: a position statement for nursing education.* London: Royal College of Nursing; 2002.

Royal College of Nursing. *A Framework for Adult Cancer Nursing.* London: Royal College of Nursing; 2003.

Royal College of Nursing Cancer Nursing Society. *A Structure for Cancer Nursing Services.* London: Royal College of Nursing; 1996.

Schön D. *The Reflective Practitioner.* London: Temple Smith; 1983.

Sprinthall NA, Thies-Sprinthall L. The teacher as an adult learner. A cognitive-developmental view. In: Griffin GA, editor. *Staff Development.* Chicago: National Society for the Study of Education; 1983.

Wetherall A. Core competency framework. *Cancer Nurs Pract.* 2004; **2**: 16–17.

Williams PL, Webb C. Clinical supervision skills: a Delphi and critical incident technique. *Med Teacher.* 1994; **16**: 139–55.

Wittman PP, Schwartz KB. Identifying the development needs of students. In: Crepeau EB, LaGarde T, editors. *Self-Paced Instruction for Clinical Education and Supervision: an instructional guide.* Rockville, MD: American Occupational Therapy Association; 1991.

Further reading

- Honey P, Mumford A. *The Manual of Learning Styles.* 3rd ed. Maidenhead: Peter Honey; 1992.
- Kaplan R. The balanced scorecard. In: *ACCA Study Text Paper 3.5. Strategic business planning and development.* London: BPP Publishing Ltd; 2002.
- McAllister L, Lincoln M, McLeod S *et al.,* editors. *Facilitating Learning in Clinical Settings.* Cheltenham: Nelson Thornes Ltd; 2001. This is a valuable resource for any educator considering the role and implementation of learning in the clinical setting.
- Royal College of Nursing. *Quality Education for Quality Care: a position statement for nursing education.* London: Royal College of Nursing; 2004.

Chapter 6

Approaches to multi-professional radiotherapy education

Kathryn Guyers

> *Few therapeutic modalities in medicine induce more misunderstanding, confusion and apprehension than radiotherapy.*
>
> Rotman
>
> *To teach is to understand. To learn is wisdom. To learn together is understanding wisdom.*
>
> Sid Mendenhall

Aim

The aim of this chapter is to discuss the approaches that have been used to deliver radiotherapy education to a range of professionals who work in the arena of cancer and palliative care. It is written as a reflection of the author's experience of developing and delivering multi-professional radiotherapy education as part of a BSc (Hons) degree in Cancer Care.

Learning outcomes

- Understand the importance of multi-professional education in cancer and palliative care.
- Understand the approaches that have been taken in multi-professional radiotherapy education.
- Identify the issues involved in multi-professional education.

Introduction

In the author's 25 years of experience as both a therapeutic radiographer and a radiotherapy lecturer, it has been apparent that radiotherapy as a treatment modality and a profession is understood by few professions outside therapeutic radiography. Many professional groups are involved in caring for patients with cancer throughout their cancer journey, and each group is expert in the area in which they specialise. These areas include the patient's journey from screening and diagnosis through to treatment, side-effect management, long-term follow-up and palliative care. What they all (including therapeutic radiographers) lack is an understanding of the roles of other professionals in these different areas (Wells 1998). Although the author acknowledges that we cannot and should not all be experts in all areas, what we should be able to achieve is more understanding of what the patient experiences and why, at each point in their journey, and therefore be able to offer meaningful information and advice to the patients in our care.

Many professional groups will care for the cancer patient before, during and after a course of radiotherapy, but may not be able to give information and advice to the patient about their radiotherapy treatment at the level that they would wish or at the level that the patient may require. 'Misinformation may adversely affect the decision patients ultimately make regarding their treatment' (Wong *et al.*, 2002, p. 409), so it is vital that information is accurate and up to date.

In 2003, a new BSc (Hons) degree in Cancer Care was developed at the University of Leeds as part of its post-registration provision to enable practitioners to acquire the knowledge and skills necessary to work in the rapidly developing area of cancer care services, and to enhance patient care (Ferrell *et al.*, 2002). The degree programme was developed so that it would be accessible to students from a range of healthcare professions, thereby increasing the opportunities for interaction between practitioners with different backgrounds, skills and experience. The development of the degree also fulfils the objective of the *Policy Framework for Commissioning Cancer Services* that practitioners involved in patient care should have undergone post-registration training in oncology (Department of Health, 1995).

As part of this programme, a module entitled 'Care of the Patient Receiving Radiotherapy' was developed as an optional module for those undertaking the BSc (Hons) Cancer Care degree, and also as an elective for students on other relevant degree programmes.

What is multi-professional education?

Multi-professional education has been defined as follows:

> *A process by which a group of professionals with different educational backgrounds come together to learn and interact. To work together in providing health-related services.*
>
> Council of Europe (1995)

Why is multi-professional education necessary?

> *Provision of good cancer care is dependent on the involvement of multi-disciplinary, properly trained teams.*
>
> (Department of Health, 2001, p. 200)

This statement demonstrates the importance of well-educated professions working together to provide adequate care for cancer patients. To enable proper training for multi-disciplinary teams (MDTs) to take place, it would seem logical for the professions to receive this training together in order to enhance their knowledge and understanding not only of cancer and cancer care, but also of one another's professions and the role of each profession in caring for cancer patients. The Clinical

Oncology Patients' Liaison Group highlighted cooperation and communication within MDTs to ensure that all staff involved with the patient were informed of the treatment plan and that there was consistency of information (Royal College of Radiologists, 1999).

The Department of Health and the National Institute for Clinical Excellence (NICE) have produced guidance reports relating to specific cancers (Department of Health, 2004). The NICE guidance reports include the suggestion that multidisciplinary teamworking is vital for improving the experience of cancer patients. They acknowledge that MDTs lead to improved communication between professional groups. Multi-professional education enables this communication to improve even further, allowing time for discussion and debate in a safe environment that does not have the constraints of a working environment. All participants are on an equal footing as students within a learning environment.

Traditionally, training and education in healthcare have been very profession specific, with little if any shared learning or education about the role of other professions (Harden, 1998a). 'The failure of different health professions to recognise each other's skills and possible contribution is a major obstacle to effective patient care' (Council of Europe, 1995). This is often manifested as a lack of knowledge of one another's role, and potential lack of confidence in the ability of other professional groups. With lack of knowledge there is the potential for lack of coordination of care, due to poor communication and/or teamwork (Faithfull and Wells, 2004). The sharing of skills and experience in an educational environment in turn allows the sharing of information about one another's profession, providing an insight into the similarities and differences between the different professions, and facilitating increased mutual respect and understanding. Multi-professional education in healthcare has many benefits (Pirrie *et al.*, 1998). The sharing of knowledge and skills gives rise to a flexible practitioner and enables them to develop both themselves and their practice so as to adopt a more holistic approach to patient care (Council of Europe, 1995).

The need for multi-professional radiotherapy education

There are many misconceptions about cancer and radiotherapy as a treatment (Wells, 1998). It is therefore important that practitioners who are caring for cancer patients have the knowledge that will help them to dispel these misconceptions, not just in patients they are caring for but also in fellow practitioners (Department of Health, 2000).

> *A key recommendation of the NHS cancer plan was that all patients and carers should have access to a range of information materials about cancer and cancer services throughout the course of their illness.*
>
> *(Department of Health, 2004)*

As previously stated, a range of professions will care for patients before, during and after a course of radiotherapy. Information about radiotherapy treatment may be required by patients at all stages of their cancer journey, and professionals caring for patients with cancer should have the knowledge and understanding to allow the information to be discussed with the patient at the required level.

The radiotherapy module under discussion was developed in order to give professionals caring for patients undergoing radiotherapy an insight into radiotherapy as both a treatment modality and a profession, and to allow them to:

- critically analyse the rationale for the role of radiotherapy in the treatment of cancer, including the local and systemic reactions of the commonest treatment sites and the strategies for managing them
- evaluate strategies for assessing, planning and managing therapeutic interventions in relation to the needs of the individual undergoing radiotherapy and their family
- justify the procedure for the safe delivery of radiotherapy treatments and the precautions necessary to protect patients, carers and staff
- critically analyse the professional, legal and ethical issues relevant to the administration of radiotherapy.

The following topics are covered in the module:

- radiobiology
- radiotherapy localisation and treatment planning
- systemic reactions to radiotherapy treatment
- management of interruptions to radiotherapy treatment
- radiotherapy technique and side-effects for a range of cancers
- the information needs of patients.

The rationale for multi-professional education needs to be made explicit with clear and achievable objectives for the module (Pirrie *et al.*, 1998). The content also needs to be relevant to the students so that they can engage fully with the module (Parsell and Bligh, 1998). To enable this to occur, the module is discussed with the group at the beginning, and the range of cancers to be covered is agreed with the group and lecturer to ensure that all of the specialist areas of the practitioners in the group are covered. Due to educational time constraints it is impossible to cover all cancers in this module, and therefore the number of students undertaking the module each year is kept to a level whereby if all practitioners were from a different specialty, they could all be covered in the same depth. This initial discussion allows the students and the module manager to 'break the ice' and get to know each other and the area in which they work. This begins the process of sharing information, which is then encouraged to continue throughout the module.

If the students are to achieve the learning outcomes, they have to gain a basic understanding of radiobiology so that they appreciate how radiation interacts with the body. This underpinning knowledge gives an understanding of why radiotherapy is used more successfully for some tumours than for others, and which areas of the body are more radiosensitive than others (Ferrell *et al.*, 2002). This knowledge then underpins the students' understanding of the side-effects of radiotherapy treatment and the methods that are used to try to minimise these.

The module gives the students an opportunity to learn about therapeutic radiography as a profession, the roles of the therapeutic radiographer, and the stages that the patient goes through from initial diagnosis, localisation and planning of the treatment through to treatment itself, including management of the side-effects of treatment for each area of the body. It also aims to dispel the misconception that radiotherapy is a purely technical profession. By including the role of the therapeutic radiographer, it aims to reduce the conflict that occurs between professions with regard to patient support during treatment (Wells, 1998).

Good educational practice

Much thought was given to how the learning from the module would be assessed. So that assessment could be meaningful to the students, it was decided to incorporate something that could be adapted for use in the student's own clinical area. When considering the effectiveness of multi-professional education, it is not just *whether* it is effective but also *the ways in which it can be effective* that are important. In the case of cancer care, the care of the patient can be improved by allowing professionals to gain knowledge and understanding to improve their informational needs (Harden, 1998b).

One of the main focuses of the *Policy Framework for Commissioning Cancer Services* (Department of Health, 1995) and *The NHS Cancer Plan* (Department of Health, 2004) is that patients, families and carers are given clear information. It was deemed appropriate therefore that the students be asked to prepare an information leaflet or poster for patient use, with a literature review giving the rationale for the information included in the leaflet or poster.

The aim of this assessment method was to evaluate the students' understanding of radiotherapy while conveying this information to the patient at a level that they could understand. Research has shown that the majority of patients who receive radiotherapy want more information about it (Kim *et al.*, 2002).

NICE guidance also acknowledges that patents are more likely to receive better care and advice from an MDT-based workplace. By enabling professions to learn more about the treatments and care that are part of a patient's journey, they can give patients accurate, meaningful advice that is less likely to be contradicted by others.

As *The NHS Cancer Plan* (Department of Health, 2004) states, for this to happen effectively, professionals need to have knowledge and information themselves. The information can only be of high quality if some education in their own and other areas has been undertaken. For example, if healthcare professionals are to tackle patients' misconceptions about cancer and the treatments involved, they need to ensure that they do not hold any misconceptions themselves.

Patients benefit from a knowledge of what to expect during their radiation treatment (Kim *et al.*, 2002). Ideally, this information should be given to the patient when the treatment option is first discussed. This discussion often takes place away from the radiotherapy department, and therefore it is important that the staff who are involved in the discussion and in supporting the patient have the appropriate knowledge and understanding to facilitate this process.

The information needs of cancer patients have been acknowledged and discussed in a number of publications. Not only patients but also their families and carers need information about the treatment they are to undergo in a format that they can understand. They also need this information at all stages of the cancer journey, from diagnosis to palliative care (Department of Health, 1995). Lack of information has been shown to increase anxiety and distress (Wong *et al.*, 2002). It is important that the information that is provided 'should be high quality, accurate, culturally sensitive, specific to local provision of services, free at the point of delivery and timely' (Department of Health, 2004, p. 26).

Patient satisfaction is now considered to be as important as clinical outcomes, so information needs to be tailored to their needs. Conflicting advice causes patients problems, and therefore it is essential that practitioners from all professions give the same level of information (Mills and Davidson, 2002).

Research by Mills and Davidson (2002) has shown that some information leaflets are either too difficult to understand or poorly produced. It is essential therefore that practitioners understand not only the information needs of patients but also how to convert this into patient-friendly literature. When producing patient literature specifically about radiotherapy and its side-effects, the uncertainty about radio-therapy treatment and prejudice against it mean that the information required before treatment may differ from that required during treatment for a specific cancer (Schafer *et al.*, 2000). The majority of patients feel that it is necessary to have a booklet to address their information needs (Schafer *et al.*, 2000).

For the assessment of the module, students are required to produce an infor-mation leaflet or poster for patients. However, it is acknowledged that the infor-mation needs of family and carers also need to be addressed, and these may differ from the needs of the patient (Wong *et al.*, 2002).

The students are allowed to choose the topic of their information leaflet in discussion with the module manager, so that it meets the needs of their clinical practice. Some students who are working in more general areas of cancer care will choose to produce a general information leaflet about radiotherapy and what the patient can expect, while others working in a specialist area (e.g. breast cancer) will elect to produce a leaflet on radiotherapy for that specific cancer. Students may also choose to produce an information leaflet on dealing with specific side-effects (e.g. skin care). The students who have already successfully completed this module have chosen a topic area in which they perceive there is a lack of information resources in their clinical environment, and leaflets have been adapted by some students for use in their clinical area.

One problem with multi-professional education is assessing the level of delivery. Some practitioners will already have completed some post-registration education or have been working in the cancer and palliative care arena for some time, sometimes to the level of specialist practitioner. As stated in the introduction to the module, the range of specialties of the students taking the module will enable group discussion. The varied experiences that practitioners bring to the module are invaluable and form an important part of the group learning process. Discussing with the group the learning objectives of the module and their own educational requirements helps to overcome some of these problems (Pirrie *et al.*, 1998). Some practitioners will already have a degree-level qualification, and therefore a post-graduate qualification is needed to meet their educational needs. Each professional group represented in postgraduate qualification will bring its own learning skills and expectations of learning styles and delivery (Hall and Weaver, 2001). It is important that these are recognised, especially in a subject which contains more hard science than the students have been accustomed to.

So far this discussion of multi-professional education has focused on the learners being from different backgrounds. However, for the education to be truly multi-professional, consideration should be given to the educators. For the module under consideration, the teaching was delivered wholly by a therapeutic radiography lecturer after being developed by a programme team that was multi-professional. It has been suggested that teachers of all participating professions should be involved in the planning and implementation of programmes such as this (Council of Europe, 1995). However, it can be difficult to know which professions will be involved as students, and also to get qualified teachers from the possible range to agree on the curriculum content. It should be possible to resolve most of these difficulties by advanced planning and careful implementation.

Key points

- Multi-professional education can help to break down the barriers between professional groups.
- The assessment methods of multi-professional education should enable the student to link theory to practice.
- Patients, families and carers will benefit from accurate, non-conflicting advice.
- The learning objectives of the module need to be discussed and matched to the learning needs of the group.

Conclusion

Multi-professional practice is becoming an essential part of cancer and palliative care, and to encourage this multi-professional working relationship, multi-professional education, particularly at post-registration level, is essential. Practitioners who are learning together will gain a better understanding of one another's role in cancer and palliative care, which will in turn help to break down the barriers between professional groups and enhance holistic patient care.

Implications for the reader's own practice

1 How do you facilitate your patients' need for information about radiotherapy?
2 How would you develop your own knowledge of radiotherapy?
3 If you work as part of a multi-professional team, do you fully understand one another's roles?
4 How could you improve other healthcare professionals' knowledge about your role?
5 How could you improve the information literature that is available for the patients under your care?

References

Council of Europe. *Multiprofessional Education of Health Personnel. Report and recommendations.* Strasbourg: Council of Europe; 1995.

Department of Health. *A Policy Framework for Commissioning Cancer Services: a report by the Expert Advisory Group on Cancer to the Chief Medical Officers of England and Wales, 1995*; www.doh.gov.uk/cancer/calmanhine.htm

Department of Health. *The Nursing Contribution to Cancer Care*. London: Department of Health; 2000.

Department of Health. *Manual of Cancer Service Standards*. London: Department of Health; 2001.

Department of Health. *The NHS Cancer Plan and the New NHS*. London: Department of Health; 2004. www.nice.org.uk

Faithfull S, Wells M, editors. *Supportive Care in Radiotherapy*. Edinburgh: Churchill Livingstone; 2004.

Ferrell BR *et al*. Strategies for effective continuing education by oncology nurses. *Oncol Nurs Forum*. 2002; **29**: 907–9.

Hall P, Weaver L. Interdisciplinary education and teamwork: a long and winding road. *Med Educ*. 2001; **35**: 867–75.

Harden RM. Multiprofessional education: the magical mystery tour (editorial). *Med Teacher*. 1998a; **20**: 395–8.

Harden RM. Effective multiprofessional education: a three-dimensional perspective. *Med Teacher*. 1998b; **20**: 402–8.

Kim Y *et al*. The effects of information and negative affect on severity of side-effects from radiation therapy for prostate cancer. *Support Care Cancer*. 2002; **10**: 416–21.

Mills EM, Davidson R. Cancer patients' sources of information: use and quality issues. *Psycho-oncology*. 2002; **11**: 371–8.

Parsell G, Bligh J. Educational principles underpinning successful shared learning. *Med Teacher*. 1998; **20**: 5229.

Pirrie A *et al*. Promoting cohesive practice in healthcare. *Med Teacher*. 1998; **20**: 409–16.

Royal College of Radiologists, Clinical Oncology Patients' Liaison Group. *Making Your Radiotherapy Service More Patient-Friendly*. London: Board of the Faculty of Clinical Oncology; 1999.

Schafer C *et al*. Patient information in radio-oncology. *Strahlenther Onkol*. 2000; **10**: 562–71.

Wells M. What's so special about radiotherapy nursing? *Eur J Oncol Nurs*. 1998; **2**: 162–8.

Wong RKS *et al*. What do patients living with advanced cancer and their carers want to know? A needs assessment. *Support Care Cancer*. 2002; **10**: 408–15.

Further reading

- Faithfull S, Wells M, editors. *Supportive Care in Radiotherapy*. Edinburgh: Churchill Livingstone; 2004.
- Griffiths S, Short C. *Radiotherapy Principles to Practice: a manual for quality in treatment delivery*. Edinburgh: Churchill Livingstone; 1994.

Useful website

- National Institute for Clinical Excellence; www.nice.org.uk

Chapter 7

Taking the pain out of pain management teaching

Sharon Wood

> *Pain suffered by patients with cancer is improved through the education of patients and health care providers.*
>
> *Ferrell et al. (1994)*

Aim

The primary aim of this chapter is to provide healthcare professionals with an understanding of the role of education in cancer pain management.

Learning outcomes

- Describe why education is a necessary component of cancer pain management.
- Identify the ideal essential components of a pain management programme.
- Appreciate the issues surrounding current and future pre-registration cancer pain education.
- Discuss a range of innovative approaches to clinical and academic cancer pain education.

Introduction

How did cancer pain education evolve?

The management of cancer pain was a largely neglected problem until the development of the hospice movement in the 1960s. Despite this early recognition of the importance of cancer pain management, it is only over the last two decades that there have been major advances in this area. This started with the first ever cancer pain management guidelines, which were developed by the World Health Organization (WHO) in 1982 (Sykes *et al.*, 2003) and later published as *Cancer Pain Relief* (World Health Organization, 1986).

The WHO *Cancer Pain Relief* guidelines (World Health Organization, 1986, 1996) identify cancer pain as an international problem, and they are still regarded as internationally accepted standards for the principles governing the management of cancer pain (Sykes *et al.*, 2003). Since the development of the guidelines, the WHO has instigated pain relief programmes on a worldwide basis through the establishment of governmental policies and the education of physicians, policy makers and the public (Sykes *et al.*, 2003).

A wide variety of clinical, educational and strategic guidelines for cancer pain management have since been published at a local, national and international level. The guidelines that have been developed over the past decade have endorsed education as an imperative component of improving cancer pain management. Education is therefore considered to be an integral component in the development, implementation and evaluation of cancer pain management at all levels, from direct individual patient care to strategic international initiatives.

Why is cancer pain education important?

Pain is the most feared consequence of cancer for many patients (Grond *et al.*, 1994), and with good reason, as it is estimated that over 25% of all cancer patients worldwide die without any pain relief (Foley, 1985, cited by Sykes *et al.*, 2003). This situation may escalate, as it is estimated that the incidence of cancer is set to rise by 50% in the twenty-first century (Stannard and Booth, 2004), coupled with the fact that increasing numbers of people are living to older ages.

With this potential rise in the number of patients, the number of patients living longer, and the number of patients living longer with cancer and possibly with cancer-related pain, it is essential that education and guidelines are implemented and evaluated now, so that they become standard practice for the future. The need to improve cancer pain control makes reducing the prevalence of pain at any stage of the cancer disease process of paramount importance (Sykes *et al.*, 2003), in order to prevent patients from suffering needlessly.

For a variety of reasons, it is difficult to ascertain how many cancer patients experience pain. However, pain is reported to be present in 20–25% of cancer patients and in up to 60–90% of patients with advanced cancer (Breivik *et al.*, 2003), with almost two-thirds experiencing pain at some point. There are multitudes of potential physical and psychological problems associated with unrelieved cancer pain, including impaired functional status, physical exhaustion, needless suffering, anxiety and depression.

Despite the fact that adequate pain control can be achieved in up to 88% of patients, many still experience inadequate pain management (Breivik *et al.*, 2003). One of the main reasons why cancer pain is often under-treated is inadequate cancer pain education of healthcare professionals (Sykes *et al.*, 2003). There is inadequate provision and also a lack of quality of undergraduate education in pain management (Paradise and Raj, 2004), despite the creation of many recommendations for pain management curriculum development, such as the *Core Curriculum for Professional Education in Pain* (International Association for the Study of Pain, 1997a) and *Recommendations for Nursing Practice in Pain Management* (Pain Society, 2002). This situation has evolved despite the presence of specialist teams and services for cancer, palliative care and pain management, to name but a few. It may be postulated that the inadequate preparation of healthcare students in terms of cancer pain education has contributed to a lack of knowledge, skills and attitudes encountered in clinical practice, which in turn has left patients to suffer unnecessary cancer pain.

In order to improve cancer pain management and reduce the number of patients who suffer from cancer pain and who die with unrelieved cancer pain, education should be incorporated into all aspects of healthcare training and development. Education provision should consequently commence in pre-registration healthcare programmes, at all levels, and should continue throughout professional careers. This should ensure that all patients with cancer have access to a healthcare professional who is not only aware of local, national and international cancer pain guidelines, but is also adequately qualified with regard to cancer pain and effective pain management (Royal College of Physicians of Edinburgh, 2000).

When should cancer pain education for healthcare professionals start?

Education alone is not sufficient to improve cancer pain relief. Most experts have recognised that healthcare professionals cannot practise what they do not know, and that they could be unconsciously incompetent. Unfortunately, most healthcare professionals are poorly prepared by their formal education programmes to assess or treat pain (Sykes *et al.*, 2003). It is therefore essential that cancer pain education of healthcare professionals reflects this principle, from the onset of student training, and continues throughout professional careers as an integral component of lifelong learning.

Considering the number of patients who suffer unrelieved cancer pain, it is morally questionable that, in general, a low priority is given to education about cancer pain management in undergraduate and postgraduate education (Sykes *et al.*, 2003). This is reflected in healthcare professional attitudes to the importance of cancer pain relief, deficiencies in knowledge of cancer pain management, and lack of awareness and implementation of cancer pain guidelines. Pain associated with cancer is complex and requires a multi-faceted and multi-professional approach to its assessment and management. Without appropriate education of healthcare professionals to address these issues, patients in the future are unlikely to receive optimum cancer pain management.

Patient education is a cornerstone of achieving effective cancer pain management, especially as patients are becoming more aware of their rights via multimedia resources, including television and the Internet. As a result, patients want more information about their cancer pain and its management. The American Pain Society (2005) encourages healthcare professionals to educate the families of cancer patients in their pain management. It recommends that patients and families be given accurate and understandable information about the importance of cancer pain management, the use of analgesic medications and other methods of pain relief, and how to communicate effectively with clinicians about unrelieved cancer pain. Consequently, healthcare professionals need to be educated to meet patients' increasing information needs and to offer appropriate advice and information about cancer pain and effective pain management (Royal College of Physicians of Edinburgh, 2000).

Cancer pain management should therefore be a compulsory component of healthcare professionals' pre-registration education, and should continue throughout their professional careers. This should ensure that healthcare professionals have clinically relevant knowledge, skills and attitudes that will ultimately improve cancer pain management. Sykes *et al.* (2003) propose that a core curriculum content for cancer pain education should include a general overview of pain, pharmacological management of pain and non-drug management of pain. This outline needs to be expanded further to incorporate other aspects, including psychological aspects of pain and its management, and invasive and behavioural approaches to pain management.

Pre-registration education

Undergraduate pre-registration curricula for healthcare professionals should place greater emphasis on pain management education (Royal College of Physicians of Edinburgh, 2000), as early education about cancer pain may play an important role in improving pain control for patients with cancer (Wilkes *et al.*, 2003). The WHO recommends that pain should be included as a compulsory subject in courses leading to basic professional qualifications, and that it should be recognised by universities and professional bodies (World Health Organization, 1997). This will promote high levels of professional competence and commitment that are fostered and sustained by specific training throughout professional careers, and which are transferred into clinical cancer pain care.

In the author's experience, cancer pain education was given little credence in pre-registration nursing courses until the development of diploma training. Since that time the University of Leeds has recognised and endorsed the impact that cancer pain education has on patients' care, and pain management has now moved from an optional 12-week pain management module within a diploma programme to a compulsory 12-week pain management module. To enhance the quality of the education delivered, multi-professional lecturers and researchers with a specialist interest in pain, cancer and palliative care have been appointed. It should be noted that the impact of this change in educational provision in terms of students' skills, knowledge and attitudes towards pain and cancer pain management has not yet been evaluated. A similar change has taken place at the University of Kentucky, where final-year medical students now undertake a compulsory course in pain management, although this is only part of a 1-month course that also covers anaesthesia and pharmacology (Sloan *et al.*, 2004).

However, there is unlimited scope for incorporating a compulsory model into pre-registration programmes for all healthcare professionals.

Post-registration education

Post-registration education within clinical practice is usually referred to as continuing professional development. Clinical education increased in the 1980s with the introduction of one-off sessions on pain for healthcare professionals, which were usually delivered by healthcare professionals. By the 1990s it was recognised that these sessions were having a minimal impact in changing practice. New models of professional education in the 1990s incorporated traditional education with other more novel ideas, such as pain link nurse practice, education and support groups. These groups have a variable success rate in enhancing cancer pain care, and good results depend on a multitude of factors, including the size of the group and the clinical area to be covered, management support and available resources. For nurses, a one-week course in cancer pain management can be adequate, provided that the teaching is given by experienced educators and it includes a clinical, hands-on component. The WHO has made it clear that such teaching requires experienced clinical teachers, and that the focus of teaching should be on the appropriate administration of a basic range of drugs in the management of cancer pain (World Health Organization, 1997). Continuing professional develop-ment ensures that clinical skills and knowledge are kept up to date with rapidly changing clinical strategies, and that healthcare professionals are competent to manage cancer pain.

Postgraduate education in pain management for healthcare professionals has developed rapidly, both nationally and internationally, over the past 15 years. A variety of formats are available, including one-off pain management modules, pain management modules that are integrated into degree pathways, and specific Masters degrees in pain management. These can be studied on a full-time or part-time basis, and by distance or open learning. The cancer pain component is usually incorporated as an integral part of the module or programme. However, in some cases it may be a discreet cancer pain module. Postgraduate cancer pain education should build on the basic framework of cancer pain knowledge gained in pre-registration programmes and continuing professional development, and should also deliver clinically relevant and intensive skills training (Plymale *et al.*, 2001). It is absolutely essential that a strong partnership arrangement exists between the healthcare professional who is undertaking education, the manage-ment team responsible for the healthcare professional, and the education centre (European Association for Palliative Care, 2005), so that the education can be translated into everyday practice. Cancer pain management and education are also recognised as an appropriate basis for scholarships, fellowships and grants (World Health Organization, 1997).

Multi-professional education

The WHO is committed to the view that the education of nurses in cancer pain control is essential when implementing a cancer care programme in acute and primary care environments (www.whocancerpain.wisc.edu). However, effective cancer pain relief is multi-dimensional and demands a collaborative, organised, multi-disciplinary approach to meet the diverse quality-of-life concerns of patients who are in pain (International Association for the Study of Pain, 1997b). This needs to be addressed in all aspects of education.

Interdisciplinary cancer pain education in acute and primary care benefits both healthcare professionals and patients (Leslie, 2003). This approach to learning and teaching may improve upon traditional uni-professional educational formats and thus promote effective cancer pain management. Interdisciplinary education pro-grammes that promote more effective cancer pain relief are being given a higher priority by governments and policy makers (European Association for Palliative Care, 2005). Influencing institutional policy and reforming systems of cancer pain care is an interdisciplinary process, the ultimate goal being to create policies, procedures, education strategies, and an environment in which cancer pain relief is expected and uncontrolled pain is viewed as an emergency (Sykes *et al.*, 2003). Effective interdisciplinary education can improve healthcare professionals' competence in managing pain and thus minimise substandard treatment of cancer pain (Plymale *et al.*, 2001). It helps students to gain a deeper and richer understanding and appreciation not only of cancer pain, but also of patients' and other healthcare professionals' perspectives of given situations, and it fosters collaboration and teamwork between professionals. Postgraduate education is more likely to use a multi-professional format than are pre-registration programmes, although some of the latter are developing a multi-professional foundation year.

Traditional methods of pain management education (i.e. lectures and case discussions) have not proved to be fully effective, and alternative approaches need to be considered if pain management behaviour is to be altered significantly (Royal College of Physicians of Edinburgh, 2000).

What teaching methods can be used for cancer pain management education?

Educators are required to be innovative and person-centred in their development of education initiatives that value prior learning and enhance practice knowledge (European Association for Palliative Care, 2005). A multitude of professional education models for cancer pain management have been developed and studied, in both clinical and educational settings, or indeed in a combination of both where appropriate. In addition to the teaching methods illustrated below, four other teaching methods (work-based teaching, experiential teaching, reflective practice and multi-professional education) can be integrated into these models. They are discussed in greater detail in Chapters 2 and 21 respectively.

Clinical setting

Cancer pain link group/network

A pain resource nurse (PRN) programme was developed in the USA and involved the education of all nurses throughout one hospital (Sykes *et al.*, 2003). The nurses were trained to create an awareness of pain and to provide commitment to pain management in every patient care area. The new knowledge and attitudes gained from the initial training were sustained in the short term and therefore influenced good cancer pain management. However, this change gradually became less marked over time. This model has since been developed in many hospitals in the USA (Ferrell *et al.*, 1993) and the UK (where it is usually termed a pain link group), and is now often a multi-professional group. However, it is unsuccessful in the majority of areas for a variety of reasons, including too large a clinical area and lack of management and resource support. Consequently, it is necessary to provide ongoing education for nurses who have been initially trained in pain management, and to recognise the value of rewarding commitment to pain management (Sykes *et al.*, 2003).

An ongoing education programme requires commitment and resources from the management, clinical and cancer pain teams if it is to be successful and indeed to influence cancer pain management. The cancer pain teams need to be in regular contact with the cancer pain link members and to be supportive in their clinical and educational capacity. It is important for the link members to feel part of a diverse, supportive and influential group. Arranging regular time out as a group can encourage the commitment and enthusiasm necessary for achieving good cancer pain management in their own clinical areas. Through this group the members encourage their clinical staff to be involved directly not only with day-to-day patient care but also in influencing clinical guidelines, patient information, audit and research, change management and clinical education.

Many link group members develop their own resource areas for cancer pain management for all staff and students to access. The range of formats that these can take is limitless. They can be very innovative or consist of a simple file of interesting articles, poster displays (some of which are rotated regularly), up-to-date research articles, student projects, trials of new equipment (usually with the cancer pain team), video recording patient care, project development as part of postgraduate education, regular ward teaching sessions, and so on.

The educational strategies used in the clinical areas need to reflect the specific needs of the individual clinical areas and be responsive to their individual environments. The sessions may be formal and involve a group of up to 10 professionals, or it may be necessary to initiate one-to-one teaching sessions while, for example, nurses are conducting a ward drug round or a dressing change. Link members can also be trained to assess competencies for a variety of clinical cancer pain management strategies, such as patient-controlled analgesia systems or nitrous oxide. The link members themselves should be encouraged to take an active role, and should participate in cancer pain ward rounds and be encouraged to advance their knowledge through, for example, conference attendance or presentations, and by advancing their postgraduate cancer pain education.

Clinical guidelines

A study by Du Pen *et al.* (2000) used an educational intervention to transfer knowledge on implementing a previously tested algorithm for cancer pain management into community outpatient oncology clinics. The educational intervention involved training physicians and nurses to use a clinical guideline (cancer pain algorithm). The algorithm is a flow chart of decision-making choices about drug management of cancer pain, based on comprehensive pain assessment and re-assessment. The algorithm encompasses a reference guide containing additional highly specified flow charts and information about drugs, such as side-effect management, titration and equi-analgesic doses. It was intended that all appropriate healthcare professionals and caregivers within the outpatient team should use the cancer pain algorithm on an individual patient basis.

The educational intervention used an expert role model approach. This involved a 5-hour study day led by cancer pain experts, and it included an overview of the algorithm, pain assessment and re-assessment, pharmacology, and case discussion. The most significant effect in cancer pain management occurred within the first 5 months, and was followed by a gradual return to baseline cancer pain practice. This indicates that algorithms do work in practice, but that methods must be implemented for retaining knowledge and maintaining improved outcomes for cancer pain management (Du Pen *et al.*, 2000).

The methods that can be used for retaining knowledge and sustaining improved cancer pain management are varied, and can be initiated either by individual professionals or on a larger healthcare scale. The cancer pain link group could be involved as illustrated above, and could also contribute to the development of algorithms, clinical guidelines and documentation to foster a sense of ownership, which may enhance motivation to use them in the clinical areas. Clinical guidelines should be easy to follow, readily accessible to all healthcare professionals and available in all clinical areas. They could have the format of cancer pain clinical guideline folders, or be presented as published information on the local intranet or on the Internet as appropriate. Roadshows about the clinical guidelines could be taken to all relevant clinical areas and placed in a prominent position so as to capture a wider audience. Again, the cancer pain link members could be involved in this process. Displaying posters of the clinical guidelines in all clinical areas can be a useful way of displaying visual information and providing an aide-memoire for staff, as well as serving as an educational tool for new and visiting staff and students in the clinical areas. Similarly, laminated copies of the clinical guidelines (e.g. assessment tools, algorithms) may be placed by each patient's bedside or in their home setting.

Small (A5) standardised leaflets of the individual clinical guidelines (or summaries/diagrams of them) are an easy way to present important information that can be instantly recognised across a large clinical environment. The leaflets can then be used in one-to-one teaching sessions, pre- and post-registration education programmes, and even large-scale conferences, acting as a constant reminder of the clinical guidelines.

Ideally, after an initial training course on cancer pain management, an annual update would endeavour to maintain up-to-date clinical knowledge and sustain improved clinical practice. This could be provided by various means, including the pain link group, cancer pain management teams and clinical educational units, in combination with universities or as part of a national cancer pain network group.

Benchmarks for pain management

The *Royal Marsden NHS Trust Benchmarks for Pain Management* (Royal College of Nursing, 2003) are an example of best practice in pain benchmarking. They are endorsed by the Royal College of Nursing and are considered to be a thorough, informed and clinically useful attempt to tackle the difficult issue of pain management. The benchmarks are based upon the best available evidence and have been developed with an expert multi-disciplinary pain management team. They can be used in clinical practice to measure the delivery of pain management to patients against indicators for best practice, such as pain assessment, patient information, pain management plans, education for healthcare professionals, patient safety, and so on. A plan can then be developed to further improve pain management as highlighted by the benchmarking exercise. Benchmarks can be specifically written for cancer pain management, and measurement of the benchmarks, staff education and implementation of change could be undertaken by link members, pain teams and/or audit departments. The findings of a benchmarking exercise can be used to educate healthcare professionals at a local or national level – for example, by means of presentations to clinical areas and departments, cancer pain network meetings, study days, conference posters and presentations, or journal and newsletter publications.

Patient education

Patients need to be aware of what treatment strategies are available to manage their cancer pain, as this will encourage them to communicate about their cancer pain and continue treatment strategies as appropriate. Standardised patient information leaflets about pain assessment and treatment strategies can be easily developed in a variety of formats (e.g. large print, Braille, audio recording, video recording, translated into other languages, etc.), and can be displayed in clinical areas and be freely available for patients to take home. Non-pharmacological strategies for managing cancer pain should be available for patients to try as appropriate in a supportive, educative environment. Many of these interventions are evidence based, cheap and easy to use. They include relaxation strategies, music, heat and cold and sensory environment equipment. Clinical guidelines, patient information leaflets and staff education should be developed to support these interventions.

Lasch *et al.* (2000) used focus groups (healthcare professionals, cancer pain societies and community representatives) to develop a culturally sensitive, linguistically appropriate cancer pain education booklet in 11 languages, for 11 different ethnic groups. Patients were involved in the focus group in order to empower them to participate in their cancer pain management. The booklet was devised as a guide for patients and as a teaching tool for healthcare professionals.

Educational setting

Outcome-based curriculum

Cancer pain management curricula should be interprofessional and dynamic in order to reflect the evolving standards of cancer pain management (Paradise and Raj, 2004). Shumway (2001, cited by Paradise and Raj, 2004) suggests that pain management curricula and assessment should be outcome based. This approach has several advantages, including performance-based learning outcomes that define assessment approaches, interprofessional and holistic learning, adaptation to local context and needs, and a focus on personal professional development. The International Association for the Study of Pain (2002) also recommends that nurses working in pain management should follow a working framework that encompasses the explicit use of competencies, standards, case histories, reflective practice and role development through the acquisition of new knowledge and skills across a range of practice and competency levels.

Cancer Pain Objective Structured Clinical Examination (OSCE)

A cancer pain OSCE is a performance-based tool to test individual skills in the essential components of cancer pain assessment and management (Sloan *et al.*, 2001). OSCEs have been used to assess the effectiveness of different cancer pain education methods, including structured clinical instruction modules (SCIM), structured home visit courses and a CD-ROM self-instruction module (Sloan *et al.*, 2004). Sloan *et al.* (2004) used an expert cancer pain multi-disciplinary approach to develop a four-component OSCE. This involved students rotating around four patient stations, allowing 5 minutes per station, where they had to perform tasks. The tasks were designed to assess the student's cancer pain management skills of taking a pain history, physical examination, analgesic management and communication of opioid myths (Sloan *et al.*, 2004, pp. 336–7). Each student was observed and graded against a predetermined checklist.

Structured Clinical Instruction Module (SCIM) in cancer pain

When administering OSCEs it was noted that immediate feedback about performance was also a very effective means of instruction. Plymale *et al.* (2000, 2001) acted on this observation and developed a SCIM by a multi-disciplinary group to meet the increased emphasis on cancer education among medical students and hospice nurses. A SCIM is an educational strategy developed for the teaching of clinical and interpersonal skills. It is a hands-on method of skills training, designed to teach important clinical and interpersonal skills concerning overall cancer pain. It involves an intensive 2-hour skills training course on the assessment and management of cancer pain. During the SCIM, small groups of trainees rotate through a number of stations, spending approximately 15 minutes at each station. A multi-professional instructor is present at each station, and at many of the stations an actual or simulated standardised patient is present with whom trainees interact. At each station students are given brief instructions and they then conduct an interview with or examination of the patient. Afterwards there is opportunity for education – by discussing the case further, asking questions and/or repeating the interview or examination. The topics covered include cancer pain history, communication of the treatment plan, pharmacological management of cancer pain, alternative routes of opioid administration, and physical therapy treatment for cancer pain.

When it was piloted, the cancer pain SCIM was found to be a valuable and novel instructional form of education for teaching essential skills in the assessment and management of cancer pain (Plymale *et al.*, 2000, 2001). The SCIM format shows durability as assessed at 4 months post instruction. The cancer SCIM is unique in its potential to substantially improve the quality of cancer pain education (Sloan *et al.*, 2004).

The cancer pain SCIM could be used as a refresher course by experienced healthcare professionals, or as an introductory educational programme on pain management for healthcare professionals new to cancer pain management, and it could also be a valuable addition to both pre- and post-registration programmes.

Structured home visit course

A cancer pain education course for medical students using a structured home visit was developed and piloted. The visit consisted of medical students taking a cancer pain history, performing a focused physical examination and receiving feedback and teaching on the essentials of cancer pain management from the hospice nurse. It was concluded that medical students benefited from the education, patients enjoyed their role as teacher, and senior hospice nurses provided excellent instruction in the management of cancer pain (Sloan *et al.*, 2001).

CD-ROM self-instruction cancer pain module

Sloan *et al.* (2004) used a self-instruction CD-ROM on cancer pain in a study designed to compare different methods of education about cancer pain. The CD-ROM contained information about the magnitude of the problem of cancer pain, assessment of cancer pain (including history and physical examination), pharmacological and non-pharmacological management of cancer pain, psychosocial approaches to pain relief, WHO guidelines on cancer pain, and three video clips of a real patient history and physical examination. There was also a section that allowed students to perform an interactive self-assessment in order to test their knowledge.

Cancer pain CD-ROM packages and appropriate Internet resources can be utilised in academic lecture and small group sessions and in clinical settings as part of clinical education sessions, as part of the link group meetings, as annual staff updates, or as part of personal professional development, and in academic settings to enhance the taught element of cancer pain modules and as an avenue to support different student learning styles.

Structured educational programme

Vallerand *et al.* (2004) have discussed a programme of structured educational interventions on the management of pain in home care patients with cancer. The programme was developed and implemented for home care nurses. The findings indicated that nurses showed a significant increase in their knowledge, a more positive attitude overall with regard to pain management, with fewer perceived barriers to pain management, and an increase in control over pain was recognised.

Case-based cancer pain management modules

Wilkes *et al.* (2003) developed and implemented a case-based cancer pain management module for graduate nursing students. It was demonstrated to be effective in improving students' knowledge of cancer pain management. On assessment of knowledge retained 24 months later, the results suggested that this knowledge was lasting.

Role model programme

A 1-day role model interdisciplinary workshop presents the principles of cancer pain management (Janjan, 1996). Team members identify barriers to effective cancer pain management in their clinical areas, and develop action plans to improve pain management and professional education. Significant improvements in healthcare professionals' attitudes to and knowledge of cancer pain management principles were observed immediately after the workshop.

National and international pain initiatives

Academic and clinical cancer pain teams can work in partnership to promote local, national and international pain initiatives (e.g. the International Association for the Study of Pain annual campaigns against pain in specific groups of patients). These can be as innovative as possible, and can incorporate expert lectures, clinical sessions, roadshows within academic, clinical, community and public settings, poster displays, self-help groups, workshops, publications and media coverage, sessions on academic modules, research and audit initiatives, development of multimedia resources, implementation of a new pain management strategy – the list is endless.

Summary of possible future developments

Educational interventions can successfully improve healthcare professionals' knowledge of and attitudes to cancer pain, although this change may deteriorate over time (Du Pen *et al.*, 2000), and it may not necessarily have an impact on patients' pain levels (Allard *et al.*, 2001). These areas are under-investigated, and further studies are required to clarify the issues and thereby reform future educational strategies in cancer pain management, in order to improve cancer pain relief for patients.

It is of paramount importance that the assessment and management of cancer pain becomes a core component of the curricula for all healthcare professionals if cancer pain is to be managed effectively for patients. This training and education in cancer pain management should then be ongoing as part of lifelong learning at all stages of the healthcare professional's career.

More research on cancer pain is needed to improve current techniques, because even established treatment programmes cannot always relieve pain at the end of life (Breivik *et al.*, 2003). This will inevitably have an impact on educational provision, and may require innovative approaches to training. Overall further research is needed to evaluate the impact of pain management education programmes for healthcare professionals on clinical practice and patient outcomes (Royal College of Physicians of Edinburgh, 2000).

Key points

- Under-treated cancer pain is unacceptable in the twenty-first century, as it has a multitude of significant and distressing consequences for patients, and affects 20–25% of cancer patients.
- Education should be an integral component of pre- and post-registration education and should continue throughout the healthcare professional's career in order to ensure that staff maintain their competencies with regard to managing cancer pain. It should incorporate as a minimum standard a general overview of cancer pain, psychological perspectives of cancer pain, assessment of cancer pain, and pharmacological and non-drug interventions for cancer pain management. Ideally it should be delivered to multi-professional students by a range of academic and clinical experts with an up-to-date knowledge of cancer pain and its management.
- A variety of professional education models have been developed for cancer pain management. The pain resource nurse (PRN) programme was one of the first to be documented, but has had a limited sustained effect on managing cancer pain. The cancer pain Structured Clinical

Instruction Module (SCIM) is a more recent development, it has received positive reports about students' knowledge and skills acquisition, and it has great potential.

• The recent development of pain benchmarks has had multi-professional involvement, and education has been intrinsic to their development and implementation. They will no doubt have a positive impact on patients' cancer pain management.

Conclusion

There have been major improvements in pain control and provision of education over the past two decades. However, cancer-related pain continues to be a significant public health concern (Sykes *et al.*, 2003). Despite investment initiatives in cancer pain educational programmes, it is indicated that the change in staff attitudes and knowledge may only be retained for a limited period of time. It is therefore evident that new, innovative approaches to learning and teaching in cancer pain are required. These should be implemented from the inception of the new healthcare professionals in training and be continued throughout each professional's career. By expanding, improving and evaluating the education that we currently provide, we will enable patients with cancer pain to receive the optimum level of pain management from healthcare professionals.

Implications for the reader's own practice

1 The available body of knowledge on the appropriate assessment of pain is not applied in the routine treatment of cancer patients. The main future challenge is to ensure that patients have access to these evaluations on a regular basis (Sykes *et al.*, 2003). Can you identify and describe a range of cancer pain assessment tools that you could use in your educational programme?
2 Reflect upon education that you have delivered on cancer pain management. Did it have a lasting impact on students and consequently on your professional practice?
3 Would you use this strategy to educate students or colleagues?
4 Could you develop an innovative method for teaching about cancer pain management that would have long-lasting effects on patient care?

References

Allard P, Maunsell E, Labbe J *et al.* Educational interventions to improve cancer pain control: a systematic review. *J Palliat Med.* 2001; 4: 191–203.

American Pain Society. *Guidelines for the Management of Cancer Pain in Adults and Children;* www.ampainsoc.org (accessed 19 September 2005).

Breivik H, Campbell W, Eccleston C. *Practical Applications and Procedures. Clinical Pain Management Series.* London: Arnold Publishers; 2003.

Du Pen AR, Du Pen S, Hansberry J *et al.* An educational implementation of a cancer pain algorithm for ambulatory care. *Pain Manage Nurs.* 2000; **1:** 116–28.

European Association for Palliative Care. *A Guide for the Development of Palliative Care Nurse Education in Europe*; www.eapcnet.org/projects/nursingeducation.asp (accessed 19 September 2005).

Ferrell BR, Ferrell BA, Ahn C *et al.* Pain management for elderly patients with cancer at home. *Cancer.* 1994; **74:** 2139–46.

Grond S, Zech D, Diefenbach C *et al.* Prevalence and pattern of symptoms in patients with cancer pain: a prospective evaluation of 1635 cancer patients referred to a pain clinic. *J Pain Symptom Manage.* 1994; **9:** 372–82.

International Association for the Study of Pain (IASP). *Core Curriculum for Professional Education in Pain.* 2nd ed. Seattle, WA: IASP; 1997a.

International Association for the Study of Pain (IASP). *Pain Clinical Updates. Cancer pain management in the home.* Seattle, WA: IASP; 1997b; www.iasp-pain.org/logomedblack.gif (accessed 19 September 2005).

International Association for the Study of Pain (IASP). *Recommendations for Nursing Practice in Pain Management.* Nursing Focus in Pain Management Working Party of The Pain Society, the British chapter of the IASP. London: The Pain Society; 2002.

Janjan NA, Martin CJ, Payne R *et al.* Teaching cancer pain management: durability of educational effects of a role model program. *Cancer.* 1996; **77:** 996–1001; www.whocancerpain.wisc.edu/eng/10_1/education.html (accessed 16 January 2006).

Lasch KE, Wilkes G, Montouri LM *et al.* Using focus group methods to develop multicultural cancer pain education materials. *Pain Manage Nurs.* 2000; **1:** 129–38.

Leslie K. Education to achieve symptom control for patients with cancer; www.nursingtimes.net/nav?page=nt.print&resource=396088 (accessed 19 September 2005).

Pain Society. *Recommendations for Nursing Practice in Pain Management.* London: Pain Society; 2002.

Paradise LA, Raj PP. Competency and certification of pain physicians. *Pain Pract.* 2004; **4:** 235–44.

Plymale PA, Sloan PA, Johnson M *et al.* Cancer pain education: the use of a structured clinical instruction module to enhance learning among medical students. *J Pain Symptom Manage.* 2000; **20:** 4–11.

Plymale PA, Sloan PA, Johnson M *et al.* Cancer pain education: a structured clinical instruction module for hospice nurses. *Cancer Nurs.* 2001; **24:** 424–9.

Royal College of Nursing. *The Royal Marsden NHS Trust Benchmarks for Pain Management. Pain points 3–6.* London: Royal College of Nursing; 2003.

Royal College of Physicians of Edinburgh. *Control of Pain in Patients with Cancer*; www.rcpe.ac.uk/guidelines/fulltext/44/index.html (accessed 19 September 2005).

Sloan PA, LaFountain P, Plymale PA *et al.* Implementing cancer pain education for medical students. *Cancer Pract.* 2001; **9:** 225–9.

Sloan PA, Plymale PA, LaFountain P *et al.* Equipping medical students to manage cancer pain in a comparison of three educational methods. *J Pain Symptom Manage.* 2004; **27:** 333–42.

Stannard C, Booth S. *Pain.* London: Churchill Livingstone; 2004.

Sykes N, Fallon MT, Patt RB. *Cancer Pain. Clinical Pain Management Series.* London: Arnold Publishers; 2003.

Vallerand AH, Riley-Doucet C, Hasenau SM *et al.* Improving cancer pain management by homecare nurses. *Oncol Nurs Forum Online.* 2004; **31:** 809–16.

Wilkes G, Lasch KE, Lee JC *et al.* Evaluation of a cancer education module. *Oncol Nurs Forum Online.* 2003; **30:** 1037–43.

World Health Organization. *Cancer Pain Relief.* Geneva: World Health Organization; 1986.

World Health Organization. *Cancer Pain Relief.* 2nd ed. Geneva: World Health Organization; 1996.

World Health Organization. *Nursing Education in Pain and Palliative Nursing;* www. whocancerpain.wisc.edu/engl10_1/education.html (accessed 19 September 2005).

Useful websites

- Agency for Health Care Policy and Research; www.ahrq.gov/consumer
- Association for Palliative Medicine of Great Britain and Ireland; www.palliative-medicine.org
- British Pain Society; www.britishpainsociety.org
- Pain Relief Foundation; www.painrelieffoundation.org.uk
- Website on pain medicine and palliative care; www.Stoppain.org
- World Health Organization Cancer Pain; www.whocancerpain.wisc.edu

Chapter 8

Teaching symptom management

Sarah Callin and Fiona Hicks

> *In the practice of medicine more mistakes are made from lack of accurate observation and deduction than through lack of knowledge.*
>
> George Howard Bell, 1905

Aim

The aim of this chapter is to explore the challenges of teaching symptom management, and to provide an overview of the range and quality of teaching methods currently available.

Learning outcomes

- Understand the challenges of teaching symptom management.
- Recognise the importance of an ongoing, integrated approach to teaching.
- Be aware of current methods of teaching symptom management.
- Understand the benefits and limitations of current methods.

Introduction

Patients with advanced progressive diseases frequently experience multiple, complex symptoms. Although pain is often reported as the most prevalent and most feared symptom, non-pain symptoms are common in palliative care patients. Grond *et al.* (1994) reported that 94% of patients with advanced cancer and intractable pain suffered from additional symptoms, with 80% experiencing more than one and 15% experiencing more than five further symptoms. Insomnia, anorexia, constipation, sweating and nausea were most frequently reported. Many of the symptoms experienced by cancer patients are also reported by patients with advanced, non-malignant diseases such as heart failure.

Physical symptoms are associated with varying degrees of distress. Symptoms are often seen only as clues to the diagnosis of a disease process, and the distress that they cause is sometimes overlooked. Although patients receiving hospice care are likely to die with their symptoms controlled, recent reports have shown that a substantial proportion of patients dying in hospital are receiving inadequate symptom management.

The current focus on increasing access to palliative care for all patients with chronic, life-threatening illnesses means that all healthcare professionals are now expected to provide palliative care as a core part of their practice. Appropriate training in skills such as symptom assessment and management is required. However, undergraduate medical and nursing education has been criticised for not providing adequate teaching on end-of-life symptom management (Field, 1995; Lloyd-Williams and Field, 2002), and there is an urgent need to improve training at all levels in this area of care (Toscani *et al.*, 2005). In addition to the complex nature of the subject, meeting the learning needs of such a large and diverse population of healthcare professionals provides significant challenges for palliative care educators.

In this chapter we shall explore current practice in symptom management education and identify those methods that have been found to be most successful.

The challenges of teaching symptom management

Attitudes to symptom management

> *In palliative care, the greatest challenge to educate is not for trainees where efforts are in place, but for people in established practice.*
>
> Currow and Abernathy (2005)

Different priorities in patient management, as well as lack of knowledge and skills, individual opinions and the culture of the workplace, can create barriers to the provision of good symptom management. Many staff fail to recognise the importance of symptom control to patients. Doctors in particular are trained to diagnose underlying disease processes on the basis of a number of factors, including patterns of presenting symptoms, yet few simultaneously consider symptoms as signs of distress that in themselves need to be assessed and managed. Even when the need is recognised, there can be a reluctance to implement available treatments due a lack of robust evidence of their efficacy. Although the practice of pain control has an increasing evidence base, management strategies for other symptoms such as shortness of breath, which are equally common and distressing, have less supporting evidence. Consequently, significant unmet needs arise from practitioners either failing to identify or ignoring symptoms that they consider to be insignificant or non-treatable.

Different professional approaches can also affect success in symptom control. Preliminary studies looking at the incorporation of palliative care into heart failure management identified important differences in the outcomes of patient and carer assessments between heart failure and palliative care nurses. They demonstrated that cardiac nurses tended to be more medically focused, concentrating on the management of physiological variables, whereas the palliative care nurses took a holistic approach and identified a wider range of issues (Segal *et al.*, 2005).

The complexity of symptoms and the palliative care approach

The assessment and management of symptoms are often complex. For the individual patient, multiple factors, including past experience and culture, can impact on the nature and severity of their symptoms. Similarly, poorly controlled symptoms have far-reaching consequences. The successful management of these patients frequently requires multi-professional input and a variety of treatment modalities. A comprehensive patient-centred assessment is of fundamental importance. Practitioners must ask patients directly about the presence of all potential symptoms, rather than merely concentrating on those that they feel confident about treating. Teaching must emphasise the multi-dimensional nature of symptoms, including a full assessment of each symptom and consideration of pathophysiology in addition to its psychological, social and spiritual impact.

Educators often separate physical, psychological, social and spiritual aspects in an attempt to clarify management. This may reinforce medical models of care, with the physical elements tending to take priority and the psychosocial and spiritual elements being overlooked.

The changing face of palliative care and skills confidence

Palliative care practitioners have considerable experience in managing symptoms in patients with cancer, but their experience of symptom management in non-cancer patients is often more limited. With the expansion of palliative care services to include other conditions as well as cancer, some practitioners lack confidence in managing patients with non-malignant conditions. This lack of confidence will create difficulties when teaching others how to manage symptoms in patients with non-malignant disease. Currow and Abernathy (2005) highlight the fact that palliative care will remain a dynamic area with practice being directly influenced by advances not only in palliative care but also in other clinical disciplines. They emphasise the need for palliative care practitioners to engage in ongoing self-directed continuing education.

When should we teach healthcare professionals about symptom control?

Opportunities to teach arise at both undergraduate and postgraduate levels, and include the following:

- formal programmes of study (undergraduate and postgraduate training)
- continuing professional development
- opportunistic teaching within clinical practice.

Formal programmes of study

There are wide variations in the content of different nursing and medical undergraduate and postgraduate curricula. A survey of undergraduate nursing education showed that entry-level students received little teaching in palliative care and that the provision was mainly theoretical (Lloyd-Williams and Field, 2002). A survey of UK medical schools in 2000–2001 (Field and Wee, 2002) showed that all clinical schools provided some palliative care teaching, but the amount and content varied widely. Although there had been an increase in the amount of teaching about the management of physical symptoms since previous surveys conducted in 1983 and

1994 (Field, 1995), junior doctors still reported that they felt unprepared with regard to this area of care (Tiernan *et al.*, 2001).

Early exploration of the general concepts of symptom management within undergraduate programmes should ensure that healthcare professionals are introduced to the basic principles, providing a basic framework to which further knowledge can be added. Sessions dedicated specifically to palliative care and symptom management are important, but integration with other elements of the curriculum is also required to help students to apply their learning to other contexts. This should promote positive attitudes to symptom control and joint working in future clinical practice. Integration of symptom management education into sub-specialty training programmes is crucial for the delivery of the palliative care approach to all areas of healthcare.

Continuing professional development

Continuing professional development is essential for all healthcare professionals if high-quality healthcare is to be delivered. Palliative care educators must be engaged in developing and promoting appropriate formal educational opportunities both within and outside the NHS. Examples of this include the organisation of symptom control study days and the development of link nurse programmes. Educators must also fulfil their own continuing professional requirements in order to enhance their skills and keep up to date with changing practice.

Opportunities for teaching in clinical practice

Informal teaching can be delivered through routine clinical practice. Joint working allows fuller exploration of complex symptom issues through role modelling and targeted teaching. Opportunities for one-to-one interactions allow teaching to be adapted to an individual learner's needs. Inter-specialty and multi-professional working brings diversity into clinical practice, providing scope for cross-professional education.

Opportunistic teaching has become a major part of palliative care education in hospital and community settings. The main challenge lies in identifying, creating and capitalising on available opportunities. The advisory roles of many of the palliative care services, along with the recognition that complex cases can provide excellent motivation for learning, mean that many opportunities arise in day-to-day clinical practice.

Methods of embedding good symptom management into practice include the following.

- *Routine use of patient assessment techniques.* Techniques such as the Edmonton Assessment Scale can highlight the degree of symptom distress experienced by patients and motivate exploration of how this can be managed.
- *Use of clinical decision support systems.* These support the process of clinical diagnosis and formation of a treatment plan, educating professionals and highlighting learning opportunities.
- *Implementation of clinical guidelines/pathways.* The National Institute for Clinical Excellence guidance for improving supportive and palliative care for adults advocates the use of the Liverpool Integrated Care Pathway for the Dying Patient

(LCP). The degree to which integrated care pathways succeed in improving patient care is still uncertain. However, their implementation undoubtedly creates scope for both structured and opportunistic teaching, and promotes collaborative working between teams. It also improves collection of audit data, highlighting gaps in knowledge and providing an impetus to seek educational opportunities.

- *Audit.* Auditing clinical practice provides a means of changing attitudes and motivating learning. Audits reviewing symptom management have demonstrated an improvement in patient care and prescribing (McQuillan *et al.*, 1996).
- *Research.* Research highlighting new developments in symptom management provides a positive motivation for learning and changing practice where opportunities exist within teams to discuss and evaluate research outcomes.

How should we teach symptom control?

Formal programmes of study previously used more traditional 'passive' methods of teaching, such as the delivery of lectures. Increasingly, however, more 'active' problem-based, self-directed and experiential learning methods are now being used in healthcare education. Studies comparing traditional and newer methods of teaching pain management show that self-directed learning improves performance (Sloan *et al.*, 2004). Case-based learning in small groups and small-group discussion are now widely used in the UK. Some medical schools involve terminally ill patients directly in their teaching, and most include hospice participation (Field and Wee, 2002). Experiential attachments and clinical practice provide opportunities for role modelling, reflection and targeted teaching in the context of shared working. Healthcare professionals are often influenced to change their practice after observing approaches that have positively or negatively influenced patient outcome.

It is important to recognise that students and teachers have different learning and teaching styles, and that teaching is likely to be most effective when a range of methods are used. Sloan *et al.* (2004) have demonstrated that a combination of traditional and newer methods of teaching pain management is more effective in improving clinical performance than the use of either method on its own.

Teaching methods that should be considered include the following:

- work-based teaching
- experiential teaching
- reflective practice
- multi-professional education
- case-based scenarios/problem-based learning
- discussion groups/bulletin boards
- multimedia teaching/resources
- assessment.

Work-based teaching

Learning in a clinical setting has many advantages. It is focused on real problems in the context of actual practice and takes into account the practitioner's own anxieties and emotions, a dimension less easily accessed by simulated situations. It has been found to be highly effective (Schulman-Green, 2003). Palliative care educators who are also in clinical practice need to be aware that their normal day-to-day work has the potential to influence attitudes and practice, and they should aim to be positive role models and teach by example. Other more specific teaching opportunities are also available, and shared working or consultation on clinical issues helps to motivate learners at a time when they recognise the need for – and welcome – specialist input. Projects that have integrated specialist knowledge into clinical practice have shown that supporting and working with non-specialist physicians improved the quality of both symptom control and education (Kloke and Scheidt, 1996).

Effective teaching within clinical practice must balance the competing clinical demands for both learners and teachers. The inherent variety of clinical work makes planning the delivery of a whole syllabus more difficult, and practitioners will vary in the extent and quality of the teaching that they provide.

Experiential teaching

Experiential teaching allows students to observe palliative care practitioners at work, to interact with patients and carers and to learn a multi-disciplinary approach to care. Many undergraduate medical and nursing programmes now include short hospice visits for all students. Some also include longer optional attachments (student-selected components) for those with a special interest. These provide an opportunity to explore issues for patients in a range of settings. A project in Australia, in which medical students were attached to experienced nurses, reported positive experiences by both nursing staff and medical students, and evaluations showed an improvement in confidence when dealing with symptom control (Barrington and Murrie, 1999).

In the postgraduate setting, clinical attachments in palliative care are being used increasingly to develop knowledge, attitudes and skills. Short attachments are encouraged in higher specialist training rotations such as geriatric medicine and oncology. Evaluation of such programmes has shown a positive impact on patient care (Von Gunten *et al.*, 1995).

Medical students generally prefer experiential teaching methods (Schulman-Green, 2003). However, it is important to remember that the quality of learning is only as good as the skills of the person or the practice being observed. Organising attachments requires considerable time commitment, because of the need to arrange appropriate patient contact with regular clinical supervision and meet the learning needs of the individual students. These organisational responsibilities can be disruptive to the host service.

Reflective practice

Reflective practice has become an important part of palliative care education. This approach involves reflecting on and critically analysing actions with the objective of improving professional practice. A reflective practice session could entail multi-disciplinary reflection about a patient with complex symptom management issues. This involves assessing the situation from different perspectives, exploring the positive and negative aspects as well as speculating about how different courses of action could have affected care. A number of courses now include experiential or reflective elements. Adriaansen *et al.* (2005) showed that a post-qualification course in palliative care for nurses, which included sessions with reflection on daily practice, increased knowledge and insight – particularly in relation to pain and symptom management.

Individuals can also use a reflective diary or log to record their own practice as a basis for in-depth reflection on cases. The *Record of Reflective Practice* for specialist trainees in palliative medicine (www.jchmt.org.uk) includes a structured grid for educational supervisor feedback on the quality of reflection in the context of appraisal, and is subject to evaluation as a formative assessment method. However, reflective practice can be time-consuming for all those involved and, in a group setting or within appraisal, it requires that practitioners be open to examination of sensitive issues. When used as an assessment method, care must be taken to credit and not to penalise students for reflecting on practice.

Multi-professional education

Multi-professional working is central to the palliative care ethos, and the management of symptoms frequently involves input from team members from different professional backgrounds. It promotes teamwork, encourages professionals to have respect for and understanding of one another's expertise, and helps to promote coordinated care. Wee *et al.* (2001) developed inter-professional workshops (including medical, nursing, social work, physiotherapy and occupational therapy students) which involved an interdisciplinary group of teachers and family carers. These workshops were rated very highly by participants.

Difficulties include the different learning needs of individuals. Material for these sessions must be developed carefully and pitched appropriately to meet the different needs of the group members.

Case-based scenarios/problem-based learning

Case-based scenarios are now widely used for teaching in both formal and less formal settings, providing a way to explore difficult symptom management problems. A case is described, highlighting the issues to be covered, and students are invited to discuss different approaches to management. This allows the educator to simulate complex clinical situations and it helps students to learn to look at the physical, psychosocial and spiritual aspects of care.

Problem-based learning (PBL) involves solving a problem presented in the form of either a case scenario or a more focused question on symptom management. The problem is used to define the students' learning objectives, and each student is required to undertake independent, self-directed study before returning to the group to discuss and develop their knowledge and understanding.

Simulated problem-solving approaches are not designed to allow full exploration of all dimensions of difficult symptom control, but aim to encourage a deeper understanding, making it more likely that students will be able to recall the material later in the clinical setting. They also allow sharing of experiences and the development of other attributes, such as communication skills, teamwork, problem solving and self-directed learning. Both methods are most suited to small group sessions, ensuring active involvement of all participants and addressing individual learning needs. The sessions require experienced and sensitive facilitation by a skilled teacher, as well as high-quality scenarios or problems.

These techniques do not suit every student's learning style, and some may find this learning environment uncomfortable. This problem may be reduced if group membership remains unchanged for a period of time. This method is discussed in much more depth in Chapter 3.

Discussion groups/bulletin boards

Group discussion is a useful method for developing knowledge and understanding of symptom management issues, allowing collective examination of a problem. It is used in both formal and less formal settings, including clinical practice (e.g. in multi-disciplinary team meetings). Since the development of the Internet and e-learning there is now access to online discussion groups and bulletin boards which allow learners who are geographically separated to engage in discussion and share ideas. Group discussion helps to develop skills in presenting ideas, listening, negotiation and teamwork. Different group structures and processes can be used when facilitating group discussions to ensure the participation of all group members. Negative aspects of group discussion can include the anxiety experienced by some contributors to the discussion, and lack of participation of less confident members. Most group discussions will therefore require a skilled facilitator to ensure a well-organised and purposeful discussion. Many of the problems associated with leading a small group will be accentuated in larger groups.

Multimedia resources

Various resources are available to support educational initiatives, and Web-based tools make self-directed learning feasible for all. Written materials include journals reporting the latest research findings, and textbooks. Difficulties relate to the vast quantity and varying quality of the information available. Education must now focus on teaching skills in information searching, critical analysis of the quality of the information provided, and how to apply findings in clinical practice.

Assessment

The process of assessment is a useful educational tool. In-training assessment (ITA) is now an integral part of specialist medical training in the UK, and has been shown to enhance clinical teaching. ITA aims to map the learner's progress towards set teaching objectives by using multiple assessments over time in both a systematic and an opportunistic way. New work-based assessment techniques such as the Mini Clinical Evaluation Exercise (Mini-CEX) consist of an assessor observing student performance – for example, a focused history and physical examination – as part of their normal practice, with subsequent discussion of the diagnosis and management plan. This process also provides opportunities for feedback and continuous learning.

Assessment runs the risk of highlighting only the readily measurable rather than promoting the essential aspects of care. The learner's awareness that they are under assessment may also affect their performance and may limit learning opportunities.

Key points

- Successful management of a patient's symptoms is dependent on a detailed assessment of symptoms relevant to the patient.
- The recognition that skills in symptom assessment and management are relevant to many areas of healthcare means that increasing numbers of diverse healthcare professionals will require access to education.
- In order to be successful, symptom management training will need to recognise different attitudes and professional approaches, and tailor teaching accordingly.
- With the widening scope of palliative care, educators will need to find ways to keep up to date with advances in many areas of healthcare in order to develop and maintain skills and confidence.
- The complexity of symptom assessment and management provides a challenge to palliative care educators, and it is likely that a range of teaching methods will need to be employed to ensure effective training for different healthcare professionals at different stages in their careers.

Conclusion

To ensure that all healthcare professionals develop adequate skills in symptom management, it is important that teaching is included and integrated at both undergraduate and postgraduate levels. The importance of assessment and management of symptoms as well as an awareness of specialist services and the benefits of joint working need to be the main focus of teaching. The content and quality of education will need to be continually re-evaluated.

Although the inclusion of symptom management education in formal programmes of study is important, palliative care educators also need to identify further opportunities to develop practitioner knowledge and skills. Teaching symptom management in the clinical setting either within experiential attachments or in actual clinical practice, although often labour-intensive, has many advantages. Educators can capitalise on the fact that learners are motivated by real symptom control challenges. Shared working also promotes inter-specialty and inter-professional sharing of ideas.

The use of integrated care pathways is likely to increase, due to their potential to reach large numbers of healthcare professionals and assist in the dissemination of locally and nationally agreed guidelines. Educators can create educational opportunities around the implementation of pathways and use them to identify further learning needs. More research is needed into both their impact on the quality of patient care and their role in education.

Implications for the reader's own practice

1 How do you assess the scope of your current teaching and identify additional areas that you could cover?
2 Are you reaching multi-professional groups? If not, who is reaching them?

3 How could you influence 'hard-to-reach' groups with teaching on symptom management?
4 Do you use a wide variety of techniques and capitalise on the opportunities that are available to you in your teaching?
5 Would the routine use of assessment tools, pathways or guidelines generate more opportunities for teaching in your workplace?

References

Adriaansen MJM, Van Achterberg T, Borm G. Effects of a post-qualification course in palliative care. *J Adv Nurs*. 2005; **49:** 96–103.

Barrington D, Murrie D. A preceptor model for introducing undergraduate medical students to palliative medicine. *J Palliat Care*. 1999; **15:** 39–43.

Currow DC, Abernathy AP. Quality palliative care: practitioners' needs for dynamic lifelong learning. *J Pain Symptom Manage*. 2005; **29:** 332–4.

Field D. Education for palliative care: formal education about death, dying and bereavement in UK medical schools in 1983 and 1994. *Med Educ*. 1995; **29:** 414–19.

Field D, Wee B. Preparation for palliative care: teaching about death, dying and bereavement in UK medical schools, 2000–2001. *Med Educ*. 2002; **36:** 561–7.

Grond S, Zech D, Diefenbach C *et al*. Prevalence and pattern of symptoms in patients with cancer pain: a prospective evaluation of 1635 cancer patients referred to a pain clinic. *J Pain Symptom Manage*. 1994; **9:** 372–82.

Kloke M, Scheidt H. Pain and symptom control for cancer patients at the University Hospital in Essen: integration of specialists' knowledge into routine work. *Support Care Cancer*. 1996; **4:** 404–7.

Lloyd-Williams M, Field D. Are undergraduate nurses taught palliative care during their training? *Nurse Educ Today*. 2002; **22:** 589–92.

McQuillan R, Finlay I, Branch C *et al*. Improving analgesic prescribing in a general teaching hospital. *J Pain Symptom Manage*. 1996; **11:** 172–80.

Schulman-Green D. How do physicians learn to provide palliative care? *J Palliat Care*. 2003; **19:** 246–52.

Segal DI, O'Hanlon D, Rahman N *et al*. Incorporating palliative care into heart failure management: a new model of care. *Int J Palliat Nurs*. 2005; **11:** 135–6.

Sloan PA, Plymale M, LaFountain P *et al*. Equipping medical students to manage cancer pain: a comparison of three educational methods. *J Pain Symptom Manage*. 2004; **27:** 333–42.

Tiernan E, Kearney M, Lynch AM *et al*. Effectiveness of a teaching programme in pain and symptom management for junior house officers. *Support Care Cancer*. 2001; **9:** 606–10.

Toscani F, Di Ginlio P, Brunelli C *et al*. How people die in hospital general wards: a descriptive study. *J Pain Symptom Manage*. 2005; **30:** 33–40.

Von Gunten CF, Von-Roen JH, Gradisher W *et al*. A hospice/palliative medicine rotation for fellows training in haematology-oncology. *J Cancer Educ*. 1995; **10:** 200–2.

Wee B, Hillier R, Coles C *et al*. Palliative care: a suitable setting for undergraduate interprofessional education. *Palliat Med*. 2001; **15:** 487–92.

Further reading

- General Medical Council. *Tomorrow's Doctors: recommendations on undergraduate medical education.* London: General Medical Council; 1993.
- Jeffrey D, editor. *Teaching Palliative Care: a practical guide.* Oxford: Radcliffe Medical Press; 2002.
- Lloyd-Williams M, MacLeod RD. A systematic review of teaching and learning in palliative care within the medical undergraduate curriculum. *Med Teacher.* 2004; **26:** 683–90.
- MacLeod RD, James C, editors. *Teaching Palliative Care: issues and implications.* Penzance: Patten Press; 1994.

Chapter 9

Teaching ethics in cancer and palliative care

Janet Holt

> *The true lover of knowledge naturally strives for truth, and is not content with common opinions, but soars with undimmed and unwearied passion till he grasps the essential nature of things.*
>
> Plato, The Republic

Aim

The aim of this chapter is to consider the reasons for including ethics in cancer and palliative care education, including the subjects that may be included and appropriate learning and teaching strategies.

Learning outcomes

- Explore the reasons for teaching ethics in cancer and palliative care education.
- Discuss the subjects, learning and teaching methods used in ethics learning and teaching.
- Evaluate the contribution made by ethical theory and the law to ethics learning and teaching.

Introduction

There can be no doubt that the learning and teaching of ethics is an important part of the healthcare curriculum. Healthcare professionals in all areas of clinical practice face ethical dilemmas that challenge ways of thinking, the values they consider important and their beliefs about what they consider to be good or bad, or right or wrong. Patients who have cancer or who are receiving palliative care present healthcare professions with a multitude of ethical problems, including questions about treatment options, withholding and withdrawing treatment, the use of advance directives, and euthanasia. Broader ethical issues such as informed consent and confidentiality are also important in these client groups, as they face difficult decisions about their treatment and care in a health service with competing demands on its resources. Healthcare professionals will want to act in the patient's best interests, but the morally correct course of action is not always obvious in complex clinical situations. In addition, members of the patient's family or friends may influence decision making, causing conflict for (and within) the multi-disciplinary team.

This chapter will address some of the important issues in learning and teaching ethics in healthcare. Three reasons for teaching ethics are identified, and these will be discussed in the context of the type of subjects that should be taught. The inclusion of ethical theory and legal perspectives in the curriculum will be explored along with the range of learning and teaching methods suitable for ethics teaching. Finally, the question of who should teach ethics will be addressed.

Why teach ethics?

There are at least three clear reasons for learning and teaching ethics:

- to prepare healthcare professionals to address the ethical dilemmas that they will encounter in clinical practice
- to allow discussion of contentious issues
- to help students to make their own moral judgements.

The professional bodies that govern the regulation and registration of healthcare professionals usually require ethics to be formally addressed in courses that lead to professional registration. For example, the Nursing and Midwifery Council identifies ethical and professional practice as a proficiency to be achieved for entry to the nursing register, and ethical issues are also addressed in the post-registration curriculum, either formally in post-registration degrees or less formally in study days and through self-directed learning.

Ethics is the study of morality and moral issues, and is about trying to decide what is right or wrong or what is good or bad about a particular course of action (Fletcher *et al.*, 1995). People are accustomed to making these kinds of judgements in everyday life over matters of honesty, telling the truth, and what may be considered to be the right thing to do. People also think about and form opinions on broader issues in society, such as decisions made by the government that have a moral dimension (e.g. the organisation of and funding arrangements for education and health), or decisions about whether to go to war with another country. People may react in different ways to these kinds of issues. Some may simply ignore them, others may discuss and debate them with family and friends, and strong feelings may be generated in others to take some form of action (e.g. campaigning or demonstrating) to support or reject the course of action that has been suggested.

While there is familiarity with discussing and evaluating ethical problems that are faced in society, this may not be carried out in a particularly systematic way, and people may choose to ignore the issues altogether. However, healthcare professionals face dilemmas that not only cannot be ignored, but also have to be fully explored in order to determine the course of action that must be taken. In cancer and palliative care, inevitably many of these dilemmas are of a very serious nature involving decisions about matters of life and death.

Ethics deals with questions of value that need to be answered with reference to value judgements. For the major ethical issues in healthcare, such as those that raise questions about withdrawing treatment, there is a broad range of views about their morality, and such questions can rarely be answered with a simple yes or no. Hence the second reason for teaching ethics – the discussion of contentious issues. Ethics by definition deals with controversial issues, and some arguments can be distasteful or distressing, but in order to address a subject fully, all possible lines of argument need to be examined. For example, a discussion about euthanasia would need to examine arguments both in support of and against its use. One argument in the literature that supports the practice of euthanasia examines the issue in the context of healthcare rationing (Ward, 1997). This is clearly a controversial line of reasoning, but one that should be examined in order to formulate arguments for either supporting or rejecting the proposition. To disallow the proposition or to refuse to discuss it solely on the grounds that it is a distasteful notion impedes debate and, more importantly, does not give students the opportunity to achieve the third reason for teaching ethics, namely to facilitate the formation of moral judgements.

Teaching ethics is therefore not about giving moral guidance to healthcare professionals on how to act, but rather it involves developing the students' skills in critically evaluating beliefs and arguments. Essentially these are philosophical skills, and although it is not necessary for healthcare professionals to become moral philosophers, selective use of philosophical methods can be useful in helping students to acquire skills in critical analysis when trying to resolve ethical dilemmas (Holt, 2002).

What subjects should be taught?

As many of the ethical issues in healthcare arise when caring for patients and clients at the end of life, cancer and palliative care is fraught with ethical dilemmas. As well as the more general issues that occur in other areas of healthcare, such as informed consent and confidentiality, there are several other issues of direct relevance to cancer and palliative care, such as questions about withholding and withdrawing treatment, resuscitation, assisted suicide, advance directives and euthanasia. Problems with access to care are also a highly relevant subject for consideration. The so-called 'postcode lottery', the way in which this affects treatment choices, and the recent cases in which women have legally challenged their denial of treatment with Herceptin (Dyer, 2006) raise important ethical questions for practitioners. From these broad subject areas ethical questions can then be identified for discussion, and while these may again be broad in nature (e.g. 'Is euthanasia morally justified?'), they may also be more focused on particular cases or circumstances (e.g. 'Was it morally right to discontinue feeding Tony Bland?'). As discussed above, the objective is for students to examine the issues and develop their own moral arguments, and ethical theories may be referred to in order to help with this.

Ethical theory

There is some debate about the usefulness of ethical theory in applied ethics. In a paper examining the application of theory to particular moral problems, Friday (2004) argues that a process whereby a theory-driven applied ethicist comes to moral conclusions does not involve any moral thinking at all. Meanwhile, Harris (2003) sounds a note of caution about the application of the four principles of

Beauchamp and Childress (2001), a popular theoretical approach in biomedical ethics, which Harris believes, if followed by everybody, would 'lead to sterility and uniformity of approach of a quite mind-boggling kind' (Harris, 2003, p. 303).

The theoretical basis of ethics is both long and varied. Nevertheless, it is worth giving some consideration to the use of ethical theories for learning and teaching in ethics.

There has been a need to formulate codes of behaviour within societies from the fifth century BC and theories have developed from the Sophists, Plato and Aristotle through medieval Christian writers such as Aquinas, British moralists such as Hume, Bentham and Mill, and European philosophers such as Kierkegaard, Kant and Hegel. In the twentieth century, writers such as Rawls, Dworkin and Williams have been influential in moral thinking, and various disciplines in applied ethics have emerged.

One of the most prominent developments in applied ethics has been that of healthcare ethics, encompassing medical, nursing and other profession-specific ethics. This has given rise to a substantial literature specifically devoted to consideration of ethical issues in healthcare practice, such as informed consent, confidentiality, organ donation and transplantation, end-of-life and beginning-of-life issues, and resource allocation. There are many well-known contemporary writers in the discipline of healthcare ethics (e.g. Singer, Harris, Kuhse, Steinbock, Beauchamp and Childress) numerous introductory texts, and several journals (e.g. *Nursing Ethics*, *Bioethics* and the *Journal of Medical Ethics*) which publish papers on a variety of ethical subjects of relevance to healthcare.

A theoretical basis is important in contemporary healthcare, as great emphasis is placed on the need for practice to be evidence based rather than carried out on the basis of guesswork, hunches or intuition. In some respects, ethical theories provide the evidence base for ethics – not by providing findings from empirical research on which to base decision making, but by providing reasons to support taking one particular course of action over another. However, what is crucially important is how theory is used in the decision-making process.

Suppose two students, Jack and Jill, are considering the dilemma of whether to tell a patient the truth about their poor diagnosis. The patient's family have asked the healthcare professional not to reveal the diagnosis, and although the patient has not yet asked any direct questions, the healthcare professional is worried about what they should do if the patient does start to question them. The first thing that Jack and Jill must do is identify the ethical question on which this scenario rests, which they agree is 'Is it morally permissible to lie to patients?' To help them to resolve this question, Jack and Jill may be encouraged to look at how particular theorists might answer it. Jack may look at consequentialist theories, while Jill may tackle the deontologists. They would not have to consult the original texts of nineteenth- and eighteenth-century writers like John Stuart Mill or Immanuel Kant, but they could read about these types of theories in any one of a number of introductory healthcare ethics texts. However, using ethical theory in this way is of limited benefit in learning about ethics. As Allmark (2005) points out, how are Jack and Jill to know which theory (out of a considerable number) they should choose, and what is to stop them simply deciding what to do and then selecting a theory that happens to fit?

What Jack and Jill should do is to look again at the question 'Is it morally permissible to lie to patients?' and identify what they think should be done and why. Having done this, they may find it helpful to look at theories and the ethics literature. Allmark goes on to suggest that, when studying ethics, students read the structured arguments of others, which may challenge their own beliefs, and help them to discard those which are insubstantial and develop new and better ways of reasoning about the dilemma (Allmark, 2005). So if Jack thinks that the right thing to do is to lie to the patient, by reading the positions advanced by ethicists in the literature about truth telling, he can develop and refine his own arguments to defend the course of action that he thinks is morally correct.

Ethical theories are not useful as problem-solving devices, but rather they are ways of thinking about situations and events, and people with diverse ethical beliefs may actually come to the same conclusion about how to act, but have very different reasons for doing so. So in Jack and Jill's dilemma, a consequentialist and a deontologist both come to the conclusion that the best thing to do is to tell the truth. The deontologists would probably argue that it is the healthcare pro-fessional's moral duty to tell the truth, but while reaching the same conclusion, the consequentialist may argue that only by telling the truth will the best conse-quences be produced for the patient, their family and/or society in general. Therefore ethical theory is an important part of learning and teaching ethics, but skilful facilitation is needed to enable meaningful application to develop the student's skills in reason and argument.

The law

A further consideration in the learning and teaching of ethics is how much consideration should be given to legal issues – and including legal perspectives is not without some difficulties. First, legal decisions are not, and may not even concur with, ethical decisions. So, for example, if a nurse stands accused of aiding and abetting suicide by obtaining the lethal substance that the patient subsequently takes and which then causes them to die, what the courts must decide is whether the nurse's actions were legally right or wrong, and what she should have done morally will be of little consequence. On the rare occasions when healthcare professionals are brought before the criminal courts, it is the lawfulness or other-wise of the act that has to be decided, and if it is proven (beyond reasonable doubt) that a criminal act has taken place, what sentence the person should serve. There is also the possibility that students may look to decided cases in law and use the judgements as a basis for their moral decision making. There may be some rational defence for this course of action – for example, in the interests of keeping one's licence to practise – but this will not help students to develop their moral thinking. If one of the objectives of students learning about ethics is to develop skills in making moral judgements, then they must be able to defend the course of action that they decide upon on moral (not legal) grounds.

Therefore, suppose that in the suicide example given above, the nurse is found guilty in law of the crime she has committed. Does it follow that her actions are also morally wrong? Suppose that in her defence the nurse states that she believes that she did the right thing, because the patient (about whose capacity there was no doubt) had asked her to do it, she had been closely involved with the care of the patient for some months and she therefore knew her well. The patient was terminally ill with no chance of recovery, and had reached the stage where her quality of life was so compromised that she did not want to go on living. The nurse therefore puts forward a moral argument for her belief that what she has done is morally the right course of action.

Whether or not you agree with the nurse's actions will of course depend upon your moral beliefs, how highly you value patient autonomy, and whether you think in some circumstances helping a patient to end their life is morally defensible, and working through these arguments is beyond the scope of this chapter. However, you cannot defend answering 'yes' to the question 'Are the nurse's actions morally wrong?' simply because she has been found guilty of a criminal act. In the same way, you could not say that the nurse's actions were morally correct if she had been found to be not guilty and was exonerated by the court. To propose that the nurse's actions are morally wrong, you need to evaluate the reasons that she has put forward to defend her actions, show why her claims are untenable and put forward counter-arguments to support your own line of reasoning. In this example, the nurse has acted unlawfully, but opinion will be divided as to whether her actions are unethical, and any claim that the nurse's actions were ethical or unethical needs to be defended with moral (not legal) arguments.

However, even acknowledging the problems involved in taking legal judgements into consideration, it is a mistake to exclude the legal perspective from ethics teaching altogether, for two reasons. First, it is important that ethics teaching for healthcare professionals is grounded in clinical practice. Therefore consideration needs to be given to the views and regulations of professional bodies and the law. Several pieces of legislation in England and Wales govern aspects of clinical practice that are ethically problematic, such as the Human Fertilisation and Embryology Act 1990 and the Human Tissue Act 2004. In addition, often in clinical practice where there is conflict over a course of action, legal judgements are sought on how to proceed – for example, in *Airedale NHS Trust v Bland* or *The Queen on the Application of Mrs Dianne Pretty v Director of Public Prosecutions and Secretary of State for the Home Department*.

The second reason for including the law in ethics teaching is that it provides rich and varied material dealing with real cases where the ethical issues can be considered in the light of the legal judgements. The Tony Bland case cited above is an example of this, as it can be used not only to illustrate the lengthy judicial process that major judgements like this must go through, but also to explore the reasons given by the Law Lords for allowing Mr Bland's feeding to be discontinued. In the same way that it is not necessary for healthcare professionals who are studying ethics to become moral philosophers, it is not incumbent upon them to become medical lawyers either. However, having received the decision on the legally correct course of action, further useful discussion can be had on the morality of the decision and what ethical arguments can be effected to support or contest the legal arguments. The cases are often widely discussed in the media, and therefore not only are they easily accessible to students, but also the arguments put forward by journalists can themselves serve as useful learning and teaching materials for students to evaluate and critically analyse.

Learning and teaching methods

A wide range of methods can be used for learning and teaching ethics. As well as traditional methods, such as lectures, tutorials and seminars, other methods – including case study analysis (Holland, 1999), drama (Illingworth, 2004), games (White and Davis, 1987), and reflective practice (Leppa and Terry, 2004) – are discussed in the literature, but there is very little evidence as to which method is most effective either in terms of learning and teaching or for preparing practitioners to address ethical issues in practice. Pragmatic decisions may need to be taken depending upon student numbers, the amount of time allowed for the subject in the timetable, and the number of teachers and facilitators in the teaching team. This is undoubtedly more of an issue in programmes leading to registration, where there may be large groups of students. Also, when teaching pre-registration students there is usually a need to introduce a broad spectrum of ethical and legal aspects of care.

More in-depth evaluation of ethical issues in cancer and palliative care can meaningfully take place with post-registration students. Such students are likely to have received some introduction to ethics and/or law in their initial programmes of study, but more importantly will have observed and been involved in ethical decision making in clinical practice. The previous experiences of the students may well influence the learning and teaching strategies to be used.

Sessions may be teacher or student led, and while there are some strengths in formal teacher-led sessions, particularly to present theoretical approaches, Allmark argues that 'there is no crucial piece of ethical knowledge which the educator must pass on to the students' (Allmark, 1995, p. 377).

Therefore it is important that students are able to fully engage in discussion and analysis of ethical issues relevant to their practice.

An important starting point is to ensure that the actual ethical issues to be addressed are identified, rather than the clinical issues in which they may be presented. A useful learning and teaching strategy is to ask students to think about the ethical issues they face in their current practice (this can be done either individually or in small group discussion), and then to collate the responses centrally. When asked to do this, students often come up with broad subjects such as resuscitation, withdrawal of treatment, or organ donation. It is important to explore such examples in order to ascertain what the actual ethical questions are. For example, resuscitation is not on the face of it an ethical issue. However, of interest ethically are questions such as who makes the decision to resuscitate or not, how much the patient him- or herself should be involved in decision making, and on what grounds a decision not to resuscitate should be made. Underlying all of these questions are further matters relating to the value of life, autonomy and informed consent. Similarly, decisions about withholding treatment in cancer care may include not only questions about informed consent and autonomy, but also consideration of the use of experimental treatment and the quality of life of the patient.

It is important to ensure that the ethical questions are identified and that they are then used as the focus of discussion, rather than the clinical cases or issues themselves. If this is not done, it is either extremely difficult to maintain the focus of the discussion and critically analyse the issues in sufficient depth, or else the discussion becomes repetitive. For example, informed consent is an important issue that underpins many specific and more general ethical issues in healthcare. Initially it can be useful to explore such concepts separately from the context in which they may have arisen, and to consider what is meant by informed consent, what conditions are need to make consent informed, how consent is obtained, what kind of information is required, and the role of third parties. Once these more general issues have been debated, the variations or specific influences from the individual clinical contexts can then be focused upon more meaningfully.

Reason and emotion

While emphasising the importance of embedding ethics teaching for healthcare practitioners in practice, a note of caution is needed about the use of reflective learning and teaching strategies. Illingworth suggests that it can be dangerous to allow students to personalise the issues under discussion, and that what she terms 'a degree of emotional distance' should be kept (Illingworth, 2004, p. 88). Learning and teaching methods that encourage self-reflection should therefore only be used in ethics teaching by educators who are skilled in the use of such methods and who have the resources for debriefing if necessary. This does not mean that difficult and contentious issues should not be explored, but rather that students should not be expected to voice their *personal* beliefs which may directly challenge or offend the views of others. For example, Rachels (1997) notes that ethics can be considered a subject like any other, such as history or mathematics, with its own distinctive problems and its own methods of solving them, and Thomson proposes that:

> In order to make moral judgements we do not need to try to become like computers, removing all tendencies to experience sympathy and resentment, but we do need to know whether in a particular situation, they are the appropriate emotions to feel.
>
> Thomson (1999, p. 147)

Inter-professional learning

The use of inter-professional learning is addressed in the literature, and is identified as one of the key elements essential to the modernisation of education and training in *The NHS Plan* (Department of Health, 2000). However, an inter-professional approach to ethics teaching can be a contentious issue for those who view the ethical issues faced by different professional groups as essentially dissimilar. For example, are medical ethics different to nursing ethics, or are they, as Fry and Veatch (2000) believe, both part of a larger general system of bioethics?

Those who argue for the uniqueness of their disciplines are unlikely to be persuaded by the arguments, but if healthcare professionals do not collaborate in the learning and teaching of ethics, an important educational opportunity will be missed. Glenn argues that 'It should be apparent to anyone who thinks about the issue, even for a moment, that health and social care today is no simple matter involving single practitioner and individual clients, patients and users' (Glen, 1995, p. 202).

Inter-professional learning is considered to be important for developing mutual respect and collaboration on ethical issues so as to improve patient care (Hanson,

2005), and ethical issues that arise in clinical practice may be accompanied by disagreement between members of the multi-disciplinary team on how to proceed. Such disagreements do not of course always divide along professional lines, but responsibility for the final decision may do so. Therefore it seems crucially important that the decision maker is able to explain their decision to other participants in the care of the patient, and that those participants in turn are able to make their views known to the decision maker.

Support for inter-professional learning in ethics is evident in the literature (Gallagher, 1995; Glen, 1995), but often practical difficulties of timetabling, student attendance and facilitation are difficult to overcome (Edward and Preece, 1999). There is also a danger that in striving to find ethical issues that are important to a range of professional groups, some important contextualisation may be lost. Midwives perhaps have more to learn about informed consent from obstetricians, neonatologists and ultrasonographers than from oncologists, palliative care nurses and therapeutic radiographers. However, healthcare professionals who specialise in cancer and palliative care clearly face similar ethical dilemmas and are by definition representatives of the multi-disciplinary team where disputes may occur. Therefore teaching ethics to a multi-professional group can provide a wealth of meaningful learning opportunities that are rooted in clinical practice.

Who should teach ethics?

Ethics is no different to other subjects in healthcare in that those who have the necessary skills, education and aptitude to do so should teach it. However, as discussed above, we are all familiar with ethical debate in our everyday lives, and some individuals may feel that this level of understanding is sufficient teaching in this area. For others, years of exposure to ethical issues in practice may be the only foundation they consider necessary to be effective educators. A comprehensive survey of ethics teaching undertaken by a working party of the Institute of Medical Ethics (IME) with the Royal College of Nursing (Gallagher and Boyd, 1991) indicated that there was little formal preparation of staff to teach ethics in 96% of the participating institutions. A more recent survey of learning and teaching ethics in the pre-registration nursing curriculum found that, in contrast to the findings of the IME study, ethics was taught mainly by specialist lecturers within nursing and healthcare departments, and 81% of participating institutions had between one and ten members of staff with taught Masters degrees in either ethics or law (Holt, 2006).

There are a number of postgraduate degrees in ethics and/or law available in higher education institutions across the UK. Such courses are popular among healthcare practitioners and those working in healthcare education, and provide an excellent theoretical foundation for ethics teachers. Although a further degree in ethics cannot be the sole requirement for ethics teachers, it is important that those involved in ethics teaching have sufficient grounding in the theoretical aspects of ethics and moral philosophy to facilitate effective learning and teaching. The IME study (Gallagher and Boyd, 1991) found that teachers who had little preparation in ethics were mainly comfortable with less formal learning and teaching strategies, such as discussions and debates. However, without skilled facilitation by individuals well versed in the subject matter, such discussions can be circuitous, repetitive and fail to reach any meaningful conclusions. The suggestion that ethical decision making is merely common sense is an entirely spurious argument (Holt and Long, 1999).

Conversely, ethics should be taught by those with knowledge of the practice issues and with a clear vision of why healthcare professionals need to learn about ethical issues. Again, it is not always necessary for the person teaching ethics to be a registered practitioner of some kind, or a specialist in a particular field. It may be argued that a teacher who does not have a clinical background may be more objective than one who does, and will therefore be less likely to be hindered by clinical details –there are many effective ethics teachers who have never been practitioners. Clearly a balance needs to be struck, but students (particularly those who are experienced practitioners) are often well informed about the practical and clinical complexities of cases. What they lack are skills in reason and argument to help them to resolve the dilemmas. Therefore the importance of a secure theoretical foundation for ethics teachers should not be underestimated.

Conclusion

To prepare healthcare professionals to address the ethical dilemmas that they encounter in clinical practice, learning and teaching in ethics should allow discussion of contentious issues and facilitate students in forming their own moral judgements. To achieve this, ethics should be firmly rooted in the context of professional practice and should explore relevant and contemporary issues. A range of learning and teaching strategies can be used, but there should be opportunities for students to identify the ethical questions underlying dilemmas in practice, and to discuss the courses of action they may take, appropriately supported by moral argument. Ethics should be taught by those with the necessary skills to do so, but a theoretical foundation in ethics is important, as well as an appreciation of the clinical context in which ethical dilemmas occur. Therefore an interwoven approach to the learning and teaching of ethics is recommended that is underpinned by ethical theory and that integrates legal perspectives with those of the professional bodies. Opportunities for inter-professional learning between practitioners in cancer and palliative care should be encouraged in order to facilitate mutual respect and collaboration on ethical issues, with the aim of improving patient care.

Implications for the reader's own practice

1 How might you change your teaching of ethics in cancer and palliative care in the light of this chapter?
2 In what new ways might you apply the theory to practice?
3 What approaches will you identify and utilise to ensure that inter-professional teaching and learning are implemented in your environment?

References

Allmark P. Uncertainties in the teaching of ethics to students. *J Adv Nurs.* 1995; **22**: 374–8.

Allmark P. Can the study of ethics enhance nursing practice? *J Adv Nurs.* 2005; **51**: 618–24.

Beauchamp TL, Childress JF. *Principles of Biomedical Ethics.* New York: Oxford University Press; 2001.

Department of Health. *The NHS Plan: a plan for investment, a plan for reform.* London: Department of Health; 2000.

Dyer C. Trust's refusal to fund trastuzumab was 'arbitrary.' *BMJ.* 2006; **332**: 747.

Edward C, Preece PE. Shared teaching in health care ethics: a report of the beginning of an idea. *Nurs Ethics.* 1999; **6**: 299–307.

Fletcher N, Holt J *et al. Ethics, Law and Nursing.* Manchester: Manchester University Press; 1995.

Friday J. Education in moral theory and the improvement of moral thought. *J Moral Educ.* 2004; **33**: 23–33.

Fry ST, Veatch RM. *Case Studies in Nursing Ethics.* Sudbury, MA: Jones and Bartlett; 2000.

Gallagher A. Medical and nursing ethics: never the twain? *Nurs Ethics.* 1995; **2**: 95–101.

Gallagher U, Boyd KM. *Teaching and Learning Nursing Ethics.* Harrow: Scutari Press; 1991.

Glen S. Educating for interprofessional collaboration: teaching about values. *Nurs Ethics.* 1995; **6**: 202–13.

Hanson S. Teaching health care ethics: why we should teach nursing and medical students together. *Nurs Ethics.* 2005; **12**: 167–76.

Harris J. In praise of unprincipled ethics. *J Med Ethics.* 2003; **29**: 303–6.

Holland S. Teaching nursing ethics by cases: a personal perspective. *Nurs Ethics.* 1999; **6**: 434–6.

Holt J. Philosophy and nursing: a useful transferable skill. *Nurs Philosophy.* 2002; **1**: 76–9.

Holt J. *Exploring Learning and Teaching Ethics in the Nursing Curriculum.* London: Higher Education Academy; 2006.

Holt J, Long T. Moral guidance, moral philosophy and moral issues in practice. *Nurse Educ Today.* 1999; **19**: 246–9.

Illingworth S. *Approaches to Ethics in Higher Education.* Leeds: Philosophical and Religious Studies Subject Centre, Learning and Teaching Support Network; 2004.

Leppa CJ, Terry LM. Reflective practice in nursing ethics education: international collaboration. *J Adv Nurs.* 2004; **48**: 195–202.

Rachels J. *Can Ethics Provide Answers?* London: Rowan & Littlefield; 1997.

Thomson A. *Critical Reasoning in Ethics: a practical introduction.* London: Routledge; 1999.

Ward PR. Health care rationing: can we afford to ignore euthanasia? *Health Serv Manage Res.* 1997; **10**: 32–41.

White GB, Davis AJ. Teaching ethics using games. *J Adv Nurs.* 1987; **12**: 621–4.

Further reading

- Holt J. *Exploring Teaching and Learning Ethics in the Nursing Curriculum.* London: Higher Education Academy; 2006; www.health.heacademy.ac.uk/sig/ethics

Chapter 10

Information for service users: educational implications

Sally-Ann Spencer Grey

> *The two words 'information' and 'communication' are often used inter-changeably, but they signify quite different things. Information is giving out; communication is getting through.*
>
> *Sydney J Harris (1917–1986)*

Aim

The aim of this chapter is to provide the reader with an overview of the key issues that require consideration when developing quality cancer and palliative care information for service users, which should subsequently ensure effective communication. Throughout the chapter these issues are presented as topics and strategies which can be converted into educational opportunities for those developing information. Potential educational strategies for those providing support when delivering this information are also outlined. The roles of the cancer/palliative care educator and service users (patients and carers) in promoting the development and use of effective, high-quality information will also be discussed.

Learning outcomes

- Explore the key issues with regard to cancer and palliative care information for service users.
- Highlight the need for and importance of education for those involved in the use and development of user information to support effective, high-quality information.
- Identify the educational topics and strategies that need to be addressed in order to effectively support the use and development of effective, high-quality service user information.
- Analyse the roles of the cancer/palliative care educator, patients and carers in promoting the development and use of effective, high-quality service user information.

Introduction

In practice there is an assumption that healthcare professionals have acquired, through experience, the knowledge, skills and ability to develop and support quality information and information services for service users (Spencer-Grey, 2005). This assumption may in many cases be correct, but is seldom certain, as this knowledge, skill and ability is rarely assessed or quantified. The evidence from service users from the national patient and cancer patient surveys (Department of Health, 2002, 2004; Swain, 2003), and from evidence obtained from user focus group meetings in the author's locality (Spencer-Grey 2005), suggests that the quality, accessibility and support with regard to information vary significantly. This variation is found across the UK, within different healthcare regions (e.g. a Cancer Network or a single healthcare setting such as a cancer unit). Variations are also found between healthcare professions (e.g. between radiographers and nurses) and between individual patients. It is generally agreed that these differences are unacceptable, but what is perhaps less well appreciated is that such variations contribute to poor service user experience, and may affect health and care outcomes.

Quality service user information and information services endeavour to communicate with and support individuals (patients and carers) throughout the cancer and palliative care journey and assist their decision making. Information and information services must contribute positively to the quality of care and the care experience for service users to facilitate the best possible outcome.

Patients and carers feel that a suitably knowledgeable healthcare professional could support the provision of information by being in attendance or being available via the telephone.

The notion of a suitably knowledgeable healthcare professional has come from patients' and carers' experiences of meetings with staff who were only able to provide them with minimal information about their situation and in some instances no relevant information at all. This is often due to poor communication between healthcare professionals and poor transfer of information, especially from acute to community settings (Spencer-Grey, 2005). It is also recognised that the knowledge base of generalist healthcare staff regarding cancer and palliative care can be limited, a prime example being general practitioners (GPs), who 'specialise in their patients', but 'it is a speciality of generalists' (Thomas, 2003, p. 32). The knowledge base for the more common cancers may be stronger, particularly in those with a specialist interest. It may be appropriate to identify the formal and informal education opportunities available locally with regard to cancer and palliative care.

Involvement in developing quality service user information provides unique education opportunities through its multi-disciplinary approach and collaborative partnerships with cancer and palliative care patients, carers and members of the local community. Not only does it stimulate learning for the individual, but it also creates opportunities to be involved in the education of others.

The results of a project conducted by the author during 2004–5, and commissioned by the Humber and Yorkshire Coast Cancer Network (HYCCN) Cancer Services Users Information Project (Spencer-Grey, 2005), explored cancer information provision for service users in acute and community settings across the network, and will be used here to supplement the literature.

Adult learning in the context of user information

An understanding of adult learning and the role of information in learning is fundamental to developing appropriate user information and establishing effective education opportunities to support this activity.

Those responsible for developing user information need to appreciate that information not only has intrinsic worth in providing knowledge, but is also a medium for learning. It is this learning – the understanding, interpretation and meaning attributed to the information by the individual – that enables them to use it to make decisions about their care and influence healthcare outcomes. Equally, an understanding of how adults learn and how information supports this learning can inform information development and support.

A clinician's knowledge and understanding of adult learning are crucial, as without these the ability to impart information and the ability of the patient to receive it may be impaired. Those responsible for delivering information development education must therefore have a very good understanding of the principles of adult learning and the nature and use of information.

Adult learners are autonomous and self-directed. They have accumulated a foundation of life experiences and knowledge, and are goal oriented, relevancy oriented and practical. Adult learners need to be shown respect, the wealth of their experiences must be recognised, and they should be treated as equals in experience and knowledge, and allowed to voice their opinions freely.

The following adaptation of Knowles' nine key principles of adult learning (Knowles, 1980) to include information could be used in information development education. Consideration of how each of these principles may be achieved can help to direct the information development process.

1   Adults need to control the information that they receive and their learning – to be provided with information choices to include timing, content, complexity, medium, quantity and the opportunity to discuss their hopes and fears.
2   Adults need to feel that the information and learning have immediate utility – they must be relevant to them and their situation at that particular point in their illness journey.
3   Adults need to feel that the information and learning focus on issues that directly affect them – specific to their disease, their treatment, their social situation, and their side-effects.
4   Adults need to be able to use this information and learning as they go along, rather than receiving background theory and general information – it is therefore suggested that a 'little and often' approach to information giving is adopted. The information provided must also be specific and timely and, when possible, anticipate immediate (short-term) future needs. Additional information can also be identified for the more long-term future.
5   Adults need to anticipate how they will use this information and learning – it must have immediate relevance and give practical and realistic options or alternatives.
6   Adults need to expect better coping and adaptation to result from this information – the information must be clear and straightforward, with no ambiguities, and should clearly state what it will endeavour to enable them to do and how, and what it cannot do.

7   Adult learning is optimal when it maximises the available resources. It should be realistic and practical, relevant to the learner's social setting, and build upon psychological and spiritual wealth (holistic approach).

8   Adult learning requires a climate that is collaborative, respectful, mutual and informal, and information must be provided under similar conditions. Information is a shared process, is accessible, understandable and supported, and builds on existing knowledge (Von Glasersfeld, 1990).

9   Adult learning relies on information that is appropriate to what is known at a given time. Knowledge, awareness, and familiarity with healthcare terms and systems, etc., will vary throughout the illness pathway, as may the individual's ability to cope, their levels of distress and their need to take or abdicate responsibility.

Quality information will enable the transfer of this learning to a new setting or situation (Knowles, 1980) – for example, when the disease progresses, new treatments are introduced or care is provided in a new setting.

The Cancer Services Users Information Project and evaluations from patient and carer courses undertaken by this author have established that there are commonalities in the information needs between patients and carers, and it is important that they receive the same information – engendering trust and valuing each equally. The service users also acknowledge that the information needs of individuals and between patients and carers could vary. Each service user will also value information that is tailored to their specific needs and being able to make some choices with regard to the nature of the information they receive and when they receive it (Spencer-Grey, 2005).

Education and educators

The Cancer Services Users Information Project (Spencer-Grey, 2005) highlighted wide variation in information provision for cancer and palliative care patients and their carers, and also identified educational needs for healthcare staff and for service users. Healthcare staff who are developing service users' information are doing so because it is deemed to be part of their role or they are interested in the topic, although it is rarely defined in their job description. There is little if any assessment of skill and ability with regard to information development, and few of these staff have attended or been offered any appropriate training. However, many felt that training would be beneficial. Service users also felt that such education would be beneficial to them as well as to staff (Spencer-Grey, 2005).

Staff education

Education provided for healthcare staff in this context needs to address the integration of theory and practical issues. It will provide information, raise awareness and develop skills. It is important to identify the following:

- the drivers for quality information
- how individuals may access, interpret and use information – patient and carer differences

- the support that individuals may need to enable them to make the best use of information
- what elements contribute to quality and effective information
- why and how quality and effectiveness may be assured and evaluated
- the needs of those from black and minority ethnic (BME) communities, those with English as a second language and those with literacy, cognitive or developmental difficulties or other disability
- the consequences of poor-quality, ineffective and unsupported information.

The processes involved in initiating and implementing an information project are complex. In addition to considering how to set up a cancer information development group and who to involve, the reader may like to address the following:

1 digital literacy – computer and Internet skills
2 how to offer patient information – the use of information menus or other decision-making tools
3 how to support information giving – by telephone, email, face-to-face meetings, support groups, etc.
4 the use of patient information templates and toolkits, and what constitutes good-quality format and layout
5 the differing needs of patients and carers
6 awareness of the needs of those with disabilities or low literacy or who are members of a BME community, and how to develop appropriate information resources
7 proof reading and guidance for proof and lay readers
8 how to map cancer patient and carer information provision, and identify gaps and overlaps
9 how to assess cancer patient and carer information (written and Internet based), with an introduction to the assessment tools agreed for use
10 guidance on how to develop content – what to include, evidence base, etc.
11 the use and development of other media
12 evaluation of the 'usefulness' of cancer and palliative care information – how to develop a robust and comprehensive evaluation process
13 how to access translation and interpretation services, and guidance on how to use bilingual material and conduct a 'consultation' using an interpreter or telephone interpretation service.

Education that is made available for service users under the tenets of adult learning will provide practical, immediately usable information and skills (Knowles, 1980). Topics 1 to 7 in the above list for healthcare staff may be appropriate for service users.

Educational opportunities

When preparing teaching sessions on information for service users, consideration needs to be given to a number of issues. The way in which information development education may be provided, its duration, who will deliver it, and also whether academic accreditation is viable or necessary could be discussed and agreed locally.

A flexible approach, taking advantage of new technology, is probably most effective. Course development for healthcare staff could include the following:

- defining the target audience and entry criteria (if any)
- defining competence elements and assessment of competence
- mapping to existing relevant competence documents, e.g. Royal College of Nursing competencies for the nurses' contribution to cancer (Department of Health, 2000a), specialist palliative care nurses (Royal College of Nursing, 2002), Skills for Health competencies, Information Nurse competencies (CancerBACUP, 2003), clinical assistant/specialist palliative care practice competencies, etc.
- mapping to the Knowledge and Skills Framework (KSF) levels and dimensions is now essential. Those aspects associated with service user development are outlined below:
  - some of the elements of all six core dimensions will be covered (communication, personal and people development, health, safety and security, service improvement, quality, equality and diversity)
  - some of the specific dimensions in health and well-being, information and knowledge, and in the general section, might also be covered
- defining the evaluation of learning (learners' reactions, changes in attitudes/perceptions, knowledge and skills (Taylor, 2005) and the learning experience, etc.)
- defining ways of evaluating practice and care outcomes.

Educational delivery

In the Cancer Services Users Information Project there was a clear consensus among staff, patients and carers that a multi-disciplinary team approach to developing user information was needed to ensure that service users' views and the relevant health and social care disciplines were represented as appropriate. Other contributors included local support groups and voluntary organisations such as hospices. It was agreed that information development needs to be coordinated and managed within a group with an appointed leader, with tasks and responsibilities allocated to team members (Spencer-Grey, 2005).

In the light of the results from this project, an educational model that reflects the information development processes and which can adapt to group dynamics and will enhance both learning and practical application is encouraged.

A host of options are available for delivery of this education. The chosen route should of course reflect local need and resources, and should not be confined to cancer and palliative care staff, although other healthcare areas will have their own specific issues. Mandatory training for staff and users may emerge in this topic following discussion with local managers. This should be supported by policy, strategy, protocols and investment. It may also be advisable to have this role defined within appropriate job descriptions. This will extend, support and perhaps provide greater recognition of its importance.

Education could be provided as one-off study days or a short course. A rolling programme of topic-specific half or full study days, each with discrete outcomes, may be an alternative. These sessions can be accessed by staff and users flexibly as appropriate to their needs. Compulsory attendance at these sessions within a defined period of time, such as 6 months or 1 year, would ensure competence. Satisfactory completion of study days could be evidenced by a portfolio. This would also provide opportunities for more experienced staff to prove acquired prior education and learning (APEL). Facilitation of such a 'drop-in' approach would of course depend upon numbers and resources. A newly established development group could, as part of their induction, have their meetings established around education topics.

The educator's role in information for service users

Cancer and palliative care educators are eminently suitable for facilitating such education. By its very nature and complexity, cancer and palliative care requires a multi-disciplinary approach. The term 'multi-disciplinary' is used here to denote the coming together of more than two different health and social care professional groups (Wilson and Pirrie, 2000) with a range of skills, who are attempting to work together to deliver a 'client-focused' service.

Many of the issues brought together in this type of learning environment overlap with cancer and palliative care teaching – for example, communication, policy and practice, holistic care, person-centred care, problem-solving approaches, symptom management, psychological, social and spiritual support, and quality. Educators are often experienced in engaging other disciplines and 'experts', healthcare professionals and others (e.g. funeral directors) to deliver elements of a subject area, and in involving patients and carers as educators. User involvement in cancer and palliative care education has a long, if anecdotal history. Improvements in cancer and palliative care information are dependent upon healthcare staff's awareness, knowledge and skills, but just as importantly they depend upon user involvement and users as educators.

The rest of this chapter explores in more detail the key issues and topics already mentioned, and further defines the educational topics and strategies that need to be addressed.

Policy and people

Policy initiatives and the key people involved in their development and implementation have the potential to impact upon the growth and expansion of information for service users.

Current drivers and policy (both national and local) impact upon everyday practice, and an understanding of these will help staff to capitalise upon available resources and initiatives. In order to balance these with known and anticipated constraints, a practical and sustainable approach needs to be ensured, incorporating local information needs.

The drivers for health information and more particularly cancer and palliative care information, as with any aspect of healthcare provision, are a mixture of demand, need, social trends, current health priorities, funding, and government and health policy.

National policy guidelines need to be incorporated into the educational programme and should be current and relevant. Educationalists should be up to date and aware of the latest policy initiatives and relevant target measures. An awareness and understanding of the national, and particularly local, population profile is essential for developing appropriate community links, securing representative involvement and meeting the information needs of the local cancer and palliative care population.

Demographics and epidemiology

Knowledge of demographics and epidemiology should include definitions of the local cancer and palliative care population and agencies. This is a great opportunity to invite speakers from the local communities and agencies to give a talk on what may work more effectively. In order to engage learners, practical activities that highlight issues regarding individual information needs and that focus on disability, poor literacy, cultural differences and learning difficulties should be integrated into the course curriculum. Learners may want to spend time with different communities as a result, and although this may be in their own time, it is to be encouraged.

Some issues in the creation and production of user information require special attention. For instance, identifying the national and local adult literacy situation is crucial to the production of information materials. In 2000, nearly 4 out of 10 adults in England were 'functionally illiterate' (Working Group on Post-School Basic Skills, 1999), with an additional 4% of the adult population severely affected by dyslexia, and it has been estimated that 10% 'show some signs' of the condition (Zabell and Everatt, 2001).

The creators of information also need to understand the implications of poor literacy and dyslexia. Dyslexia can adversely affect concentration and short-term memory. Poor literacy ability is also associated with deprivation and limited educational achievement that may further affect comprehension. Staff will require education about these issues, and need to develop tactful ways of dealing with poor literacy (Hixon, 2004) and dyslexia. Identification, liaison and collaboration with local and national agencies and organisations that specialise in adult literacy, plain English and dyslexia will help to inform this education, and such networking can only help to widen the avenues for promoting cancer and health awareness.

Many patients and carers may be affected to some extent by a learning disability. According to the national and local disability profile figures, there are an estimated 8.6 million disabled people in the UK (14.7 % of the population), with disabilities affecting sight, hearing, mobility, cognition (learning disability) and mental health.

Information can be tailored to the needs of these individuals. Understanding that disabilities are not mutually exclusive and that the incidence of most of the disabilities also rises with age is particularly important, as more than 80% of the cancer patient population are over 60 years of age (Quinn *et al.*, 2001).

This should lead educationalists to encourage their course participants to profile the problems associated with clients in the older age group in their locality. There is a potential for elderly patients and carers (spouses are commonly of a similar age) to acquire physical and cognitive disabilities. This is relevant if the local population has a high density of elderly patients. Some areas of the country have particularly high concentrations of people over 60 years – for example, Eastbourne and Harrogate, which tend to be favoured areas to which to retire.

Cultural awareness is a core issue when training staff to develop information for service users. Staff need to acquire a knowledge and understanding of their clients' cultural background and explore the influences that make them seek information. It is crucial that NHS staff identify different cultural communities – this should encompass black and minority ethnic groups as well as asylum seekers and refugees – to ensure that they 'not only access healthcare services but also receive quality of care which takes into consideration the cultural and religious aspects of healthcare' (Greater Glasgow Primary Care Trust, 2004).

Educationalists should also highlight the fact that language can often be a barrier that inhibits black and minority ethnic groups from accessing information. Teaching strategies can include highlighting the different information sources they may have from other members of their indigenous population, via such media as newspapers, cinemas and community groups.

Education can also include awareness of the local Race Equality Scheme and, particularly with regard to information and policy development, the Race Impact Assessment (Commission for Racial Equality, 2006) process and assessors.

Educational activities on this topic can provide a golden opportunity to investigate attitudes and behaviours with regard to age, disability, literacy and culture. Occasional insensitivity coupled with a lack of alternative formats, particularly written materials, and a shortage of interpreters, all combine to prevent disabled people (French, 1994; Steinberg *et al.* 2002) from accessing health information and services. These barriers also apply to those with poor literacy, the elderly, and black and minority ethnic communities.

Maintaining and improving quality in user information

There are moral, ethical and legal obligations in the provision of quality information in cancer and palliative care, and the full weight of that responsibility must be recognised and used to ensure quality.

Quality begins with ensuring that the right people are engaged in the development of users' information, with an inclusive rather than exclusive approach being adopted. Group members must have or be able to access education to ensure that they have the appropriate knowledge, skills and abilities. As stated before, a multi-disciplinary approach is advocated to ensure representation from patients and carers, different local communities, relevant health and social care disciplines and voluntary organisations, and criteria regarding membership could be established. A collaborative approach with designated roles would constitute effective use of resources. Consideration must also be given to how the group will monitor its effectiveness and efficiency.

Professional writers may help to improve the quality of the information and smooth the process of development. Whether or not the writer has a background in or awareness of the healthcare setting, the content must come from the development team, and the writer will always be heavily reliant on a good brief to be able to meet the necessary requirements (Duman, 2003).

Issues that 'quality' education would need to address

An understanding of the principles of quality assurance, clinical governance and local quality and clinical governance systems is essential. The approach to quality assurance of information must be systematic and enable clinical audit. It will support the delivery of high-quality healthcare and a system of continuous improvement, promoting patient-centred care and reducing variations in process and outcomes.

Moral, ethical and legal obligations are inherent in providing quality user information. The use of anecdotal, outmoded, unsupported or non-evidenced information by healthcare professionals does not fulfil their ethical duty to patients and could, at worst, be deemed negligent. An example of outmoded information would be advice to patients not to wash their hair during cranial radiotherapy. Research now shows that there is no increase in adverse skin reactions with normal hair washing (Westbury *et al.*, 2000). Information has clinical consequences, so due consideration must be given to legal liability when developing patient information, especially if patients and carers rely solely upon this information to make treatment decisions (Duman, 2003).

Most importantly, it is essential to identify evidence, resources and tools that can be used to inform quality assurance and clinical governance systems for information, and to develop or improve local policies, protocols and procedures.

The *NHS Toolkit* for producing patient information is available from www. nhsidentity.nhs.uk/patientinformationtoolkit/patientinfotoolkit.pdf. This is very helpful for providing trust-level protocols and templates, but it is not cancer/ palliative care specific. Another useful tool is *How to do a Race Impact Assessment*, which is available from www.cre.gov.uk/duty/reia/flowchart.html.

Employing a systematic approach to identifying the nature and strength of evidence is also advocated by using a recognised referencing scheme (e.g. Harvard) and applying a hierarchy of evidence. For example, the National Institute for Clinical Excellence currently employs a hierarchy that is an adaptation of a system developed by Eccles and Mason (2001) and Mann's *Clinical Guidelines: using clinical guidelines to improve patient care within the NHS* (Mann, 1996) (Spencer-Grey, 2005).

Central to quality assurance is the ability to assess the quality of the existing materials and the process of development of information resources and the ensuing final product. Where specific tools have not been identified for use within local policies and protocols, the development group needs to decide, using the available evidence, which tools and processes they advocate and why. Information-related education must include details of how to implement or use the chosen tools. The Cancer Services Users Information Project (Spencer-Grey, 2005) showed that just making tools available will not guarantee their use. Staff have access to some quality assurance tools (e.g. DISCERN), but have little time to familiarise themselves with them and consequently do not feel confident about using them. Tools and toolkits are very useful but they do have limitations, so the process of development should encompass different methods of evaluating and assessing information throughout.

A useful and interesting way of teaching an understanding of the different tools and processes is to address this in a practical manner, providing learners in the classroom with the opportunity to experiment with them on real user information, enabling a comparison of approaches as well as assessment of current resources. In addition to layout and readability, learners will also be looking for review dates, content, evidence base, authors, contact information, and evidence of the tool or process having been through a quality assurance system.

Helpful sources of information include the following:

- a policy-into-practice guide, entitled *Producing Patient Information*, produced by the King's Fund (Duman, 2003).
- DISCERN, described as 'a brief questionnaire which provides users with a valid and reliable way of assessing the quality of written information on treatment choices for a health problem' (an introduction can be found at www.discern. org.uk).
- Readability assessment tools are available, such as the McLaughlin 'SMOG' Formula (McLaughlin, 1969), but they have limitations as reading is a complex process and 'testing with patients should also be done' (Smith *et al.*, 1998). Readability encompasses all of the factors that affect success in reading and understanding a text.

Matching reader ability and text may require the use of a literacy screening tool. Readability formulae help to identify the reading grade of the information, but do not help to assess the patient's reading age. In order to match the reader and the text one must be able to identify the reader's ability. Very few adults with low literacy regard their skills as below average, and it is also recognised that shame often accompanies illiteracy (Parikh *et al.*, 1996). Therefore healthcare professionals require education about literacy and tactful ways of dealing with the problem (Hixon, 2004). Individuals with marginal difficulties cannot be easily assessed. Therefore written information must always accommodate the potential for poor literacy and dyslexia.

As previously mentioned, cancer terminology can be confusing and disabling. Attention should be paid to eliminating unnecessary and complex medical language. Similarly, the effects of anxiety on learning as motivating or disabling are well recognised (Mandler and Sarason, 1952). Distress is a common phenomenon associated with a cancer diagnosis, but is also evident in cancer patients and carers across diagnoses and across the disease trajectory (Carlson *et al.*, 2004). The disabling effects of bereavement on carers and family members are also recognised. Anxiety may motivate patients and carers to take steps to reduce this by obtaining information (Massie and Holland, 1989), whereas the stress of the increased demands of cancer and its treatment can impair attention, with a resulting loss of concentration. Situational stress and its effects may be particularly evident at significant points in the illness journey (e.g. diagnosis and recurrence), and can be exacerbated as the disease progresses (Spencer-Grey, 2005), in which case there is an argument that information given at these significant times may need to be 'simplified.' Consideration should therefore be given to developing information on each topic available in incrementally more complex versions to accommodate differing needs.

Involving lay readers other than cancer patients or their carers can enhance the quality process, providing additional validity and diversity. Individuals can be invited from a range of backgrounds, cultures and age groups, and include those with learning, cognitive and physical disabilities. This approach was supported by patients and carers in the Cancer Services Users Information Project. These patients and carers recognised that their 'expertise' was essential to the information development process, but equally that familiarity with the cancer setting could result in a failure to recognise confusing and complicated language and the impact that the way in which information is presented may have on newly diagnosed patients (Spencer-Grey, 2005).

Recent evidence suggests that there is and will continue to be a need both to develop local cancer service information and to tailor information to individual needs. However, it has also become clear that there is a wealth of information about cancer and palliative care available from national organisations and via the Internet, which is easily available and widely used (Spencer-Grey, 2005). This challenges the concept of information development locally when other resources are readily available.

In the light of all the issues raised so far, the educator needs to encourage the learner to consider the following.

- Systematically mapping current information resources, identifying locally developed information and information from other sources.
- Identifying gaps in provision – gaps can be identified through staff, patient and carer focus groups, by mapping the patient care pathway (e.g. Network Site Specific Groups or NSSGs), developing patient information lists, etc. Are the gaps specific to the locality and therefore needing to be developed locally, or could these information gaps be filled with information from elsewhere?
- Using information from national organisations, which is mainly accessed through the Internet or requested by telephone from a directory of resources. A number of well-respected organisations provide this service. Points to consider with regard to using such information include the following:
  - How relevant is the information provided to your client group? Most often it provides a comprehensive overview of a disease, treatment or topic. How would you assess this?
  - There is often an assumption that the information is good quality because of the source. How could this be confirmed? As good practice this information should be sponsored through the same approval and governance system as information developed locally.
  - How will these resources be funded and will the source of funding affect their distribution and equity of access?
  - How is the decision to use this information made – that is, how is it decided that this 'external' information is to be used routinely as part of a given information pathway?

Evaluation: usefulness and effectiveness

Quality assurance should also include a robust audit and evaluation process, and education will be needed to support this.

Measuring the usefulness and effectiveness of information requires clarity with regard to expected outcomes and what should be measured. For instance, users' satisfaction with the resources may encompass knowledge, degree of decision making, degree of involvement, and psychosocial and clinical outcomes (Duman, 2003). However, satisfaction surveys are subjective, and satisfaction measurement reflects three variables – personal preferences, expectations, and the realities in their opinion. Measuring patients' experience is more useful, and interviews and focus groups are recognised methods for doing this (Picker Institute for Europe, 2005).

A combined approach to evaluation, using a range of different evaluation methods, can be an integral part of the quality system. Evaluation may include formative evaluation through continuous feedback on the draft material. Summative evaluation should be conducted once the work is completed. The results can be audited against standards set as part of the quality process and used to inform the information review process.

Information choices and supporting information

It is recognised that once patients receive a diagnosis of cancer they are bombarded with information from all directions (Center for Advancement in Cancer Education, 2005; Spencer-Grey, 2005), but studies have shown that they still often find that their information needs are not being met (Department of Health, 2000b; Healthcare Commission 2005; Spencer-Grey, 2005).

There is also a consensus in the literature that overloading the cancer patient with irrelevant, unhelpful information will ultimately hinder the process of selecting the useful information, resulting in the patient giving up the search for the information that they want or need, and this may lead to their disengagement from the decision-making process.

Key points

- The development and support of a user information service are complex and often difficult to define and deliver.
- To help the reader to produce their own service user information strategy and develop supportive education opportunities, the key points have been displayed in a user-friendly table (*see* overleaf).
- This information will assist the reader in developing this important type of service in a way that is appropriate to their locality and to meet service users' needs.

Conclusion

Information and information services must contribute positively to the quality of care and the care experience for service users in order to facilitate the best possible outcome.

Patients and carers feel that most information is available for the acute situation at the early stage of the cancer pathway, when someone is first diagnosed and prior to treatment. They also feel that information for those who have advanced cancer or are living with long-term cancer is very limited. These patient and carers feel left out of the 'information loop' and unsupported. They also feel that the nature of long-term illness implies to healthcare professionals that they are 'self-sufficient' regarding

Table 10.1   Key points for developing an information strategy

Topic	Education: what and why	Theory to practice: who and how
Adult learning	Understanding of adult learning and transference in this context.	Define a process to ensure that information developed accommodates the key principles of adult learning and facilitates transference.
Who to involve	How to establish, lead and maintain an information development group to ensure inclusivity and best practice. How to educate and support those involved. How to monitor the group's effectiveness and efficiency.	Establish a clear process and criteria regarding the development and quality assurance, etc., of cancer and palliative care information. Ensure that all those involved in information development are aware of the processes and criteria and education available. Identify the best ways to 'audit' the process.
People and policy	Relevant health, cancer and palliative care and information policy and guidance recommendations and targets are known and understood. User involvement – principles and practice are understood.	Local cancer information development group, policies and practices established. User involvement in information development established and supported.
Quality assurance	Understanding of clinical governance, clinical audit and the quality assurance and governance processes and systems controlling patient information. Are issues regarding readability, poor adult literacy and disability understood? Are the potential effects of stress, distress, poor health and fear on the request for, use of and comprehension of information understood? How can complex terminology, ideas and interventions be tackled? Ensure user involvement. How is this achieved? How is user involvement to be supported? How are lay readers to be recruited and supported?	Review of the process to ensure that quality assessment and evaluation are integral to information development. Set standards and methods of review and audit. Education and training in the use of quality assessment tools. The evidence base and strength of evidence must be confirmed – implement the use of a recognised reference scheme and hierarchy of evidence. Decide which readability and literacy assessment tools, if any, are to be used, and instigate training. Establish a system to recruit and support user and lay person involvement. Develop information for significant events /points on the illness journey to accommodate situational stress.
Evaluation	Is quality assurance and clinical audit understood? How is evaluation tackled? Is there formative and summative evaluation? How are usefulness and effectiveness measured? What standards have been set? What results are to be measured? How will the results of audit be used?	Review evaluation and create a robust approach to evaluation. Ensure that staff are trained appropriately. Ensure that users are involved in the evaluation process.
Information needs	Understanding of information needs and appropriate health outcomes for the client group (patients and carers) and the role of quality information in supporting these.	Clearly define the client group and canvass them about their perceived information needs.

Topic	Education: what and why	Theory to practice: who and how
Resources	Internet skills and awareness – website assessment, facilitating searches, etc. How is information (all media types) from non-NHS sources to be chosen and assessed? How is media other than written information to be developed and assessed? Are disability issues understood and accommodated? Are attitudes and behaviours with regard to disability examined? Cultural competency – awareness and understanding competency frameworks can be employed.	Obtain information on the local BME communities and the languages used. Approach BME communities and form partnerships with them. Establish a system that will detail media other than written information and points along the illness journey that can be used instead of or in addition to existing information. Ensure that media from all sources and of all types are assessed by the same quality assessment process.
Information Choices	What choice of information is provided (style, media, complexity and support)? What is the rationale for each item? When is this information most pertinent/significant in the care journey? How is information held and where? How can current systems be used to facilitate production of information menus and recording of patient information choices and preferences? Who needs to be involved in developing such a system?	Establish a system to facilitate information choice (checklists and menus, flagged items, etc.), and educate staff in the use of this system.
Information support	Overview of information support strategies – pros and cons and the need for flexibility and individuality. Are the needs of long-term patients considered? Ensure that there is an appropriate knowledge base, access to resources and skills to access resources for those providing support.	Mechanisms are established to ensure that patients and carers are involved in determining how best to support them both as a client group and also on an individual basis. Clear lines of responsibility and points of contact for all patients and carers with regard to information and support are determined, agreed, recorded and adhered to. Mechanisms are established to ensure access to a central information resource or to similar resources by all parties supporting patients and carers and their information needs.

the need for and access to information and support, when this is not always the case (Spencer-Grey, 2005).

Given the importance of service user information to healthcare decision making and health outcomes, the quality of service user information and information services cannot be left to chance, and policies and systems must be established to support them (Department of Health, 1998, 2000c; National Institute for Clinical Excellence, 2004). The knowledge base, skills and abilities of those involved in developing user information must be assured, and provision of appropriate education opportunities can help to address this. Involvement in developing quality service user information provides unique education opportunities through its multi-disciplinary approach and collaborative partnerships with cancer and palliative care patients, carers and members of the local community. Not only does it stimulate learning for the individual, but it also creates opportunities to be involved in the education of others.

Training should not apply solely to NHS service provision. Support provided by voluntary organisations needs similar consideration. Access to information by voluntary organisations must be integrated into health service provision. Voluntary services need to have an awareness of and access to the same cancer and palliative care information as their NHS colleagues, ensuring consistency and continuity. This will improve communication and help to maintain quality.

The development of quality cancer and palliative care information is a complex issue and process, but if it is tackled from an informed position using a collaborative, systematic and accountable approach, great things can be achieved.

Implications for the reader's own practice

1 How will you find out what is available and being taught locally with regard to information for service users?
2 How will you map current information resources and ensure that they are all quality assured?
3 How will you produce a strategy that includes the delivery of appropriate and timely information?
4 Are your staff educated in information development, delivery and support?
5 What will you do to produce a quality educational/training programme appropriate to your local needs?

References

CancerBACUP. *Competencies for the Cancer Information Nurse Specialist;* www.cancerbacup.org.uk/Healthprofessionals/Workingincancercare/CISnursecompetencies (accessed 10 December 2004).

Carlson LE, Angen M, Cullum J *et al.* High levels of untreated distress and fatigue in cancer patients. *Br J Cancer.* 2004; **90:** 2297–304.

Center for Advancement in Cancer Education. First accessed in March 2005 from the Patient Services page at www.beatcancer.org

Commission for Racial Equality. *Race Equality Duty;* www.cre.gov.uk (accessed 8 May 2006).

Department of Health. *A First-Class Service: quality in the new NHS.* London: Department of Health; 1998.

Department of Health. *The Nursing Contribution to Cancer Care: a strategic programme of action in support of the national cancer programme.* London: Department of Health; 2000a.

Department of Health. *The NHS Cancer Plan: a plan for investment, a plan for reform.* London: Department of Health; 2000b.

Department of Health. *The NHS Plan.* London: Department of Health; 2000c.

Department of Health. *National Surveys of NHS Patients. Cancer Network Report 1999/2000, Humber and Yorkshire Coast.* London: Department of Health; 2002.

Department of Health. *The Manual of Cancer Services: standards.* London: Department of Health; 2004.

Duman M. *Producing Patient Information. How to research, develop and produce effective information resources.* London: The King's Fund; 2003.

Eccles M, Mason J. How to develop cost-conscious guidelines. *Health Technol Assess.* 2001; **5:** 1–69.

French S. Attitudes of health professionals towards disabled people. *Physiotherapy.* 1994; **80:** 687–93.

Greater Glasgow Primary Care Trust. *Asylum Seekers and Refugees;*

www.show.scot.nhs.uk/ggpct/Equality_and_Diversity/useful_info/asylum_seeker.htm (accessed 3 February 2005).

Healthcare Commission. *National Patient Surveys;* www.healthcarecommission.org.uk (accessed 4 February 2005).

Hixon AL. Functional health literacy: improving health outcomes. *Am Fam Physician.* 2004; **69.** Accessed 25 February 2005 from the American Academy of Family Physicians at: www.aafp.org/afp/20040501/medicine.html

Knowles MS. *The Modern Practice of Adult Education: from pedagogy to andragogy.* Revised ed. New York: Cambridge University Press; 1980.

McLaughlin H. SMOG grading – a new readability formula. *J Reading.* 1969; **22:** 639–46.

Mandler G, Sarason SB. A study of anxiety and learning. *J Abnorm Soc Psychol.* 1952; **47:** 166–73.

Mann T. *Clinical Guidelines: using clinical guidelines to improve patient care within the NHS.* London: Department of Health; 1996.

Massie MJ, Holland JC. Overview of normal reactions and prevalence of psychiatric disorders. In: Holland JC, Rowland JH, editors. *Handbook of Psycho-Oncology: psychological care of the patient with cancer.* New York: Oxford University Press; 1989. pp. 273–82.

National Institute for Clinical Excellence (NICE). *Guidance on Cancer Services. Improving supportive and palliative care for adults with cancer.* London: NICE; 2004.

Parikh NS, Parker RM, Nurss J *et al.* Shame and health literacy: the unspoken connection. *Patient Educ Counsel.* 1996; **27:** 33–9.

Picker Institute for Europe. *Measuring a Patient's Experience of Health: the Picker approach;* www.pickereurope.org/about/approach.htm (accessed 25 February 2005).

Quinn M, Babb P, Brock A *et al. National Statistics. Cancer trends in England and Wales, 1950–1999.* London: The Stationery Office; 2001.

Royal College of Nursing. *A Framework for Nurses Working in Specialist Palliative Care.* London: Royal College of Nursing; 2002.

Smith H, Gooding S, Brown R *et al.* Evaluation of readability and accuracy of information leaflets in general practice for patients with asthma. *BMJ.* 1998; **317:** 264–5.

Spencer-Grey SA. *Cancer Services Users Information Project.* Hull: Humber and Yorkshire Coast Cancer Network; 2005.

Steinberg AG, Wiggins EA, Barmada CH *et al.* Deaf women: experience and perceptions of healthcare system access. *J Womens Health.* 2002; **11:** 729–41.

Swain D. Information and communication on the process of care. In: *January Newsletter;* www.nhssurveys.org (accessed 25 October 2003).

Taylor V. Palliative care education: establishing the evidence base. In: Foyle L, Hostad J, editors. *Delivering Cancer and Palliative Care Education.* Oxford: Radcliffe Publishing; 2005.

Thomas K. *Caring for the Dying at Home.* Oxford: Radcliffe Medical Press; 2003.

Von Glasersfeld E. An exposition of constructivism: why some like it radical. In: Davis PB, Maher CA, Noddings N, editors. *Monographs of the* Journal for Research in Mathematics Education. Reston, VA: National Council of Teachers of Mathematics; 1990. pp. 19–29.

Westbury C, Hines F, Hawkes E *et al.* Advice on hair and scalp care during cranial radiotherapy: a prospective randomized trial. *Radiother Oncol.* 2000; **54:** 109–16.

Wilson V, Pirrie A. *Spotlight 77. Multidisciplinary teamworking indicators of good practice;* www. scre.ac.uk/spotlight/spotlight77.html (accessed 8 May 2006).

Working Group on Post-School Basic Skills. *The Moser Report. Improving literacy and numeracy: a fresh start.* London: Working Group on Post-School Basic Skills; 1999.

Zabell C, Everatt J. Subtypes of dyslexia in dyslexic teenagers and adults. *Proceedings of the Fifth British Dyslexia Association (BDA) International Conference*, University of York, 18–21 April 2001. Reading: BDA.

Further reading

- Spencer-Grey SA. *Cancer Services Users Information Project.* Hull: Humber and Yorkshire Coast Cancer Network; 2005. This comprehensive report is cancer specific and tackles all of the topics discussed in this chapter in depth through discussion and analysis, as well as providing a wealth of information and direction to additional resources. The executive summary is available at www.saspencergrey.co.uk. Further information and copies of the full report are available from the author by emailing sally@saspencergrey.co.uk
- Duman M. *Producing Patient Information. How to research, develop and produce effective information resources.* London: The King's Fund; 2003. This a comprehensive policy-into-practice guide produced by the King's Fund. It is healthcare specific and primarily aimed at those working in the NHS, although it is not specific to cancer or palliative care.

Chapter 11

Pre-registration nursing: cancer and palliative care education

Julie MacDonald and Tracey McCready

Suffering and joy teach us, if we allow them, how to make the leap of empathy, which transports us into the soul and heart of another person. In those transparent moments we know other people's joys and sorrows and we care about their concerns as if they were our own.

Fritz Williams

Aim

The aim of this chapter is to look at the challenge of cancer and palliative care education within pre-registration nursing curricula.

Learning outcomes

- Appreciate the recent influences on pre-registration nurse education.
- Reflect on the recent history of cancer and palliative care education within pre-registration nursing education.
- Explore how health and social policy impacts upon cancer and palliative care education within pre-registration curricula.
- Appreciate the importance and benefits to patients that result from educating student nurses in cancer and palliative care.

Introduction

Nurse education is central to enabling skilled expert nursing to improve outcomes for patients and their families (Royal College of Nursing, 2002). The position statement of the Royal College of Nursing (2002) on *Quality Education for Quality Care* highlights pre-registration nursing as one of four key areas where challenges lie, the others being continuing professional development and lifelong learning, professional regulation and higher education workforce issues. The key issues relating to pre-registration nursing include a review of the current four branches of nursing as highlighted in the *Fitness for Practice* report (United Kingdom Central Council for Nursing, Midwifery and Health Visiting, 1999), the level of the award given on completion being commensurate with other professions, recruitment strategies achieving cultural diversity, and programme content ensuring cultural competence. The position statement by the Royal College of Nursing (2002) builds on the work undertaken in the *Fitness for Practice* report (United Kingdom Central Council for Nursing, Midwifery and Health Visiting, 1999), which highlighted issues of student nurses being fit for practice at the point of registration. Other key issues highlighted by that report included the variable nature of practice placements, variable support for students in practice, and a perceived imbalance between theory and practice. The report recommended that standards for registration should be based on competencies, with the balance between theory and practice promoting the integration of knowledge, skills and attitudes.

Standards of proficiency for nursing define the overarching principles of being able to practise as a nurse. The student at the point of registration should meet these standards, which include the following (Nursing and Midwifery Council, 2004):

- practising in an anti-discriminatory way
- acknowledging the differences in beliefs and cultural practices of individuals engaging in therapeutic relationships through the use of appropriate communication and interpersonal skills
- being able to undertake a comprehensive assessment of the physical, psychological, social and spiritual needs of patients, clients and communities
- being able to demonstrate knowledge of effective inter-professional working practices.

The *Standards of Proficiency for Pre-Registration Nursing Education* of the Nursing and Midwifery Council (2004) build on recent government and nursing initiatives, and suggest guiding principles to meet proficiency standards and enable nurses to be fit for practice (Department of Health, 1999; United Kingdom Central Council for Nursing, Midwifery and Health Visiting, 1999; Royal College of Nursing, 2002). The Nursing and Midwifery Council (2004) highlights the importance of balancing theory and practice, utilising the best available evidence to inform practice, and providing care that is responsive to the needs of different client groups and which is holistic in nature. The Nursing and Midwifery Council also suggests a framework for the pre-registration curriculum which includes professional, legal and ethical issues, theory and practice of nursing, the context in which care is delivered, organisational structures and processes, communication, social and life sciences relevant to practice, and frameworks for social care provision and care systems. The standards of the Nursing and Midwifery Council (2004) are based on a backdrop of directives from Europe which have mandatory requirements for pre-registration programmes and include programme content directives and practice experience, both of which are based on some of the key points highlighted and both of which are generic in nature.

For those of us practising within cancer and palliative care, where does this leave the preparation of student nurses to care for patients and clients with cancer or a life-limiting illness, and their families? The following information aims to set cancer and palliative care within the context of current pre-registration education by looking back at some of the influences on and evidence in this area.

Cancer care education

One in three people will be diagnosed with cancer at some point in their life, and one in four will die from the disease (Department of Health, 2000b; Cancer Research UK, 2005). The needs of cancer patients, their families and friends will change as the disease develops, and in order to deal with this effectively, nurses need the knowledge and skill to understand the care that is required (Royal College of Nursing, 2003). Health and social policy has, over the last decade, attempted to shape nurse education in cancer care at both pre-registration and post-registration levels (Department of Health, 1995, 1999, 2000a, 2000b; Royal College of Nursing, 1996a, 1996b, 2003). Unfortunately, the key challenges in cancer care education are the same now as they were over a decade ago, when Corner and Wilson-Barnett (1992) highlighted reports of poor pain and symptom management in cancer care as well as ineffective communication and psychological support (Department of Health, 2000b; National Institute for Clinical Excellence, 2004). Misconceptions that were common at the time of the study by Corner and Wilson-Barnett (1992) included the gross despondency of nurses when faced with patients with a cancer diagnosis, impressions of poor cure rates, and evidence of the under-treatment of pain and symptoms. Education was advocated by some as key to changing nurses' attitudes and improving care, while other studies that were conducted at the time reported equivocal results (Craytor *et al.*, 1978; Johnson *et al.*, 1982). The research by Corner and Wilson-Barnett (1992) was aimed at newly qualified nurses, and therefore gives useful feedback on cancer care education at pre-registration level. The study set out to collect information about nurses' attitudes, knowledge, confidence and perceived educational needs in cancer care, in order to develop an educational package to meet those needs. The data revealed that nurses were generally pessimistic about cancer and had feelings of inadequacy about their care of cancer patients. Overall, nurses' knowledge of cancer and cancer care was judged to be poor. In their recommendations, Corner and Wilson-Barnett (1992) suggested that pre- and post-registration education needed to address what appeared to be a neglected area.

In the mid-1990s, a report on the state of cancer services, *A Policy Framework for the Commissioning of Cancer Services: a Report to the Chief Medical Officers of England and Wales (Calman–Hine Report)* (Department of Health, 1995), kick-started reform within cancer care services and highlighted education in cancer care as being key to moving services forward. The following year saw the Royal College of Nursing (RCN) streamline the commissioning and purchasing of cancer education with the following key suggestions (Royal College of Nursing, 1996a).

- Service providers should be represented in education-purchasing consortia.
- Specific cancer education and training needs should be promoted by a representative of the consortia at the regional education development group.
- Education providers should be provided with commissioning plans at an early stage.
- Programmes of cancer care education should be flexible and modular.
- Multi-disciplinary and multi-professional education should be promoted.

Later the same year, the Royal College of Nursing (1996b) published guidelines for good practice in cancer nursing education. They highlighted the importance of course planning and development of cancer nursing content in the pre- registration curriculum to meet the needs of the service. The standard statement highlighted the fact that course content should contribute to the development of students' knowledge skills and attitudes, to ensure that they care competently for people with cancer. In order to achieve this, the Royal College of Nursing (1996b) made the following suggestions.

- Those teaching the cancer component of the pre-registration programme should be qualified teachers holding a first degree.
- They should also hold a recordable qualification in cancer nursing.
- They should have clinical expertise in cancer nursing.
- The course content should demonstrate an evidence base and be reviewed annually.

One study that reviewed course content was the English National Board (ENB) commissioned study, which looked at cancer nursing education by utilising a literature review and documentary analysis (Langton *et al.*, 1999). Within the literature, nine key themes were identified as being significant to cancer nursing education:

- prevention/detection
- the nature of cancer
- treatment
- psychosocial aspects
- rehabilitation and survivorship
- death and dying
- organisation of care
- key skills
- the future of cancer nurse education.

It is interesting to note that key subject themes highlighted by nurses in the study by Corner and Wilson-Barnett (1992) are implicit rather than explicit in the listing (i.e. pain and symptom management, communication skills and psychological care). The English National Board (Langton *et al.*, 1999) also highlighted the importance of clinical experience within educational programmes. However, it was recognised that in reality it is very difficult to match specific theory and practice.

The NHS Cancer Plan: a plan for investment, a plan for reform (Department of Health, 2000b) set out to address the challenges of delivering high-quality cancer care with education and development of staff as a key priority. In the same year, *The Nursing Contribution to Cancer Care* (Department of Health, 2000a), a strategic programme of action in support of the national cancer programme, was published. With regard to workforce, education and training, *The Nursing Contribution to Cancer Care* highlighted the need to revise pre-registration nursing education to accommodate the need for all nurses to have an awareness of the knowledge and skills required to provide initial and ongoing care for people affected by cancer, and at the same time to link competencies to a career framework. The strategy goes on to suggest that, where possible, the good practice of exposure to a cancer care setting during pre-registration education and heightened awareness at both pre- and post-qualifying level of cancer symptoms should be encouraged. The combination of theory- and practice-based learning set out in the United Kingdom Central Council's *Fitness for Practice* proposals (United Kingdom Central Council for Nursing, Midwifery and Health Visiting, 1999), and the plans for pre-registration set out in *Making a*

Difference (Department of Health, 1999), as well as the Nursing and Midwifery Council's *Proficiency Standards* (Nursing and Midwifery Council, 2004), would suggest that enough clinical experience is provided to make the goal achievable. Yet in fact few student nurses will be placed in a designated cancer area, the reality being that experience of cancer care for most students will be in general areas.

Contrasting the experiences of England and Wales with an international perspective, an action research programme conducted by Kelly *et al.* (1999) in Ireland set out to develop the cancer content of pre-registration nurse education programmes based on the European Oncology Nursing Society's core curriculum for post-basic courses in cancer nursing. Kelly *et al.* (1999) assessed the cancer content of the pre-registration nurse education programmes in general and sick children's training hospitals in Ireland after completing a literature review which demonstrated that, in Europe and North America, cancer nursing is addressed at pre-registration level but there is wide variation in the following:

- how it is taught
- which aspects are covered
- the amount of time dedicated to the subject.

No published reports were found on the cancer content of pre-registration nurse education in Ireland. However, 52 nurse teachers with some responsibility for pre-registration cancer education from all 21 training hospitals were interviewed. The results highlighted the fact that pre-registration education is based on a syllabus which does not refer to cancer nursing as a subject area, and which allows for a very broad interpretation, with the result that there is diversity in the curriculum offered by each school. The amount of time allocated ranged from 5 to 25 hours. Thus some nurses qualify with limited knowledge, but most patients are cared for in general areas. In some schools the curriculum follows a systems approach in which cancer is not addressed as a discrete entity, and other schools had resolved the problem by developing a discrete module in cancer care. In some schools specialist cancer nurses taught on the curriculum, whereas in others this was not the case. In some schools the cancer content was felt to be adequate, although this was not always reflected in the indicative content of the curriculum. The study highlights a very disparate service.

Current influences on the cancer care input into pre-registration curricula include *The Nursing Contribution to Cancer Care* (Department of Health, 2000a) and the RCN's *Framework for Adult Cancer Nursing* (Royal College of Nursing, 2003). *The Nursing Contribution to Cancer Care* (Department of Health, 2000a) recommends that pre-registration programmes should provide education to support the initial and ongoing care of people affected by cancers. The ethos of holistic care affords opportunities to incorporate cancer-related subjects across the curricula – for example, age-related cancers in children's and older people's care, lifestyle-related cancers, and screening in health promotion modules. The RCN's *Framework for Adult Cancer Nursing* (Royal College of Nursing, 2003) suggests that it is essential that the structure, training and education of the nursing workforce provide nurses with a sound knowledge and understanding of the needs of cancer patients, their families and friends. It is also realistic about its recommendations in an arena where rapid change makes specific curriculum content difficult to recommend. The RCN highlights the importance of developing programmes that are responsive to the demands of contemporary cancer nursing provision and cancer research (Royal College of Nursing, 2003). In the light of this, it makes the following recommendations.

Generic (an awareness in common foundation programmes, leading to more targeted knowledge in branch pathways)

Cancers related to demographics

Age, gender, sexual health, ethnicity and poor socio-economic indicators.

Mental health implications

Bad news, chronic illness, the worried well, and coping with serious life changes.

Counselling and communication skills

Breaking bad news, listening to and supporting people, reflective practice, mentorship support, psychological boundaries and multi-professional collaboration.

Specific (branch pathways)

Primary focus

Health promotion, primary prevention initiatives, screening, self-examination techniques, skills and abilities with regard to improving personal poor self-health, cancer awareness in primary care, school nursing, community health and genetic counselling.

Secondary focus

Primary and acute care settings, investigations for cancer, and the patient's complete experience of cancer care service and support.

Tertiary focus

Managing difficult therapies, coping with chronic illness, body image changes, sexual and reproductive health problems, disability, rehabilitation, communication and counselling in loss and bereavement and supporting colleagues.

The work conducted over the past decade in the area of cancer care education clearly highlights the importance of theory and practice in cancer care. *The Cancer Plan* (Department of Health, 2000b) has done much to streamline cancer services, care delivery and education, but still leaves cancer education open to interpretation. Lecturers working in higher education need to utilise research evidence as well as the input of service users to inform education programmes. Educational programmes are not uniform, and guidelines are open to interpretation. The situation highlighted in the study by Kelly *et al.* (1999) in Ireland still exists today, with some pre-registration programmes having optional cancer modules, some having cancer themes, and some in which the curriculum planner might have considerable difficulty in identifying the cancer input.

Palliative care education

Nurses are the healthcare providers who are most often with individuals at the end of their lives, and as such they should be knowledgeable about end-of-life care and the provision of palliative care services. Despite this, nurses themselves have reported that key elements of end-of-life care were not covered in their under-graduate education (Robinson, 2004). Nurse educators have also identified that, historically, nurses have not been prepared for providing care for dying patients (Mallory, 2003). Over 30 years ago, studies in the USA on the education of nurses with dying patients highlighted inadequate educational provision for nurses in this area of care (Birch, 1983). These findings were supported by research undertaken by Webber (1989) in the UK. This study found that nurses received little prep-aration to help them to care for the dying, and that until the birth of the hospice movement, death education for nurses focused on practical and legal aspects of death, with little or no input on interpersonal skills and pain and symptom management (Webber, 1989).

Despite the lack of education in this area being highlighted, one survey of nurses in the USA found that almost 90% of nurses believed that end-of-life content is important for basic nursing education, yet 62% rated their undergraduate prep-aration on these issues as inadequate (Last Acts, 2002).

Zabalegui (2002) states that in Spain nearly all nursing schools offer some formal teaching about end-of-life care, although there is evidence that current diploma nursing training is inadequate, with palliative care being an under-represented area. Increasing attention to palliative care education has created major oppor-tunities for improving education about care at the end of life, and palliative care teaching is said to be received favourably by students, positively influencing their attitudes and improving communication skills (Zabalegui, 2002).

In Canada, palliative care has been identified as having fundamental develop-mental deficiencies, with professional ignorance and apathy being cited as con-tributing factors (Williams *et al.*, 2002). It is argued that education in this area needs to be enhanced, with lack of palliative care educators being seen as the second most serious critical problem in palliative care, preceded only by inadequate resources (Sellick *et al.*, 1996). In a survey of 135 non-physician service providers working in long-term care settings, it was reported that 57% felt that their formal education did not adequately prepare them for the delivery of palliative care (Robinson, 2004).

The need to provide clinically relevant, focused education programmes to meet the challenge of palliative care practice remains of major importance to educators in this field (McLeod and James, 1994).

In Europe, the UK has the widest range of courses in palliative care, and other countries also have education initiatives in this area. It is argued that it is necessary to have some guidelines on the educational preparation necessary for disciplines involved in the delivery of high-quality palliative care. In 1997, the European Association for Palliative Care (EAPC) proposed that member associations in each country should create a national education network to link with the EAPC education network. The remit was to establish minimal recommendations for training in palliative care for both nurses and doctors. The subsequent report, entitled *A Guide for the Development of Palliative Nurse Education in Europe*, was agreed in November 2003, and the document represents a body of opinion about the future structure and potential framework that could be utilised in the preparation of palliative nursing programmes across Europe (de Vlieger *et al.*, 2004).

The report emphasises the value of multi-disciplinary education, stating that it cannot be underestimated in terms of learning to work together and share responsibilities. It also argues that palliative care education should be based on the principles of adult education, namely self-directed and problem-based learning (Spencer and Jordan, 1999). These approaches are said to produce the benefits of clear critical thinking and problem solving. The report also states that education which is separated from practice is ineffectual and inadvisable.

It is argued that not everyone needs to be a specialist in palliative care, but that a palliative approach to practice provides a solid framework. In its report, the European Association for Palliative Care (2003) proposes three level of knowledge acquisition (see bellows).

As this chapter is discussing undergraduate palliative care education, a summary of the knowledge to be acquired at the undergraduate level is identified (the European Association for Palliative Care believes that this should also represent the basic knowledge and skills of a postgraduate nurse delivering palliative care). For information on the knowledge and skills expected at the other levels, the reader is referred to the European Association for Palliative Care document (*see* References section for website address).

Level A: undergraduate and postgraduate

At this level, the European Association for Palliative Care (2003) has suggested that the following knowledge and skills might be expected of the nurse. They should be able to clearly define the core values of palliative care and the relationship between palliative care and the healthcare system. In addition, they should be able to identify the impact of serious illness on all members of the family, and the possible social consequences that may follow. The normal processes of grief and loss should be understood, and the support mechanisms that are available to families identified. The roles of the different team members and their contribution to the team should also be identified. The multi-disciplinary nature of pain, the concept of total pain and the tools used to guide pain assessment should be taught, and the nurse should be able to identify common symptoms associated with patient care at the end of life, to describe the different modes of administration of medication, and to demonstrate skills in teaching the patient about their medication. The nurse should be able to anticipate problems at the physical, psychological and spiritual level. They should understand the needs of their patient, and provide culturally sensitive care up to and immediately after death, responding to the family's need for guidance around emotion, grief and any formalities which may be necessary. An understanding of the key ethical issues should also be demonstrated by the nurse.

Level B

At this level, the practitioner may fulfil the role of a resource person.

Level C

Here practice is delivered at a specialist level, including an education and research component (European Association for Palliative Care, 2003).

The decision as to what constitutes each level is left to the individual country, as is the educational preparation for each level (de Vlieger *et al.*, 2004).

The ultimate goal of palliative care education must be to influence, improve or change practice so that it benefits patients and their families. High-quality education improves knowledge, skills and attitudes and produces practitioners who are competent and confident enough to question their own and others' practice. Unless practitioners are able to put into practice what they have learned, it is argued that the education may be of little benefit (Kenny, 2003).

Kenny (2003) also argues that everyone involved in education must have a clear idea about what that education is intended to achieve. She argues that students should be involved in the planning of their education through the use of individual learning contracts, and theory and practice are highlighted as being of equal importance.

Of course palliative care education is not just about delivery. Evaluation is essential, and courses should demonstrate measurable outcome objectives to the funding provider. Failure to do so will do little to enhance the status of palliative nurse education (de Vlieger *et al.*, 2004).

Key points

- Over the last decade, health and social policy and educational initiatives have attempted to shape cancer and palliative care nurse education.
- The evidence suggests that newly qualified nurses would have liked more education in communication skills and pain and symptom management in the pre-registration nursing curriculum.
- The value of multi-disciplinary education cannot be underestimated in terms of learning to work together and share responsibilities.
- Unless practitioners are able to put into practice what they have learned, the education may be of little benefit.
- Evaluation of cancer and palliative care education is essential, and courses should demonstrate measurable outcome objectives.
- At present, although there are some published guidelines, there is no uniform framework for delivery of cancer and palliative care education in the pre-registration curricula.

Conclusion

Over the last decade, health and social policy documents have identified deficiencies in pre-registration cancer and palliative education and have developed frameworks to address the shortfalls. The areas that need to be addressed include a curriculum that highlights the key subject areas of pain and symptom management, communication and psychological support. The curriculum should be evidence based, and it should be facilitated by individuals with the relevant practice experience and skills in learning and teaching. Practice and education should be valued, as should inter-professional learning.

The evidence suggests that, despite clear guidance, cancer and palliative care education in the pre-registration nursing curricula remains disparate (Department of Health, 1995; Kelly *et al.*, 1999; Royal College of Nursing, 2003). The hope for the future must be that nurse educators, both in higher education and in practice, will work together to implement guidelines at a local level. There are those who would advocate a national inter-professional curriculum, the worry being that cancer and palliative care education is not given the time and resources within the curriculum that it deserves (Whitehead, 2005). This could have serious implications for the patient with cancer or a life-limiting illness and their family.

> *Education is for improving the lives of others and for leaving your community and world better than you found it.*
>
> *Marian Wright Edleman*

Implications for the reader's own practice

1 How do current educational developments affect your teaching/support of pre-registration students?
2 Reflect on the education that you have received in cancer and palliative care. Does this meet current guidelines?
3 Think about your practice area. Are students encouraged and supported in putting their learning into practice? If not, how can this best be achieved?
4 How can you influence the learning of pre-registration students in your own locality?

References

Birch JA (1983) Anxiety and conflict in nurse education. In: Davis BD, editor. *Research in Nurse Education*. Beckenham: Croom-Helm; 1983. pp. 26–47.

Cancer Research UK. *Cancerstats Incidence UK*. London: Cancer Research UK; 2005.

Corner J, Wilson-Barnett J. The newly registered nurse and the cancer patient: an educational evaluation. *Int J Nurs Stud.* 1992; **29:** 177–90.

Craytor JK, Brown J, Morrow G. Assessing learning needs of nurses who care for persons with cancer. *Cancer Nurs.* 1978; **1:** 211–20.

de Vlieger M, Grochs N, Larkin PJ *et al.* Palliative nurse education: towards a common language (editorial). *Palliat Med.* 2004; **18:** 401–3.

Department of Health. *A Policy Framework for the Commissioning of Cancer Services: a Report to the Chief Medical Officers of England and Wales (Calman–Hine Report)*. London: The Stationery Office; 1995.

Department of Health. *Making a Difference: strengthening the nursing, midwifery and health visiting contribution to health and healthcare*. London: The Stationery Office; 1999.

Department of Health. *The Nursing Contribution to Cancer Care*. London: The Stationery Office; 2000a.

Department of Health. *The Cancer Plan: a plan for investment, a plan for reform*. London: The Stationery Office; 2000b.

European Association for Palliative Care. *A Guide for the Development of Palliative Nurse Education in Europe;* www.eapcnet.org (accessed 12 September 2005).

Johnson J, Mosier NR, Johnson C. Registered nurses: perceptions of patients, cancer nurses and themselves. *Oncol Nurs Forum.* 1982; **9:** 27–33.

Kelly J, Furlong E, Redmond K. The oncology nursing development project: background and implementation. *Eur J Oncol Nurs.* 1999; **3:** 90–95.

Kenny LJ. An evaluation-based model for palliative care education: making a difference to practice. *Int J Palliat Nurs.* 2003; **9:** 189–94.

Langton H, Blunden G, Hek G. *Cancer Nursing Education: literature review and documentary analysis.* London: English National Board; 1999.

Last Acts. *Means to a Better End. A report on dying in America today;* www/rwjf.org/special/betterend (accessed 17 June 2005).

McLeod RD, James C. *Teaching Palliative Care. Issues and implications.* Penzance: Patten Press; 1994.

Mallory JL. The impact of a palliative care educational component on attitudes toward care of the dying in undergraduate nursing students. *J Prof Nurs.* 2003; **19:** 305–12.

National Institute for Clinical Excellence. *The Supportive and Palliative Care Needs of Adults With Cancer.* London: National Institute for Clinical Excellence; 2004.

Nursing and Midwifery Council. *Standards of Proficiency for Pre-Registration Nursing Education.* London: Nursing and Midwifery Council; 2004.

Robinson R. End-of-life education in undergraduate nursing curricula. *Dimens Crit Care Nurs.* 2004; **237:** 89–92.

Royal College of Nursing. *A Structure for Cancer Nursing Services.* London: Royal College of Nursing; 1996a.

Royal College of Nursing. *Guidelines for Good Practice in Cancer Nursing Education.* London: Royal College of Nursing; 1996b.

Royal College of Nursing. *Quality Education for Quality Care: a position statement for nursing education.* London: Royal College of Nursing; 2002.

Royal College of Nursing. *A Framework for Adult Cancer Nursing.* London: Royal College of Nursing; 2003.

Sellick SM, Charles K, Dagsvik J *et al.* Palliative care providers' perspectives on service and education needs. *J Palliat Care.* 1996; **12:** 34–8.

Spencer JA, Jordan RK. Learner-centred approaches in medical education. *BMJ.* 1999; **318:** 1280–83.

United Kingdom Central Council for Nursing, Midwifery and Health Visiting (UKCC). *Fitness for Practice: the UKCC Commission for Nursing and Midwifery Education.* London: UKCC; 1999.

Webber J. *The effects of an educational course on problems identified by nurses caring for patients with advanced cancer.* Unpublished MSc dissertation, King's College London, 1989.

Whitehead D. Nurse education in the future: will one size fit all? *Nurse Educ Today.* 2005; **25:** 251–4.

Williams A, Montelpare W, Wilson A *et al.* An assessment of the utility of formalised palliative care education: a Niagra case study. *J Hospice Palliat Nurs.* 2002; **4:** 103–10.

Zabalegui A. Palliative nursing care in Spain. *Eur J Cancer Care.* 2002; **10:** 280–83.

Further reading

- European Association for Palliative Care. *A Guide for the Development of Palliative Nurse Education in Europe;* www.eapcnet.org (accessed 21 October 2005).
- Royal College of Nursing. *A Framework for Adult Cancer Nursing.* London: Royal College of Nursing; 2003.

Chapter 12

Is nurse education in paediatric and adolescent oncology fit for purpose?

Sue Fallon and Linda Sanderson

> *An education isn't how much you have committed to memory, or even how much you know. It's being able to differentiate between what you do know and what you don't.*
>
> *Anatole France 1844–1924*

Introduction

In this chapter the issue of paediatric and adolescent oncology nurse education is analysed. The diversity of paediatric and adolescent oncology nursing is highlighted, and the extent to which education enables these nurses to be fit for purpose now and in the future is discussed.

The scene is set with a brief overview of the epidemiology of children's cancer, the emergence of paediatric oncology as a specialty, and the formation of the United Kingdom Children's Cancer Study Group (UKCCSG) and the Paediatric Oncology Nurses Forum (PONF). The literature about current provision of paediatric oncology nursing education in the UK is summarised.

The key influences on current and future paediatric oncology service developments are highlighted by considering recommendations from central government reports. From these, suggestions about how paediatric oncology nursing might evolve in the future have been developed, and the issue of how nurse education can rise to the challenges of future developing practices are discussed.

In the UK, the annual incidence of childhood cancer is 1 in 650 children under the age of 15 years. This approximates to 1,500 new cases each year. Paediatric oncology started to emerge as a separate specialty within paediatric medicine in the UK over 30 years ago, and in 1977 the United Kingdom Children's Cancer Study Group (UKCCSG) was formed. This consisted of a group of paediatric oncologists who came together having recognised the need to develop clinical trials, provide guidance and advance supportive care with the aim of improving treatment outcomes. There are now 22 UKCCSG regional centres providing diagnosis, treatment and supportive care for children with cancer.

Over 75% of children with cancer receive treatment within national and international studies or controlled trials. The philosophy is one of child-centred care in a multi-disciplinary/multi-professional team. Some centres have operated a system of shared care, whereby cancer is often diagnosed at the regional centre, but aspects of ongoing treatment and care are delivered in the patient's local district hospital or community.

During the past 30 years, the outcome for children with cancer has continued to improve, and it is now estimated that 75% of these children will be living 5 years after diagnosis, and the majority of these will become long-term disease-free survivors (Stiller, 2002).

Development of paediatric oncology nursing

In parallel with medical developments, increasing numbers of nurses have been specialising in the field of paediatric oncology. In 1984, the Paediatric Oncology Nurse Forum (PONF) was formed, the first subgroup of the Royal College of Nursing (RCN).

Nursing care of children with cancer has developed along with the specialty of paediatric oncology. Nurses in this specialty are first and foremost children's nurses, but their skills have developed with experience and education to care for children, young people and their families with a specific set of illnesses. Gibson and Hooker (2004) utilise the International Council of Nurses (ICN) framework to demonstrate the extent to which paediatric oncology nurses are specialists within the field of children's nursing.

The ICN has described 10 essential features of the organised development of specialisation (International Council of Nurses, 1991).

1 The specialty defines itself as nursing and subscribes to the overall purpose, functions and ethical standards of nursing.
2 The specialty is sufficiently complex and advanced, and is beyond the scope of general nursing practice.
3 There is both a demand and a need for the specialty service.
4 The focus of the specialty is a defined population, which demonstrates recurrent problems and phenomena that lie within the discipline and practice of nursing.
5 The specialty practice is based on a core body of nursing knowledge, which is currently being expanded and refined through research.
6 The specialty has established educational and practice standards, which are congruent with those of the profession and are set by a recognised nursing body or bodies.
7 The specialty adheres to the registration requirements for the general nurse.
8 Specialty expertise is obtained through a professionally approved advanced education programme which leads to a recognised qualification. The education programme preparing the specialist is administered by a nurse.
9 The specialty has a credentiality process determined by the profession.
10 Practitioners are organised and represented within a specialty association or a branch of the National Nurses' Association.

Gibson and Hooker (2004) describe precisely how the scope of paediatric oncology nursing matches all of these features.

In 1992, a United Kingdom Central Council for Nursing, Midwifery and Health Visiting (UKCC) document, *The Scope of Professional Practice* (United Kingdom Central Council for Nursing, Midwifery and Health Visiting, 1992) offered enormous opportunities and challenges for nurses to undertake an increasing number of tasks to enhance and expand their role. Unfortunately, this document failed to address educational, training and assessment requirements. In addition to this, there was concern that in taking on new tasks, the holistic goals of nursing care for the child and family would be fragmented and eroded (Casey, 2001, cited by Gibson and Hooker, 2004).

As the specialty has matured, nurses have been keen to develop their roles and to consider new ways of working to improve the quality of care offered to children and their families. For example, some of the new roles that have been taken on include general tasks such as venepuncture and blood sampling, more specialised tasks such as chemotherapy and antibiotic administration, and expansion of roles into community outreach and clinical research.

There have also been outside influences on these developments. One of the major influences that have affected the way in which nurses develop their roles has undoubtedly come about as a result of the changes in doctors' roles and ways of working. This has challenged doctors and nurses to work together in new ways, where their roles are often similar and thus blend and complement each other, maintaining a high-quality service for children with cancer and their families.

Developing roles and the features of specialisation, as set out by the ICN, requires that nurses must be adequately and appropriately educated to ensure they are fit for purpose and able to provide a high-quality service.

The current state of paediatric oncology nurse education in the UK

For many years the English National Board (ENB) course entitled 'The Care of the Child with Cancer' (ENB 240), run by a number of different providers throughout the country, represented a stable national benchmark of content and outcomes for the education of nurses caring for children with cancer (Sanderson *et al.*, 2004). This course normally ran over a 6-month period, and the students were assessed both academically and in practice.

With the move of nurse education into universities and then the demise of the ENB in 2002, the potential for diversity in the education of nurses who care for children with cancer has increased. Long *et al.* (2003) have praised the work of the Paediatric Oncology Nurse Educators group (PONE, a subgroup of PONF) in maintaining a national perspective on the education of nurses caring for children with cancer. However, Hollis (2005) argues that nurse educators are in broad agreement about the theoretical component of paediatric oncology nursing courses, but that there is little agreement nationally about how clinical competencies should be included or assessed for nurses completing courses in specialist practice.

In 2003, a study undertaken by Long *et al.* (2003) was completed. This study, entitled 'An evaluation of educational preparation for cancer and palliative care nursing for children and adolescents' was commissioned by the ENB and then supported by the Nursing and Midwifery Council following the demise of the ENB. This three-part study is the only research of its kind which attempts to map and analyse the current (although now dated) educational provision for nurses who care for children with cancer, so the messages from the study merit discussion in this chapter.

In stage 1 of the study curriculum, documents of all eight providers of the ENB 240 courses were analysed and mapped against the 20-point expected course outcomes for courses in paediatric and adult oncology cancer nursing as agreed by the European Oncology Nurses Society (EONS) (1999). During this stage the issue of shared learning, the inclusion of adolescents' needs and the prescribed process of assessment of clinical practice were considered.

There was widespread compliance of English courses with the EONS standards, but two areas were found to have been neglected, namely 'Prevention and early detection of cancer' and 'Understanding specific principles of cancer clinical trials.' It was suggested by the research team that the first issue may have been neglected because it is of more relevance to adult nursing. It was surprising that the second issue was neglected, and the research team suggested that the wording in the curriculum documents may have differed from the EONS standard, as 'research' and 'evidence' were generally included in all of the courses.

All of the ENB 240 courses had to demonstrate the assessment of nurses in practice. In stage 1 of the study there was found to be a range of prescribed assessment practices, the degree of direct observation varied, and indirect measures (e.g. review of critical incidents, assessment of written reflections) predominated.

The research team also found that there appeared to be little specific recognition of adolescence as a discrete topic, and shared learning seemed to be introduced for logistical reasons only.

Conclusions from stage 1 of the study

- There is a diversity of courses due to allegiance to different universities (e.g. length, number of CAT points), although there is broad compliance with EONS standards.
- The unifying link for the courses, namely the ENB, has gone. The study recognised the importance of the PONF and PONE groups in maintaining a national approach/coherence to education. The research team recommended that other specialty areas should utilise such groups.

Stage 2 of the study looked at the actual assessment of practice in practice. Perceptions of the inclusion of adolescent needs on the ENB 240 courses were sought, as were perceptions of the value of shared learning. Interviews with clinical assessors, current and former students were conducted either face to face or over the telephone.

Conclusions from stage 2 of the study

- Rigorous assessment of practice could not be guaranteed.
- The role of the student in self-assessment was unclear, as was the way of validating this self-assessment.
- Students had varying levels of starting knowledge and experience. This, coupled with the lack of rigour, calls into question a level end point of student knowledge and skills. The transferability of clinical skills/knowledge is

also questionable. An obvious example of this lack of national outcome was the administration of chemotherapy.

- Students need the opportunity to work and to be assessed while caring for adolescents.
- There is an emphasis on inter-professional, inter-agency working, so effort needs to be put into reaping the benefits of shared learning, making it useful for students.
- Developing the roles of the practice educators in the field of paediatric oncology and the ongoing activity of the RCN PONF and PONE groups may be influential in resolving the problems identified by the study.

Stage 3 was designed to establish the attributes indicative of adequate (threshold or 'good enough') and higher-level (expert) practice of children's cancer nurses. This part of the study was conducted by videotaping episodes of care provided by nurses for children who were receiving cancer nursing or palliative care nursing. Nurses, child patients or service users and carers were interviewed. Edited versions of this material were then presented to members of a multi-professional, expert panel to stimulate the identification of outcomes or attributes to be addressed in future programmes of preparation.

Conclusions from stage 3 of the study

- There were no conflicting principles of threshold level of care between users and members of the expert panel, but users put more emphasis on the personal attributes of the nurse (e.g. humour, kindness).
- Expectations of threshold level of practice include partnership with children and families, clinical skills, multi-disciplinary teamworking and personal attributes.
- Users focused particularly strongly and explicitly on the personal attributes of the nurse. This has implications for recruitment.
- Nurse educationalists need to consider training in the presentation of self to enhance the service from a user perspective.
- Expert practice was much more difficult to address by the expert panel and service users. There was an expectation that the threshold attributes would be demonstrated at a higher level, but very few specific factors were identified to define expectations of expert practice. Expert practice was associated with clinical leadership and management roles.
- Videotaped episodes of care were used in stage 3. This was innovative work, ethical approval was obtained, and it was found to be much less anxiety provoking and intrusive than had initially been predicted. The benefits and potential applications should be explored further.

Although the study discussed above provides the most up-to-date evaluation of the educational provision for nurses caring for children with cancer, it is apparent that advances have been made since the time of the study. For example, there are now several modules available on adolescents with cancer. Efforts have been made to improve access to appropriate courses (e.g. a distance learning course is available at the University of Cardiff (Davies, 2004)).

The challenge is to provide education which is relevant theoretically and which supports the development of skills that are useful, transferable and consistent from course to course. This challenge is intensified in the face of current key influences.

Context and key influences on the current and future paediatric oncology service development

If post-registration paediatric nurse education is to continue to be fit for purpose, the wider health service context needs to be considered.

Key policy influences

These include the following:

- the Children Act (Department of Health, 2004) – five key outcomes for children
- the *National Service Framework for Children, Young People and Maternity Services (NSF)* (Department of Health, 2005)
- guidance from the National Institute for Clinical Excellence (NICE) (2005).

The Children Act (2004)

There are five key outcomes for children.

1   Be healthy.
2   Stay safe.
3   Enjoy and achieve.
4   Make a positive contribution.
5   Achieve economic well-being.

National Service Framework for Children, Young People and Maternity Services (NSF) (Department of Health, 2005)

This sets out a 10-year programme intended to stimulate long-term and sustained improvement in children's care. Its aim is to design and deliver services around the needs of children and their families rather than around those of organisations and professionals. The basic aim is to offer high-quality, integrated health and social care from pregnancy through to adulthood. There are 11 standards in total, all of which will shape the health and social care that is offered to children and young people. The impact on children and young people with cancer has not yet been fully realised, but it may have implications for the place of service delivery (i.e. more care may be offered closer to the child's home), the services for adolescents may be further developed as young people should have access to age-appropriate services, and there will be a continuing emphasis on training and education of staff to ensure that high-quality, evidence-based care is available in all settings.

Although the NSF addresses the needs of children in general, the needs of children with cancer were on the whole omitted from a major document which has shaped adult oncology services, namely *The NHS Cancer Plan* (Department of Health, 2000). This omission has been addressed in the recently published NICE guidance on healthcare services for children and young people with cancer (National Institute for Clinical Excellence, 2005).

National Institute for Clinical Excellence (NICE) (2005) guidance

In their recent document, *Healthcare Services for Children and Young People with Cancer*, NICE have issued a number of key recommendations (National Institute for Clinical Excellence, 2005), many of which mirror the Children's NSF Standards but also focus on the needs of young adults. The guidance is that cancer networks must ensure that children and young people with cancer have access to the safest and most effective treatment available, as close to their home as possible (e.g. district general hospitals, community-based services). All care for children and young people under 19 years of age must be provided in age-appropriate facilities. Young people aged 19 years or older should also have unhindered access to age-appropriate facilities and support when needed. All children and young people must have access to tumour-specific or treatment-specific clinical expertise as required.

All aspects of care should be provided by staff who have received appropriate training.

It must be noted that although NICE guidance can recommend 'best practice', there is no automatic central funding. Therefore it is the responsibility of local commissioners and providers to decide how they implement and fund these recommendations.

Other influences

Greater user involvement

Within the past five years there has been growing recognition of the importance of consulting and collaborating with users about developing policy and implementing services. The importance of patient and public involvement in health services has now been recognised in the Health and Social Care Act (Department of Health, 2001). This places a statutory obligation on NHS trusts, primary care trusts and strategic health authorities to consult and involve users in ongoing service planning, proposal development and general service delivery.

Children and young people have been consulted and their opinions utilised in major government initiatives such as the *National Service Framework for Children, Young People and Maternity Services* (Department of Health, 2005) and the NICE guidance on *Healthcare Services for Children and Young People with Cancer* (National Institute for Clinical Excellence, 2005).

Recently, the Nursing and Midwifery Council (2005) began a major consultation in which young people and their families will be asked about their expectations of nurses and their concerns about the standards of care that nurses deliver. It is hoped that the opinions and ideas generated by this exercise will be utilised to inform nursing curriculum change and development.

Long *et al.* (2003) focused a major part of their study on the opinions of service users about what makes a good children's cancer nurse.

These issues must surely be taken into consideration when developing education for nurses who care for children and young people with cancer. Educational providers should also seek the opinions of service users when planning, developing, delivering and evaluating their programmes (Gallini and Hooker, 2005).

The outside influences on the specialty of paediatric oncology nursing have been discussed, but there are other issues from within the specialty that are beginning to influence service delivery and which will therefore have an impact on the education of nurses in this field. From within the specialty there are developing sub-specialties, such as adolescent oncology and paediatric palliative care.

Adolescent oncology and paediatric palliative care

The growth of the sub-specialty of adolescent oncology has been marked by a proliferation of Teenage Cancer Units in the UK (now 8 units in total, with a further 11 units under discussion) and the appointment of medical and nursing staff specialising in this field. The document *A Guide to the Development of Children's Palliative Care Services* (Association for Children with Life-Threatening or Terminal Conditions and their Families/Royal College of Paediatrics and Child Health, 2003) has raised the profile of paediatric palliative care wherever it is delivered as an area of care that needs appropriate and specific funding and expertise. Children with cancer account for 25% of children utilising palliative care services, so these services and the education of nurses within them must be considered (Long *et al.*, 2003).

Clearly this is not a comprehensive list, but rather a selection of key issues that are currently affecting paediatric oncology service development.

The following main themes are emerging:

- tension between delivering technical services in centres of excellence and the need to deliver care as close to home as possible
- the importance of appropriate, safe and effective treatment and high-quality care that is being carried out as close to the patient's home as possible
- patients and their families have a vital role in the development and delivery of services, and should therefore be consulted and remain involved in all aspects of care and service planning and delivery, and education
- the importance of age-appropriate services, especially the specific needs and communication issues of teenagers and young adults
- finally, and of most relevance to this chapter, the need for staff to be appropriately trained and for their specific training needs to be met is repeatedly stated.

What direction might paediatric and adolescent oncology nursing take in the future?

The policies and developments discussed above raise expectations and pose challenges for nurses to deliver what is considered necessary to make the recommendations a reality for patients and their families.

There is no doubt that service will be delivered in a range of environments, and it is useful to look at each in order to consider what nurses caring for children and young people with cancer may be doing in the future.

The ongoing and vital role of the paediatric oncology ward-based nurse will continue. The clinical skills and communication expertise of these nurses are key at all stages of the patient's treatment, in particular at diagnosis, initial treatment and relapse, and will remain so in the future. The challenge will be to ensure that nurses working in the field are adequately trained/educated and supported to deliver excellent, evidence-based nursing care as treatment regimes become more intensive and complex. Technical skills need to be excellent and consistent. However, alongside this, nurses need to be confident in developing their communication, decision-making, leadership, teaching and problem-solving skills, so that they can continue to make a valuable contribution to the team approach to care.

The emphasis on reduced duration and decreased number of hospital admissions also highlights the nurse's role in outpatient and day care units. In most regional centres, nurses in these areas already administer intravenous chemotherapy, but with the development of nurse practitioner and nurse specialist roles, aspects of physical examination, prescribing and increased clinical decision making could move into the nurse's domain. In the field of paediatric oncology, long-term follow-up nurses have for some time taken over many of the tasks that were traditionally performed by medical colleagues in an effort to improve the patient's cancer journey (Bicheno, 2004).

Nurses working in district general hospitals where a shared care arrangement is already established with the regional centre may find that they have to review how they might improve the patients' care if they were to take on an expanded role, such as venepuncture or cytotoxic drug administration. Conversely, where shared care arrangements are not established, it may be the nurses' role to champion this cause with local hospital management.

They will possibly need to be trained in children's community care and the delivery of complex care in the community. These nurses could be either paediatric oncology outreach nurses (POONs) or children's community nurses who would choose to expand their role to include more complex aspects of care delivery, such as intravenous antibiotics, chemotherapy and possibly transfusions.

Finally, the emphasis on age-appropriate services means that in the future nurses will have the opportunity to choose to work in the field of adolescent or paediatric oncology. It has become increasingly clear that the needs of teenagers and young adults are very different from those of younger children.

As services shift and change shape, education providers will need to be responsive in terms of the method of delivery and the content of their programmes.

How will nurse education meet these patient-centred needs?

Education needs to be aimed at all the different levels of nurses involved in caring for children and young people with cancer.

Levels of learning
Basic level 1–2 (pre-registration)

At this level it would be appropriate for the nurse to receive an overview of subjects such as childhood cancer, treatment, outcomes, basic care and palliative care. It cannot be assumed with certainty that these subjects are covered in all UK pre-registration curricula. The RCN PONE group is currently considering undertaking a national pre-registration curriculum check to address this issue. In the mean time, students can access a new website (www.cancernursing.org) which offers units of learning aimed at a basic level (pre-registration nurses or the public) on such subjects as the biology of cancer, treatment and side-effects, and palliative care.

Level 3 (degree level)

This is practice led and focused – that is, the nurse selects programmes/modules that will enhance their role or confidence in a given aspect of paediatric oncology care (e.g. adolescent cancer and care of the child receiving treatment).

Masters programmes

There are Masters level courses specifically related to paediatric or adolescent cancer care. However, general courses in clinical oncology are available which may address relevant issues, e.g. Birmingham University.

An exciting development led by Helen Langton (former Chairperson of the Paediatric Oncology Nurse Educators' Group) has been validated at Coventry University. The Postgraduate Certificate in Teenage and Young Adult Cancer Care is a web-based course aimed at an international, multi-disciplinary audience. The course is due to commence in February 2007.

All of the above forms of educational provision need to be accessible to nurses working with children and teenagers with cancer, irrespective of their work environment.

Potential modes of delivery/learning

- These include programmes, short courses, stand-alone modules or study days, and in-house training.
- Nurses need to be released from their work commitments in order to study, and must receive adequate funding.
- Multi-disciplinary/multi-professional learning is to be encouraged.
- Other modes of learning include the following:
  - distance learning
  - self-directed learning
  - Web-based learning with access to national and international links
  - blended learning (a mixture of distance, Web-based and higher education institution learning)
  - summer schools.

The content of these courses/programmes needs to be appropriate to the intended audience, but must also meet the needs of the service. A major challenge is to ensure that nurses attending study programmes can clearly identify the impact that the course will have on their practice. Course outcomes must be clearly identified and systematically assessed to demonstrate the achievement of these outcomes.

Conclusion

In this chapter the issue of paediatric and adolescent oncology nurse education has been analysed. There is no doubt that nurses working with children and adolescents with cancer have many different roles and therefore different educational needs.

Current educational provision is diverse, and is available in a variety of settings and at a range of academic levels. The work of the PONE group has been praised as they attempt to maintain a national perspective on the education offered to paediatric and adolescent oncology nurses. However, diversification of roles is set to continue as more complex regimes are developed and the pressure to deliver care in a variety of different settings increases.

Educationalists in liaison with their service colleagues and users can no doubt develop courses that enable nurses to be fit for purpose. The challenge is to ensure consistency of outcomes and transferability of skills so that nurses are actually fit for purpose wherever they may choose to work in the UK.

Key points

- Paediatric and adolescent oncology nurse education must be responsive to the changing clinical arena.
- The educational provision must be appropriate to the intended audience, and must continue to be offered at all levels.
- A variety of modes of delivery is essential in order to ensure that paediatric and adolescent oncology nurse education is accessible to the maximum possible number of nurses.
- It is important that a national perspective is taken to ensure consistency of outcomes and transferability of skills, so that nurses are fit for purpose wherever they may choose to work.

Implications for the reader's own practice

1 To what extent is the education provision that you offer responsive to the clinical environment?
2 Consider the level of education that you provide. How could you develop this to meet the needs of nurses at a higher or lower educational level?
3 What strategies do you use, or could you use, to maximise the number of nurses who access your courses?
4 To what extent do you network locally and nationally with your clinical and educational colleagues?

References

Association for Children with Life-Threatening or Terminal Conditions and their Families (ACT) and Royal College of Paediatrics and Child Health (RCPCH). *A Guide to the Development of Children's Palliative Care Services.* 2nd ed. London: ACT and RCPCH; 2003.

Bicheno S. Childhood survivors. *Cancer Nurs Pract.* 2004; **3**: 12–14.

Casey A, Gibson F, Hooker L (2001) Role development in children's nursing: dimensions, terminology and practice framework. *Paediat Nurs.* 2001; **13**: 36–40.

Davies R. Progress through education. *Cancer Nurs Pract.* 2004; **3**: 1–2.

Department of Health. *The NHS Cancer Plan.* London: The Stationery Office; 2000.

Department of Health. *Health and Social Care Act. Section 11.* London: The Stationery Office; 2001.

Department of Health. *The Children Act.* London: The Stationery Office; 2004.

Department of Health. *National Service Framework for Children, Young People and Maternity Services.* London: Department of Health Publications; 2005.

European Oncology Nurses Society. *A Core Curriculum for a Post-Registration Course in Cancer Nursing.* 2nd ed. London: European Oncology Nurses Society; 1999.

Gallini A, Hooker L. Young people's and carers' views on the cancer services they receive. *Cancer Nurs Pract.* 2005 **4**: 27–32.

Gibson F, Hooker L. Defining a framework for advancing clinical practice. In: Gibson F, Soanes L, Sepion B, editors. *Perspectives in Paediatric Oncology Nursing.* London: Whurr; 2004. pp. 5–27.

Hollis R. The role of the specialist nurse in paediatric oncology in the UK. *Eur J Cancer.* 2005; **41**: 1758–64.

International Council of Nurses. *Guidelines on Specialisation in Nursing.* Geneva: International Council of Nurses; 1991.

Long T, Hale C, Sanderson L *et al. An Evaluation of Educational Preparation for Cancer and Palliative Care Nursing for Children and Adolescents.* Manchester: Salford Centre for Nursing, Midwifery and Collaborative Research, University of Salford; 2003.

National Institute for Clinical Excellence. *Healthcare Services for Children and Young People With Cancer.* London: National Institute for Clinical Excellence; 2005.

Nursing and Midwifery Council. NMC consults young people on standards in nursing. *Paediatr Nurs.* 2005; **17**: 4.

Sanderson L, Long T, Hale C. Evaluation of educational programmes for paediatric cancer nursing in England. *Eur J Oncol Nurs.* 2004; **8**: 138–47.

Stiller CA. Overview: epidemiology of cancer in adolescents. *Med Pediatr Oncol.* 2002; **39**: 149–55.

United Kingdom Central Council for Nursing, Midwifery and Health Visiting (UKCC). *The Scope of Professional Practice.* London: UKCC; 1992.

Useful websites

- Royal College of Nursing; www.rcn.org.uk
- National Institute for Clinical Excellence; www.nice.org
- Free online courses on cancer care: www.cancernursing.org

Educational strategies to improve palliative care for learning-disabled patients

Jackie Saunders

> *We need to improve how we communicate bad news to people with learning disabilities; it is not impossible – we need to learn new skills and be brave.*
> JC, Community Macmillan Nurse

Aim

To explore the challenges and opportunities facing teachers who design and deliver learning opportunities for those who support and care for people with learning disabilities who encounter death, dying and loss.

Learning outcomes

- Understand the special needs of people with learning disabilities who are facing death, dying or bereavement.
- Understand the similarities and differences between learning disability carers and specialist palliative care staff, and the impact that this has on designing appropriate learning material.
- Understand the unique approaches needed to provide palliative care education for all those caring for people with learning disabilities.
- Understand the variety of strategies that facilitate mutual exchange of learning in order to provide quality, focused education.

Introduction

Why should 'palliative care for people with learning disabilities facing death' warrant special tailor-made education?[a]

Palliative care principles are exactly the same for people with learning disabilities[b] as they are for the 'ordinary' population. The National Institute for Clinical Excellence guidance entitled *Improving Supportive and Palliative Care for Adults with Cancer* (Department of Health, 2004) laid down the standards expected for all patients, and a White Paper entitled *Valuing People: a new strategy for learning disability for the twenty-first century* (Department of Health, 2001) established the rights of people with learning disabilities to equity of access to healthcare at a level and of a quality expected by the general population. Dying and grieving are normal processes for all, yet anecdotal stories abound highlighting the disasters and problems encountered by people with learning disabilities and the ensuing substandard care that they received. Clinical expertise in palliative care for people with learning disabilities has developed in small pockets, among staff from a variety of disciplines and among family carers who have had to problem solve in isolation. Dedicated individuals have built up personal experience and become the local unpaid experts. Alongside their 'day job' of nurse, social worker, doctor, psychologist or parent, they have become known as the person to contact for help. Beyond these dedicated few, learning disability services have not had skills or experience, and specialist palliative care teams had little to offer. Indeed, Margaret Fray illustrates with painful clarity how she encountered obstruction and discrimination rather than supportive behaviours and attitudes when she was caring for Kathleen, her sister, who was dying of end-stage Down's syndrome-associated dementia (Fray, 2000). Her short book represents uncomfortable reading for those committed to palliative care. It highlights how palliative care services failed to help a frail older woman who had encountered prejudice from birth, but who was cherished by her family.

The taboos of death and learning disability are difficult when encountered individually, but problems are intensified when they coexist. Even when there is good teamwork between learning disability, generalist and specialist palliative care staff, it is apparent that in order to achieve a good outcome for the patient, the accepted models and practice of how care is delivered have to be amended to accommodate the special needs encountered. This chapter will consider these special needs and will give examples of means by which education can be used to inform staff in order to improve the quality of care for learning-disabled people with learning disabilities, and thereby the job satisfaction of their carers.

Why is palliative care for learning-disabled patients important?

Just as this chapter needs a prefix to explain why issues of demography, epidemiology, prejudice, exclusion, communication and social care provision are 'different and other' for people with learning disabilities, so any learning material needs to encompass these points and the impact that they have on palliative care.

Around 1.2 million people in the UK have a mild or moderate learning disability, and 210,000 have a severe or profound disability, which is about 2% of the UK population (Department of Health, 2001). One hundred years ago the life expectancy for someone with a learning disability was less than 15 years. Over the last century their longevity has risen faster than that of the general population, at 1.2% per year. Improved socio-economic conditions, greater understanding of learning disability and intensive neonatal/paediatric care will ensure that this trend is set to continue (Cooper *et al.*, 2004). Learning disability organisations now routinely care for people in their sixties, seventies, eighties and even nineties. This is important, as the life-limiting illnesses associated with ageing will become more common (Carter and Jancar, 1983). A longer life means greater likelihood of experiencing the death of aged parents or friends.

People with learning disabilities have different disease profiles to the wider population. The incidence of various cancers is different, with higher rates of oesophageal, stomach and gall-bladder cancer (NHS Health Scotland, 2004). People with Down's syndrome have an increased incidence of early-onset dementia, heart disease and leukaemia. An individual may present with multiple health problems associated with their learning disability (e.g. epilepsy, respiratory disease, deafness and visual impairment). It has been estimated that 8 out of 10 people with learning disabilities have difficulties with understanding or being understood. Particular attention to methods of communication will be needed if the person has limited understanding or vocabulary, is non-verbal, or uses Makaton[c] or a unique language only understood by people close to them. The time needed to support a person with a learning disability is likely to be greater than that required for a member of the wider population. As Cathcart (1995) notes, they 'may need assistance to interpret what is happening to them.' Over their lifetime, well-meaning family or carers may have unconsciously hidden 'dying' and 'death' from the learning-disabled person in order to protect them. Major work may be needed to help the person to understand these concepts for the first time. Death is a taboo subject, and learning disability staff are unlikely to have had opportunities in the work setting to explore their own feelings and fears, let alone those of their clients. The learning material for staff and carers in the learning disability setting must take account of this.

These issues are significant when one reflects on how to convey the early symptoms of oesophageal, stomach and gall-bladder cancers (which, as mentioned earlier, have been identified as having a higher incidence than in the general population). How would indigestion, difficulty in swallowing, and pain associated with eating be expressed by people with a limited vocabulary? If pain or physical distress is expressed through changes in behaviour (e.g. withdrawal, irritability or aggression), rather than by conversation (e.g. 'I have a pain in my tummy' or 'I'm constipated'), healthcare professionals may interpret the changes as a consequence of the learning disability and not as the symptoms of a new disease. This is called 'diagnostic overshadowing', and it results in symptoms remaining undiagnosed until the disease is well advanced (Cooke, 1997). It is vital that people with learning disabilities have their symptoms identified and their emotions catered for to the same standard expected by other people. Education must enable staff and general practitioners to be vigilant with regard to new, unusual behaviour such as repetitive movements or laughter-like noises, and to enquire further in order to ascertain the reason for the change.

Although it is recognised that respiratory and cardiovascular diseases are the primary causes of death in people with learning disabilities, the principles of cancer care are eminently transferable. Similarly, much of what is specific to people with learning disabilities is of great relevance to other groups, such as people dying of dementia or neurological disease, and those with concurrent mental illnesses.

Application to cancer and palliative care education, and multi-professional implications

A learning-disabled person who is facing death will, hopefully, be cared for by the primary healthcare team, the hospital staff generalists, the specialist team (e.g. oncology, respiratory or cardiac) or the specialist palliative care staff, as well as the different disciplines involved within learning disability services (e.g. psychiatry, psychology, allied health professionals), their teachers (if they are still at school or in further education), and not least their family and friends. The development of teaching material must take account of the fact that learners are most likely to represent all or any of the service providers (private, charitable, statutory and 'for profit'), disciplines and carers involved. Learning must be designed to accommodate people from a variety of work settings and professional backgrounds. There are both differences and similarities in the learning needs of specialist palliative care staff and learning disability staff. The art is to help the two groups to share their skills with each other. Learning together and developing services together have firm foundations when one realises the similarities between the two specialiies. Both have developed a client-centred approach and strive to involve the family (Department of Health, 2002), both work with people and families who experience rejection and isolation, and both maximise achievement despite disability. The curriculum must be influenced by people with learning disabilities and their lay carers.

Katherine Froggatt discovered that specialist palliative care professionals should not aim to 'teach' palliative care topics to care home staff unless the material is adapted to take into account the different cultural and organisational ethos of nursing homes (Froggatt, 2001). This discovery should be borne in mind for the learning disability setting, too. There are some major but 'hidden' differences in the practice and provision of 'care' between learning disability and palliative care.

The learning disability focus is on living and maximising independence. Although as words this transposes directly to specialist palliative care, the essence of what is meant is different. The carers may be family members or from social care organisations rather than a healthcare background, and they may need a vast amount of support, guidance and information to enable them to continue to care. Learning disability staff will not see their work in the context of dying and, just like the lay public, they may be terrified of the implications of working in the context of 'facing death.'

There are different ratios of healthcare support workers to trained staff in each setting. Hospices are fortunate in that they often employ highly qualified, mature staff, they have a relatively low staff turnover and there is a high staff-to-patient ratio. In contrast, learning disability services rely on unqualified (but not necessarily inexperienced) younger staff with a high staff turnover and a low staff-to-client ratio. As few or no staff will have a clinical/medical background, it cannot be assumed that learning disability staff have cared for sick people before. They may feel very unskilled and anxious, but as they may have known the client for many years they may be determined to facilitate them staying in their home. Carers may be unable to recognise when dying begins, and can become terrified when death is imminent, with the resulting fear, 'Please don't let it happen on my shift!' (Brown *et al.*, 2003).

Each specialty uses terminology differently. Learning disability services have successfully moved from an oppressive medical model of care to a social model. This transition was underpinned by individuals no longer being called 'patients' but 'clients' or 'service users.' The dilemma for learning disability staff occurs when the client warrants the title 'patient' again, due to their life-threatening illness.

The staff's relationship with patients and their families can be significantly different in each specialty. Specialist palliative care staff probably know their patients and families for days or months at the most, whereas learning disability staff know their clients for years. The relationship is very different. A group home will function as a family unit with relationships which, although professional, undoubtedly incorporate modified love and respect (Cambell, 1984). Facing dying and death will raise all the natural emotions associated with loss and grief in both the staff and other residents. In their article entitled 'Death of a friend', Birchenall and Jenkinson (1993) described how the death of a person with a profound learning disability who was well known to staff 'made the staff look at themselves as individuals, as human beings.' They 'discovered the true and often painful meaning of holistic care.' Compassionate leave is available for staff who suffer the death of a close family member. However, the death of a member of a community 'family' will be viewed differently even though, for some, the sadness may be equally profound. It is vital to incorporate the basics of affective domain learning into the teaching programme. It is also crucial to agree ground rules and establish an emotionally safe environment. The discussion of loss and bereavement issues may rekindle unresolved losses experienced by participants in their workplace.

Different policies and constraints apply to these two unique settings. Specialist palliative care staff recognise the therapeutic benefit of touch, a reassuring hug or a hand on the shoulder, provided that the patient has consented to this. Implicit in learning disability care is the prevention of sexual abuse (which continues to be a real problem). Touch could be misconstrued to the extent that some organisations have policies which forbid staff from expressing such behaviour. The teaching must incorporate how compassionate caring can be expressed in the absence of touch to a client group for whom words may not be adequate to express feelings and fears. Staff must also be encouraged to challenge the established policies to ensure that they allow and promote appropriate responses.

Therefore specialist palliative care staff need to learn about the nuances associated with supporting people with learning disabilities before they teach learning disability staff about palliative care. It is not about 'telling' learning disability staff but rather about finding ways to share skills that are transferable to the other clinical setting.

Issues for practice

Communication

Telling a person with a learning disability that they are dying or that someone has died is a process, not an event, and it may take days, weeks or many months for the information to be understood (Blackman and Todd, 2005). The recommended practice of 'firing a warning shot' and 'pausing' to allow the person to ask questions is of little use to people who communicate using concrete language (as opposed to abstract language), and who have difficulty pre-empting what others are thinking. Similarly, the recommended practice of not imparting bad news unless the patient asks a leading question may be thwarted by the fact that some people with learning disabilities will be unable, or lack the confidence, to proffer questions to initiate the discussion. Likewise, the use of euphemisms such as 'he has passed away' and 'rest in peace' will lack clarity and may confuse them.

> **Breaking bad news using the gold standard cancer model (Baile *et al.*, 2000)**
>
> Carer: *'I've got some bad news for you.'* (the 'warning shot')
> Client: *'Don't tell me there won't be fish 'n' chips tonight.'*

With regard to consent, the good practice of establishing capacity, not incapacity, will be enshrined in the Mental Capacity Act as of April 2007. Documentation will have to reflect clearly how every effort has been made to help the person to understand issues that influence their choices.

Symptom control

Our ability to understand people with learning disabilities and interpret their non-verbal communication underpins sound assessment and symptom management. Regnard *et al.* (2003) describe thoroughly the many variables to be considered when assessing a person with a learning disability. There is little to distinguish the 'language of distress' from that of expression of pain. Therefore, if pain assessment tools are used, 'it is not possible to guarantee that physical pain is being measured rather than other causes of distress' (Regnard *et al.*, 2003). This is important, as analgesics are inappropriate for the treatment of emotional distress. Furthermore, Foley and McCutcheon (2004) quote Hennequin *et al.* (2000) as stating that 'there is evidence to suggest [*the people with mild to moderate learning disability*] are less accurate in localising the pain, slower to acknowledge it, and do not demonstrate recognisable pain behaviours.' This means that the range of pain assessment tools available for the general population will be of little use for people with learning disabilities. The key to assessment is meticulous observation by people who are familiar with the patient – people who can critically analyse how behaviours, noises, facial expression, posture, pallor and other indicators have changed. These observations need to be documented in a way that is unambiguous to others. The Disability Distress Assessment Tool (DisDAT), which was developed by the Northgate Palliative Care Team, enables distress to be documented but does not attempt to be a scoring tool.

The following case study can be used when teaching to illustrate the complexities of cancer and palliative care for people with learning disabilities.

Nancy's story

I was asked by a learning disability community home to provide a short focused session on breast cancer to the staff. The care team consisted of carers, some of whom had NVQs in care, and Learning Disability Nurse Team Leaders. They wanted to be fully aware of what to observe in Nancy, an older non-verbal severely disabled woman who had been diagnosed with breast cancer a year ago. Her disease appeared to be controlled on a once-a-day hormonal medication. Nancy became distraught if her daily routine was altered in any way and, through her behaviour, had made it quite clear that she did not want to go to hospital, and did not want blood tests or biopsies, let alone operations. She would have required total sedation for any investigations.

Questions arising from this scenario are listed below.

- Nancy had arthritis of her major joints and her spine. How would the learning disability staff know if bone metastases existed?
- She could only walk short distances before getting breathless. How would they know if lung metastases existed?
- She had epilepsy and fitted periodically. She had poor balance and needed two canes to help her to walk. How would they know if brain metastases existed?
- She vomited from time to time. How would they know if liver metastases existed?
- From an ethical/moral and legal viewpoint, should Nancy have full investigations like any other woman with early breast cancer?

Case study implications

This story highlights how the task of observation was very complex. However, it was inappropriate for the learning disability staff, who were not trained in cancer or specialist palliative care, to be diagnosing disease progression. By affirming their knowledge of DisDAT and their meticulous documentation of appearance and behaviours during times of contentment and distress, they were able to realise their positive contribution to the overall care. They could inform the medical team of their observations, albeit not the 'traditional' observations of bodily functions (e.g. blood pressure and pain scores). As DisDAT notes: 'If changes are recognised early, the suitable interventions can be put in place to avoid crisis.' The specialist oncology/palliative care staff would need to understand DisDAT, trust their learning disability colleagues' observations, and work together to interpret their meaning.

Bereavement

The majority of people with learning disabilities live in the community. For many of them a parent is the main carer. People with learning disabilities may be faced with the death of parents and of people they know in their community. Palliative care staff will more often experience people with learning disabilities as relatives and 'significant others' of terminally ill patients than as patients themselves. In her book, *Loss and Learning Disability*, Noëlle Blackman describes how 'loss' extends beyond bereavement, with many clients having unresolved losses – for instance, loss of physical ability with ageing, loss of intellectual ability as a result of dementia, as well as the multitude of losses resulting from inferior life opportunities (Blackman, 2003). The research of McEvoy *et al.* (2002) suggested that 'although people with a learning disability may possess an incomplete concept of death, they can attribute appropriate emotions to the context of bereavement.' It is important that the teaching helps staff to recognise that 'normal' grief includes pining, talking to the dead, searching, withdrawal, anger, and repetitive speech and repeated conversations. Traditionally, people often keep mementos of the dead (e.g. photos, items of clothing, pieces of furniture or pottery) to help them to mark the loss. However, for security reasons, residential homes need to lock away the property of the deceased, so 'evidence' of the deceased is taken away from the bereaved with whom they shared a home. Such mementos are crucially important to this user group. By appreciating the norm, staff will be less likely to misinterpret grieving as challenging behaviour, and will ensure that their place of work allows time and privacy for grief. The consequence of denying these opportunities was observed by Emerson (1977), who found that among people with learning disabilities who had been referred to her for help with apparently 'spontaneous' emotional or behavioural difficulties, 'about 50% of the time there has been either the death or the loss of an individual close to the client preceding the onset of symptoms.' Although adults with learning disabilities should not be treated like children, if they have never been taught about death, the approaches that are used to help children can be useful. The life-cycle approach of stories about leaves on trees dying in autumn and the transformation of a caterpillar into a butterfly can be used to explain death within a natural context (Hedger *et al.*, 1993).

It is important to note that all people may become dependent and needy after a death, and people with learning disabilities are no different in this respect. We have witnessed clients being the primary carers of older parents – organising the cleaning, cooking, shopping and caring. However, such complex skills were ignored by the staff who became involved after the death of the parent. This resulted in the bereaved individual being excluded from important rituals such as funeral arrangements, choosing memorials and keeping mementos, which in turn complicated the grieving process. Worden's Four Tasks of Mourning model can be used to encourage learners to explore the aspects of loss and grief for the general population (Worden, 1991). The skill lies in the teacher facilitating an appreciation of the special circumstances faced by people with learning disabilities, such as being creative in allowing expression of grief for non-verbal clients.

Evidence of good educational practice

Palliative care for people with learning disabilities is not on the national agenda yet in the UK. Pioneering work by the National Network for the Palliative Care of People with Learning Disabilities (NNPCPLD) is ensuring the provision of conferences and regional study days. Education around the country ranges from the degree module at Keele University to stand-alone study days on bereavement and palliative care for people with learning disabilities at St Nicholas Hospice and Kirkwood Hospice. For people who cannot attend study events, Amelia Jones has created comprehensive continuing professional development material for personal study (Jones, 2003). *Positive Approaches to Palliative Care* is a workbook that covers all of the learning outcomes for the Learning Disability Awards Framework (a certificated course for unqualified carers in the learning disability field) (Jones and Tuffrey-Wijne, 2004). In Dublin, St Michael's House, a community-wide organisation that supports people with learning disabilities, instigated an in-house intensive 3-day training programme to help heads of departments to develop their understanding of bereavement so as to be able to cascade the information throughout the service. By injecting laughter into their learning they make the focus on death bearable. For example, a member of staff dressed up as the grim reaper to distribute the certificate of attendance at the end of the course!

St Nicholas Hospice invited people with learning disabilities to tell their stories of death and grief to learning disability and palliative care staff who were planning to design a short course on breaking bad news to people with learning disabilities. Although this approach is ideal for capturing the views of the clients and for producing material informed by clients, it may not be possible in all organisations. Another option is to use the video *A Billion Seconds*, in which people with learning disabilities tell the story of 'cancer' and 'loss.'

Contentious/controversial issues salient to the topic

Unfortunately, although research and best practice evidence is highlighting the specific and often overlooked needs of this client group, the resources for the education necessary to change practice are not readily forthcoming. The transformation of pioneering work through to the general setting is compromised by significant funding constraints. Assuming that staff develop their understanding, one wonders whether procedures will change to support modifications in practice.

In the future, hospices may face the challenge of admitting people with learning disabilities who are noisy, display challenging behaviour, or have dual diagnoses or other mental health problems. Similarly, hospice staff may be invited to become increasingly involved directly with people with Down's syndrome-associated early-onset dementia, or indirectly via education of the staff and carers of people with learning disabilities. These challenges exist, and it remains to be seen whether hospices and specialist palliative care services will rise to meet them.

Summary of potential future developments

The field of learning disability has much to teach palliative care – not least the robust means by which service users are genuinely engaged in service planning and review. People with learning disabilities must be involved in the design and delivery of educational material. They know what is needed, as is borne out by Richard West's recommendations in his paper entitled *When My Dad Died: a relative's perspective* (www.intellectualdisability.info/mental_phys_health/DadDied_west.html).

Key points

- People with intellectual disabilities should be given the same information about death and dying that all other people are given.
- This information needs to be accessible, using pictures, photographs, easy words and/or video.
- The information should be given to everyone who works with people with intellectual disabilities (e.g. healthcare professionals, social services, voluntary workers, family, etc.).
- It is best to plan and work with people with intellectual disabilities who have cancer, and to explain to them how services can make their needs better.
- These skills can be transferred to other people who are cognitively impaired (e.g. patients with brain tumours or dementia).

Conclusion

Partnership working between learning-disabled people, learning disability services and palliative care services (including specialist palliative care) is essential to the design and delivery of the necessary education. A greater long-term impact would result from bringing together service managers, commissioners and planners of services in order to ensure that working structures are in place. This would support the new insights gained by the learners. Improved end-of-life care will need education, avenues of creative funding and committed policy makers.

One size does not fit all – each person with a learning disability will have their own unique story and experience. The education must address commonalities while at the same time promoting an individual approach. It is vital that the teaching takes into account the fact that the learning disability staff may be 'family', so will be distressed by the diagnosis and any deterioration. Indeed, they will undoubtedly grieve themselves, and sources of support need to be highlighted.

Implications for the reader's own practice

1 What links does your hospice/specialist palliative care service have to local learning disability services?
2 How does your palliative care education provider(s) inform the local learning disability staff of forthcoming courses?
3 How can you ensure that hospice/specialist palliative care staff are aware of, and responding to, learning disability models of care such as Circles of Support and Person-Centred Planning?
4 Do you know who your end-of-life facilitators are? How can you encourage further links with learning disability organisations using end-of-life principles and practice?
5 How can adult and children's hospices share good practice, thereby ensuring improved care for young people with learning disabilities who have a life-limiting illness?
6 Has your hospice/palliative care service joined the National Network for the Palliative Care of People with Learning Disabilities?

References

Baile WF *et al.* A six-step protocol for delivering bad news. *Oncologist.* 2000; **5**: 302–11.

Birchenall P, Jenkinson R. Death of a friend. *Nurs Times.* 1993; **89**: 65–6.

Blackman N. *Loss and Learning Disability.* London: Worth Publishing; 2003.

Blackman N, Todd S. *Caring for People with Learning Disabilities who are Dying.* London: Worth Publishing; 2005.

Brown H, Burns S, Flynn M. 'Please don't let it happen on my shift!' Supporting staff who are caring for people with learning disabilities who are dying. *Learn Disabil Rev.* 2003; **8**: 32–41.

Cambell A. *Moderated Love: a theology of professional care.* London: SPCK; 1984.

Carter G, Jancar J. Mortality in the mentally handicapped: a 50-year survey at the Stoke Park Group of Hospitals (1930–1980). *J Ment Defic Res.* 1983; **27**: 143–56.

Cathcart F. Death and people with learning disabilities: intervention to support clients and carers. *Br J Clin Psychol.* 1995; **34**: 165–75.

Cooke LB. Cancer and learning disability. *J Intellect Disabil Res.* 1997; **41**: 312–16.

Cooper S, Melville C, Morrison J. People with intellectual disabilities. Their health needs differ and need to be recognised and met. *BMJ.* 2004; **329**: 414–24.

Department of Health. *Valuing People: a new strategy for learning disability for the twenty-first century.* White Paper. London: The Stationery Office; 2001.

Department of Health. *Planning with People. Towards person-centred approaches: guidance for implementation groups.* London: Department of Health; 2002.

Department of Health. *Improving Supportive and Palliative Care for Adults with Cancer.* London: Department of Health; 2004.

Emerson P. Covert grief reaction in mentally retarded clients. *Ment Retard.* 1977; **15**: 46–7.

Foley DC, McCutcheon H. Detecting pain in people with an intellectual disability. *Accid Emerg Nurs.* 2004; **12**: 196–200.

Fray M. *Caring for Kathleen: a sister's story.* Kidderminster: British Institute of Learning Disabilities; 2000.

Froggatt KA. Palliative care and nursing homes: where next? *Palliat Med.* 2001; **15**: 42–8.

Hedger CJ, Dyer Smith MJ. Death education for older adults with developmental disabilities: a life cycle therapeutic recreation approach. *Activities Adapt Aging.* 1993; **18**: 29–35.

Hennequin M, Morin C, Feine JS. Pain expression and stimulus localisation in individuals with Down's syndrome. *Lancet.* 2000; **356**: 1882–7.

Jones A. Palliative care and people with learning disabilities. *Learn Disabil Pract.* 2003; **6**: 30–37.

Jones A, Tuffrey-Wijne I. *Positive Approaches to Palliative Care.* Kidderminster: British Institute of Learning Disabilities; 2004.

McEvoy J, Reid Y, Guerin S. Emotion recognition and concept of death in people with learning disabilities. *Br J Dev Disabil.* 2002; **48**: 83–9.

NHS Health Scotland. *Health Needs Assessment Report. People with learning disabilities in Scotland.* Glasgow: NHS Health Scotland; 2004.

Regnard C, Mathews D, Gibson L *et al.* Difficulties in identifying distress and its causes in people with severe communication problems. *Int J Palliat Nurs.* 2003; **9**: 173–6.

Worden JW. *Grief Counselling and Grief Therapy: a handbook for the mental health practitioner,* 2nd ed. New York: Springer; 1991.

Further reading and useful contacts

- Blackman N, Todd S. *Caring for People with Learning Disabilities who are Dying.* London: Worth Publishing; 2005. This is a small and uncomplicated book for learning disability staff who are new to the concept of caring for seriously ill people.
- McEnhill L. Disability. In: Oliviere D, Munroe B, editors. *Death, Dying and Social Differences.* Oxford: Oxford University Press; 2004. This chapter gives a very comprehensive academic analysis of learning disability in the context of society, prejudice and the ramifications for health and care.
- The National Network for the Palliative Care of People with Learning Disabilities. This is a national resource for staff, families and people with learning disabilities. Details of regional groups can be obtained by contacting LindaMcEnhill@natnetpald.org.uk, or via the Help the Hospices website at www.helpthehospices.org.uk/NPA/learningdisabilities/index.asp

Useful video

- *A Billion Seconds*. This video shows a 40-minute theatre performance by the Strathcona Theatre Company. It tells the story of Sam, a man with Down's syndrome whose father died of cancer, and Sash, a woman with learning disabilities who finds a breast lump. The video is suitable for people with learning disabilities, carers and professionals. Telephone 01562 723010 for a free copy.

Endnotes

[a] To avoid the lengthy repetition of 'people with learning disabilities who are newly diagnosed with cancer, have advanced cancer, are experiencing the worry of a friend or family member who has cancer, or who are bereaved', I shall use the phrase 'who are facing death.' I appreciate that cancer does not equal death, but know that, in our society, cancer is still strongly associated with fear of death.

[b] The term 'learning disability' describes a range of disabilities from mild to profound, which the Mental Health Act 1993 defines as 'a state of arrested or incomplete development of mind which includes significant impairment of intelligence and social functioning.' It must be acknowledged that able and competent people with learning disability will be living independently in the community without support from professional staff.

[c] Makaton is a unique language programme that offers a structured, multi-modal approach, using signs and symbols, for the teaching of communication, language and literacy skills to people with communication and learning difficulties.

Chapter 14

Palliative care in nursing homes: an educational challenge

Patricia Hirst and Anne Boyce

> *A core value for palliative care from its inception has been in enabling people to make genuine choices about their care ... improved co-ordination of palliative care provision through education can allow more service users to die in their care home, which is their home, if they so desire.*
>
> *Davies and Higginson (2004)*

Aim

The aim of this chapter is to explore the change of care setting for delivering palliative care for the elderly patient, and to identify what underlying influences have effected this change. The resulting impact on the provision of care delivered in the care home setting will be discussed. The educational strategies required to ensure safe and competent palliative care delivery by home care staff will also be outlined.

Learning outcomes

- Be aware of the factors that can limit the provision of palliative care in the nursing home sector.
- Identify the constraints that prevent care home staff from accessing education in relation to palliative care.
- Gain insight into the complexity of palliative care for frail service users with multiple pathology and polypharmacy in their treatment.

Introduction

Many nations of the world are facing a significant challenge in responding to the question of end-of-life care for the older person. The founders of modern palliative care and elderly medicine had much to say about this issue as long ago as the early 1950s. In 1990, the NHS and Community Care Act (Department of Health, 1991) resulted in a shift from institutional to community-based care. Together with the closure of long-term hospital wards, this resulted in a changed profile of older people in care homes to one of older, more frail and ill service users. Hospices are also changing the focus to more acute interventions, with the consequence that some hospices are discharging people with short life expectancy into care homes. Along with hospices, therefore, care homes have been led to assume a greater responsibility for dying people, with the additional demands for supportive and medical care that this entails. Introduction of NHS 'targets', demands and competition for funding are greater than ever before, and this has further encouraged hospitals to transfer out patients with chronic, progressive or terminal illness and to recommend their placement in care homes.

Between 2% and 5% of people aged 65 years or older now live in care homes, with one in five people dying in the care home sector (National Council for Palliative Care, 2005). It is vital that palliative care is available to the service users in these settings, and it should be a central feature of the care home provision, whatever the diagnosis. There is a growing acknowledgment that the delivery of specialist palliative care services should not be limited to the care of patients with a cancer diagnosis. The palliative care approach can be usefully applied to any patient for whom active treatment is no longer a viable option (Addington-Hall and Higginson, 2001).

In the UK it is now acknowledged that older people should receive care that is based on their individual needs, priorities and circumstances, rather than on their age (Department of Health, 2001). Service users in care homes are often older people who are frail or have chronic physical or mental disabilities, and common diagnoses include stroke, cardiac failure, chronic pulmonary disease, Parkinson's disease and dementia. In the final stages of their lives, service users in care homes are often suffering from one or more of these chronic degenerative diseases, and have a more unpredictable trajectory of dying than cancer patients, who are traditionally cared for by the palliative care services (Addington-Hall and Higginson, 2001; Hockley and Clark, 2002).

Consequently, comorbidity becomes problematic, and issues may arise in the management of medications due to the necessity for polypharmacy, with many treatment complexities arising from drug reactions and/or interactions. Such patients can therefore often present more of a challenge to achieving effective symptom control than the 'well' cancer patient (Katz, 2003).

The authors would suggest that the range of diseases and complexity of management in care homes are significantly underestimated, thereby increasing the priority and importance of specialist palliative care support in this setting. Froggatt (2004) outlines specialist areas of care provided in the care home sector, including dementia, mental disorder, learning disabilities, physical disabilities, drug and/or alcohol dependency, terminal illness, old age and sensory impairment. It follows therefore that the qualifications and educational needs of staff will depend on existing areas of expertise within the home. Although the care home population is primarily frail and elderly, there are a number of people under 65 years of age with similar pre-existing complex needs prior to the onset of the dying process, due to a variety of causes. However, many people regard a move into a care home as the 'last resting place' before death, and clearly many of the service users living in these care homes will have palliative care needs (Hockley and Clark, 2002). The status of such patients could be considered as the 'disadvantaged dying', highlighting this as an issue that needs to be urgently addressed. One approach would be to ensure that education and training are accessible for all care home staff (Katz, 2003).

Recent studies have confirmed that palliative care education results in increased knowledge, skills, confidence and competence (Froggatt, 2000a; Loftus and Thompson, 2002). Continued provision of planned palliative care education programmes in response to needs assessment may go a long way towards improving nurses' confidence in their ability to attend to the general palliative care needs of their patients. Increasing numbers of service users who would previously have been cared for within a hospice or hospital setting are being moved to care home care. It can be assumed that enhanced education relating to oncology and palliative care needs to be in place in order to facilitate effective transfer between care settings. As the incidence of cancer in an ageing population increases, especially for those over 85 years (Williams, 2000), there is an increased potential for elderly patients already diagnosed with cancer to require care home beds. Those service users already in place in the care home environment have the potential to develop a new cancer diagnosis. Therefore recognition of early symptoms and the ability to support patients through active or palliative oncological treatments requires continuing education. The effective provison of oncology and palliative care services can be enhanced by a shared educational process with care home staff (Jordhoy *et al.*, 2003), especially where there are other specialist needs, such as learning disabilities or mental health problems.

The care goals in care homes, in contrast to those in acute care settings, are more consistent with the holistic model of palliative care. Care homes emphasise the restoration and maintenance of functional status as the primary objective (Hockley and Clark, 2002). Issues of quality of life, comfort and dignity can outweigh issues of definitive treatment or prognosis. Emphasis should also be placed on advance directives and maximum autonomy for patients who are dying (Kane *et al.*, 1989). Most patients who are dying in care homes do not have cancer and may have a significant degree of cognitive impairment. Care home staff will have multiple opportunities to participate in some of the most complex ethical issues in palliative care. Staff may be required to contribute to discussions about end-of-life care and its appropriateness in a wide variety of conditions. Likewise, the dilemma of when individuals can be reasonably expected to be capable of making decisions in order to maximise their quality of life, as well as its duration, can be an issue for staff. For this reason alone, the care home setting can be a valuable learning environment for all healthcare providers when looking at the wider issue of long-term care.

The cost of education of registered nurses in the care home sector is problematic, not being covered by purchaser contracts (Royal College of Physicians, 2000). Education and training have to be paid for by the care homes or the individual practitioner. Even when funding is available from charity organisations, there is often a stipulation that the charity will pay for half of the cost and that the care home will pay the other half. Links between care homes and the providers of higher education would benefit both organisations, as has been demonstrated by work in the USA, where care homes have developed these links and this has led to the setting up of specific educational programmes for care homes (Kaesar, 1998; Metzy *et al.*, 1997). The creation of a care home that is focused upon education and is affiliated to providers of higher education could be innovative in the UK, and has the potential to have a dynamic impact on the care home sector. With the increasing size of the older population, these facilities could help to prepare pre- and post-registration nursing students for the challenges of caring for the older person.

Following research undertaken by Froggatt (2000b), recommendations were made to instigate new palliative care roles, working specifically with nursing homes. Macmillan Cancer Relief has funded a number of pilot projects in which clinical nurse specialists in palliative care have been funded to undertake local educational and clinical needs assessments. These projects are designed to enhance palliative care and specialist palliative care provision within the nursing home sector. Some post holders have concentrated on educational initiatives, while others have adopted a dual clinical and educational role. Enhanced uptake of educational opportunities and increased referral rates to specialist palliative care services have demonstrated that such posts, targeted and developed to specifically address the palliative care needs of the service users in the care home sector, are successful in improving communication. These projects also demonstrate that levels of clinical and theoretical awareness in relation to patients' palliative care needs have been improved.

An outcome of greater engagement with care home staff and residents has resulted in an enhanced understanding of staff and patient needs. Many areas have developed palliative care link nurse programmes to facilitate regular updates. By attending regular meetings with the duel agenda of educational and service development, these practitioners can become educational and clinical palliative care resources for other staff within the care home (Froggatt, 2004).

Other educational initiatives include the instigation of posts to promote and support the use of such measures as the Integrated Care Pathway for the dying (Ellershaw and Wilkinson, 2003), or the Gold Standards Framework (in palliative care) (Thomas *et al.*, 2005) within the care home sector. Many of these projects have achieved the dual objectives of identifying challenges in delivering these stategies. The next phase of these projects includes identifying their use in raising awareness of palliative care needs and enhancing provision of care.

Palliative care resource files have been provided in many areas by palliative care specialists, and have been well evaluated in their localities, as is the case in both areas where the authors practise. These files often include symptom control management advice, local contact details, information relating to educational events and even charitable funding available. A website containing this information is also being piloted in one area, and so far evaluation of this site (www.nursinghomes. cht.nhs.uk) has been positive. Such resources are available to staff within the care homes either as references in case of specific problems, or to provide information for teaching sessions.

The invitation for registered nurses to join acute trust or primary care trust educational events promotes an integrative approach between NHS and independent sector staff. This enriches overall service provision by promoting improved communication through enhanced professional relationships, and it promotes equity of care provision through a shared knowledge base.

Nurses working within the care home sector are subject to the professional development regulations laid out by the nursing regulatory body, namely the Nursing and Midwifery Council. In order to continue to practise, they must comply with the minimum professional educational development stipulated every three years (Nursing and Midwifery Council, 2002). However, the development needs of healthcare support workers specifically in relation to palliative care have been neglected (Froggatt, 2000a). The care home sector suffers from a history of employing healthcare support workers who are predominantly represent unskilled labour, frequently supervised by a lone registered nurse, and this, together with expenditure constraints and patients' high levels of dependency, leaves workers little time for paid study leave.

Several authors have identified the need for support and education directed at healthcare assistants. This is important, given that they are the largest group within the staffing of care homes (Katz *et al.*, 1999; Komaromy *et al.*, 2000; Froggatt *et al.*, 2002). A variety of initiatives have been developed for access to local care homes, with Macmillan Cancer Relief and the Open University developing a teaching package for use nationally (Macmillan Cancer Relief, 2004). This package, entitled *Foundations in Palliative Care. A programme of facilitated learning for care home staff*, designed for use with healthcare assistants, can be accessed free of charge by any care home, is interactive, and contains detailed resources for both facilitator and participants.

As mentioned previously, the care home sector has a history of employing staff who do not hold a formal nursing qualification. Mainly anecdotal evidence suggests that the care home workforce, both with and without a formal nursing qualification, is usually female, older and employed on a part-time basis (Maslin-Prothero and Masterson, 1998). In urban areas, a significant proportion of staff are non-white (Gerrish *et al.*, 1996). Many care home owners, particularly those operating independently, are forced to minimise labour costs in order to offer fees at competitive rates. Staff turnover may be high, for a variety of reasons, and one study suggests that it may be as high as 20% (Laing and Buisson, 2001). This high turnover contributes to the workforce sharing the same marginalised status as the service users to whom they deliver care.

Traditionally, qualified nurses with an interest in palliative care nursing were able to pursue national board courses such as the ENB 237, 931 or 285. With the abolition of the national boards, relevant material has been subsumed into courses leading to diploma or degree qualification. At the present time, post-registration education opportunities range from completing a module as part of a post-registration nursing degree or diploma, to completing a specialist degree or diploma comprising many core and some optional modules permitting individual choice and direction. Post-registration education in palliative care may be offered by hospices or community palliative care teams, occasionally in conjunction with a validating university. The structure of courses varies according to the provider institute, and courses range from distance learning to day release or block study time.

In April 1995, the legislation relating to post-registration education and practice (PREP) came into force, obliging registered nurses to complete five days of study activity every three years in order to maintain effective registration. Nurses working in the private sector are often obliged to contribute to the cost of PREP, and undertake study activity in their own time. This precedent disadvantages those who are on lower incomes and/or have family commitments, and also those who work for an organisation with a small or non-existent education budget.

It is worth noting that so far educational provision has been discussed in terms of care home staff. Froggatt (2000b) clearly identifies that clinical nurse specialists who intend to provide clinical and educational palliative care support in care homes will have identifiable educational needs. Care homes cover a wide range of specialties, and staff may demonstrate a significantly greater knowledge base in the management of mental health issues, learning disabilities, or the management of dementia and other specific diseases than a clinical nurse specialist specialising in palliative care. In this arena a mutual exchange of knowledge and skills can be as beneficial to the clinical nurse specialist as it is to the care home staff, and often boosts the self-esteem of the care home staff when they find that they have assumed the role of the educator.

Palliative care education is all too often specifically geared to the care of patients with malignant disease. Avis *et al.* (1999) have reported that registered nurses from care homes comment on the structure and delivery of accredited courses, the time and cost of attending educational programmes, and the lack of relevance of this education to the care home service user group. If it is not relevant to practice, education can become a paper exercise where theory may be more difficult to transfer to practice. Care home staff will continue to be marginalised if they are excluded from education by insufficient application of learning to their work environment. Good care does not just rely on the resources within the care home. It is also dependent on effective partnership with members of the multi-disciplinary team across all the healthcare settings. Often care home staff are motivated and willing to develop care practices, but may encounter professionals from other settings who are unable to engage with this. This can lead to a potential for conflict and prevent beneficial changes in clinical practice.

Both authors undertook a detailed learning needs assessment within their local care homes, on commencement of their posts, with their outcomes reflecting national findings (Katz *et al.*, 1999; Froggatt, 2004). Issues of funding, staffing levels and access to educational events were consistently identified as obstacles to education/training by care home managers and their staff. As a consequence of this, flexible approaches to education were developed, including the delivery of in-house education within the care homes offered in tandem with enhanced access to locally provided palliative care education. Some education was targeted specifically at care home staff, and the availability of other palliative care educational opportunities was advertised more vigorously than previously, with supplementary information provided on how to access alternative methods of funding. Where possible it was negotiated that care home staff should be able to access NHS study days at no cost to themselves or the care home. In some instances, money was made available to provide backfill for staff who were attending courses.

Educational events have been offered to both qualified nursing staff and healthcare assistants, with a wide range of topics, including symptom management, communication issues and syringe-driver skills. Educational/training needs are often identified during clinical intervention in the care of a resident, facilitating experiential learning within the care home setting. An example of this was a man who had had a glossectomy for cancer of his tongue, and was no longer able to manage any oral diet or fluids. Following extensive radiotherapy to his head and neck he had a dirty, offensive-smelling mouth. It was appropriate to spend time looking at the anatomy of the mouth and how it had been altered following surgery, demonstrating the appropriate mouth care techniques and discussing the effect of radiotherapy on the salivary glands. Over several weeks a variety of products were used, and eventually this patient's problems were resolved. However, it was noted that the care staff had also implemented the mouth care assessment tool with other service users. Role modelling is a useful educational tool for the Clinical Nurse Specialist (CNS), as is the use of reflective practice with staff members, where clinical events have been seen as complex, difficult or distressing (Butterworth and Faugier, 1992).

One of the authors designed and disseminated a resource file containing clinical information, contact details of specialist palliative care services and educational events, funding information and information relating to accredited courses. Although the resource file offered immediate access to information, and in theory was available for all of the care staff to access in each care home at any time of day or night, it was the experience of one of the authors that this file was occasionally kept in the manager's office or 'lost.' The other author extended the provision of an existing resource file to local care homes, and developed the website discussed previously. This was easier to keep up to date, and as the care home staff could contribute to the content more easily by responding on the web page, they could develop some 'ownership' of the information that was entered on to the site. Both authors have encouraged care home staff to access other specialist services and to liaise closely with their primary care teams. Care home staff have also been encouraged to access local hospices for training and development and to obtain 'out-of-hours' clinical advice and support.

In the current context of care, a raised awareness of the educational and support needs in care homes, both at a strategic level and as an integral component of their role, has been witnessed. These issues have therefore been highlighted at a local level within primary care and acute trusts, and also regionally at Cancer Network meetings.

Key points

- The shift from institutional to community care has resulted in a significant increase in the number of service users with complex palliative care needs approaching the end of life being cared for within the nursing home sector.
- To achieve equity of care for the 'disadvantaged dying', palliative care educational initiatives must be designed to meet the needs of care home staff and their service users.
- Factors that contribute to constraints in the delivery of care include the skill mix of staff who are predominantly healthcare support workers, the lack of government funding to support palliative care education, and the low staffing levels imposed to enable care for service users to be provided at a competitive rate.

Conclusion

The main emphasis of this chapter has been on meeting the challenges of providing enhanced palliative care provision in care homes, through the medium of increased educational initiatives. However, it should not be forgotten that there is evidence of excellent care provision in the care home sector. The needs of cognitively and physically frail patients may sometimes be better met within a care home than in any other care sector. It is therefore incumbent on any practitioner /teacher who is approaching the task of palliative care support of care home staff and patients to undertake this with a view to the exchange of mutually relevant information.

Accessibility is vital if education and training are to reach the care home staff whom they are targeting. To maximise accessibility, education needs to be flexible and tailored to the needs of those receiving it, via the appropriate methods.

In order to ensure that the most vulnerable sections of our community receive the highest possible level of care, a more flexible approach to funding education is essential. Although older adults and their nurses have moved from the NHS to the private sector, educational funding does not necessarily follow them. Without 'external' intervention in the education of staff in care homes, there is the potential for two tiers of continuing care to develop. The National Council for Palliative Care (2005) recommends actions for all key stakeholders in order to facilitate equity of care provision. These stakeholders include the care homes, primary care trusts, strategic health authorities, specialist palliative care providers, regional palliative care networks and the National Council for Palliative Care itself. Recommended actions include the active promotion of effective working relationships, improved access to clinical advice and support with regard to palliative care, equity of access for care home residents to medication and the full range of NHS services, and the consideration of issues relating to care homes at a strategic level locally, regionally and nationally.

The barriers to education and training that have been identified in this chapter present a real challenge in the current climate of staff shortages, increasing demand for training and financial constraints. Palliative care services will increasingly face the challenges of determining their responsibility in the provision of care for people who are dying from illnesses other than cancer, particularly those with the degenerative conditions that accompany old age.

Implications for the reader's own practice

1 How could you identify any specific educational needs in order to meet the palliative care requirements of a service user who is being discharged to a care home?
2 How could you identify your own learning needs in relation to care provision within your local care home sector?
3 How could you facilitate integration of care home staff into your current educational provision with regard to palliative care?
4 How do you identify your own educational requirements to reach beyond the palliative care traditionally offered to patients with malignant disease?

References

Addington-Hall J, Higginson I, editors. *Palliative Care for Non-Cancer Patients.* Oxford: Oxford University Press; 2001.

Avis M, Jackson JG, Cox C *et al.* Evaluation of a project providing community palliative care support to nursing homes. *Health Soc Care Commun.* 1999; 7: 32–8.

Butterworth T, Faugier J. *Clinical Supervision and Mentorship in Nursing.* London: Chapman and Hall; 1992.

Davies E, Higginson I. *Better Palliative Care for Older People.* Geneva: World Health Organization; 2004.

Department of Health. *NHS and Community Care Act.* London: Department of Health; 1991.

Department of Health. *National Service Framework for Older People.* London: Department of Health; 2001.

Ellershaw J, Wilkinson S. *Care of the Dying. A pathway to excellence.* Oxford: Oxford University Press; 2003.

Froggatt K. Evaluating a palliative care education project in nursing homes. *Int J Palliat Nurs.* 2000a; **6**: 140–46.

Froggatt K. *Palliative Care Education in Nursing Homes.* London: Macmillan Cancer Relief; 2000b.

Froggatt K. *Palliative Care in Care Homes for Older People.* London: National Council for Hospice Care; 2004.

Froggatt K, Poole K, Hoult L. The provision of palliative care in nursing homes and residential care homes: a survey of clinical nurse specialist work. *Palliat Med.* 2002; **16**: 481–7.

Gerrish K, Husband C, Mackenzie J. *Nursing for a Multi-Ethnic Society.* Buckingham: Open University Press; 1996.

Hockley J, Clark D, editors. *Palliative Care for Older People in Care Homes.* Buckingham: Open University Press; 2002.

Jordhoy MS, Saltveldt I, Fayers P *et al.* Which cancer patients die in nursing homes? *Palliat Med.* 2003; **17**: 433–44.

Kaesar L. Developing an effective teaching nursing home: the planning process. *Nurse Educ.* 1998; **14**: 37–41.

Kane RA, Ouslander JG, Abrass IB. *Essentials of Clinical Geriatrics,* 2nd edn. McGraw-Hill: New York; 1989.

Katz J. Training of care home staff. *Eur J Palliat Care.* 2003; **10**: 154–7.

Katz J, Komaromy C, Sidell M. Understanding palliative care in residential and nursing homes. *Int J Palliat Nurs.* 1999; **5**: 58–64.

Komaromy C, Sidell M, Katz J. The quality of terminal care in residential and nursing homes. *Int J Nurs.* 2000; **6**: 192–200.

Laing & Buisson. *Care of Elderly People: market survey 2000.* 13th edn. London: Laing & Buisson; 2001.

Loftus I, Thompson E. An evaluation of palliative care course for generic nurses. *Int J Palliat Nurs.* 2002; **8**: 354–60.

Macmillan Cancer Relief. *Foundations in Palliative Care. A programme of facilitated learning for care home staff.* London: Macmillan Cancer Relief; 2004.

Maslin-Prothero S, Masterson A. Continuing care: developing a policy analysis for nursing. *J Adv Nurs.* 1998; **28**: 548–53.

Metzy M, Mitty E, Bottrell M. The Teaching Nursing Home Program: enduring educational outcomes. *Nurs Outlook.* 1997; **45**: 133–40.

National Council for Palliative Care. *Focus on Care Homes.* London: National Council for Palliative Care; 2005.

Nursing and Midwifery Council. *Code of Professional Conduct.* London: Nursing and Midwifery Council; 2002.

Royal College of Physicians. Doubling in NHS funding for care homes needed to improve 'haphazard' services for vulnerable older people. *RCP News.* 2000; **August**. www.rcp london.ac.uk/news/news.asp?PR_id.45

Thomas K, Meehan H, Maryon K. *Use of the Gold Standards Framework in Care Homes. Report on the introduction of GSF into 12 care homes in the pilot phase 1, April to December 2004.* Birmingham: Gold Standards Framework Programme Central Team; 2005. www.goldstandardsframework.nhs.uk

Williams M. *The Transfer of Palliative Care Patients to Nursing Homes.* London: St Christopher's Hospice; 2000.

Useful website

- Nursing homes; www.nursinghomes.cht.nhs.uk

Chapter 15

Family care: sensitive and dynamic approaches to teaching

Pam Firth

> *On his way back from the K'un-lun Mountains, the Yellow Emperor lost the dark pearl of Tao.*
> *He sent Knowledge to find it, but Knowledge was unable to understand it.*
> *He sent Distant Vision, but Distant Vision was unable to see it.*
> *He sent Eloquence, but Eloquence was unable to describe it.*
> *Finally, he sent Empty Mind, and Empty Mind came back with the pearl.*
> *Lao Tzu (Hua Ching Ni, 1993)*

Aim

The aim of this chapter is to explore issues that arise for oncology and palliative care patients and their families which should be addressed by educationalists in a comprehensive and sensitive way.

Learning outcomes

- Understand the impact of family care on palliative care education.
- Understand the need to teach the assessment of families using a systemic approach.
- Explore the importance of understanding a three-generational approach to family assessment.
- Understand the value of using a genogram and an ecomap with families.

Introduction

This chapter, with its emphasis on teaching about families, demonstrates the shift in our thinking from providing palliative care for individuals to the wider focus, which includes the family. The influence of systemic thinking and social construction theories has led to the acknowledgement that we are all part of systems which interact with each other, and therefore the patient cannot be seen in isolation. Recently, with the shift in the UK and other European countries to care based in the community, there is more concern and thought about the role of the family as caregiver. There has been a growing interest in providing support services for family caregivers, which can in most cases mean offering bereavement care after the death. This has also led to concerns about the children involved when a relative or significant friend has a life-threatening illness.

What is a family? How are families organised? What happens to the children? What do health and social care professionals need to think about when talking to families both before and after a death? This chapter will address these issues, focusing on ideas used by family therapists, and will then make suggestions about how basic training in this area can be provided.

The chapter will be illuminated by short case examples. These could be used in teaching sessions to assist the learning and demonstrate specific points.

In the past, society used to regard families as the primary group, providing nurturing and socialisation (Altschuler, 2005). Now we recognise that the family is a dynamic social structure (Payne, 2004), and it is often the relationship which defines effective family (Firth, 2005). Cultural differences and ideologies in society affect the way in which people live together (Dallos and Draper, 2000). However, it is important to acknowledge that whether people remain in touch with their birth parents or not, our early experiences affect us all throughout our lives, and they influence the way in which we deal with situations.

Relationships within families have different meanings and significance, which will often determine the way that a family cares for a family member who is sick. The family history of illness, death and dying will have an influence on the way in which a life-threatening illness is experienced both by the patient and by his family. McGoldrick (1991) focuses on the family legacy of loss and how patterns become entrenched, whereas Byng-Hall (1985) describes family scripts that produce behaviours which are enacted whenever similar contexts are experienced. The work of Bowen (1991) helps the reader to understand the emotional shock waves that engulf family members following a serious event in the life of the family, such as sudden illness or a death. This again highlights the need to understand the connections between family members, and it will be explored in the section about assessments.

Smith (2004) describes both the negative and positive aspects for an individual who is caring for a terminally ill family member. The negative aspects include the effects on the carer's physical and psychological health, as well as social isolation and financial demands. The positive aspects include a closer relationship, expressions of love and affection, fulfilment of family duty and earning the respect of others. Researchers also suggest that the patient's experience and the course of the illness are determined by the involvement of the family caregivers and how they manage the stress and the effects of the illness on the patient (Wright and Leahey, 2000).

When a family member has a life-threatening illness, the family has to make major adjustments to family life. Everyone is affected.

Families as systems

Ideas about families as systems began to emerge in the 1950s (Burnham, 1999). Until then, most writers and practitioners in the helping professions were heavily influenced by psychodynamic theories which sought to understand people's early experience and history in terms of their effect on their inner world. Theories about death and dying reflected this, and were initiated by Freud's paper, published in 1914, on mourning and melancholia (Freud, 1957). Recent research and practice have focused more on interactive models (Stroebe *et al.*, 1997; Silverman, 2005), whilst Bowlby (1980) was concerned with the primary emotional attachments that children form with their parents/caregivers, and how these attachment determine the quality of subsequent close adult relationships. Bereavement researchers have examined the quality of the attachment and attachment behaviours as predictors in determining the reaction to close bereavements (Machin, 2005). In a recent publication, Tan *et al.* (2005) discuss attachment theories and the way that the style of attachment can affect the relationships formed by patients and clinicians when the patient has a serious illness.

All systems are seen as being composed of interacting parts, and there needs to be a balance in order for things to run smoothly. The family system is no different, and in families there are structures in place to maintain the balance. However, these structures need to be flexible enough to allow for some change as the family grows and moves through the life cycle. The concept of the family life cycle and the work of Carter and McGoldrick (1989) have enriched our thinking about the tasks of each stage of development in family life. The sense of outrage and the practical problems for a young family when a child or parent is dying can be understood more fully by bearing in mind the fact that this is so alien to the life-cycle stage. The tasks for a young family are to allow new members into the system, not to deal with a death.

The flexibility of families as systems can affect the way in which any change is managed. A family that communicates effectively and which has developed a range of problem-solving skills will be better able to negotiate the adaptations required when a family member is seriously ill. However, recent developments in the treatment of cancer have led to patients living longer with their disease. As a consequence, families have to problem solve this illness over time, which can lead to less flexibility. Support systems change – for example, friends who once helped may drift away, and family members age. A grandmother who helped to care for the children may herself now have health problems. Patients also lose their capacity to cope effectively due to frailty and pain, and they lead more restricted lives. Social isolation can have distressing consequences for both the patient and the family carer.

Recently, more attention has been paid to the use of family therapy to help families to adjust to the increasingly difficult circumstances that serious illness can bring. Kissane and Bloch (2002) describe their work with families prior to bereavement, and demonstrate the effectiveness of using therapeutic interventions that build on a family's positive problem-solving skills.

The organisation of family life

When people decide to live together, they work out a whole set of rules about how they will manage day-to-day tasks, and who will be responsible for earning money, paying bills, doing the household chores, caring for the children, and so on. Often these tasks are explicitly gender determined, but they are also related to past experience, and are an amalgam of value systems and issues such as power and control. The family develops a way of seeing the world and a belief system about how life should be lived. Much of this development of a belief system is unconscious, and it is important to recognise that culture also determines how the world is viewed.

> Margaret was only 40 years old when she died of an AIDS-related illness. She had become HIV positive after a blood transfusion. She infected her husband and her unborn child, both of whom subsequently died. Her elder daughter was not affected. The family came from Africa to the UK, and everybody assumed that Margaret's illness was sexually transmitted, leading to an extra burden for Margaret's daughter in both communities. Like many children in this situation, she suffered from racism and stigma and had no one to care for her. Many people blamed Margaret for her illness, and she had been shunned by friends in her own community. Eventually a second cousin took the child in.

If we are to access the family's belief systems, we need to listen and to ask sensitive questions – for example, '*I wonder what you and your family are making of your illness.*' After a home visit or a meeting in a clinic, it is important to reflect on what the illness is meaning both for the patient and for the family members. Experience suggests that there are similarities but also great differences between the cancer journey for the patient and the family's journey.

> Janet was only 40 years old when she developed cancer. She was also an alcoholic and had two teenage daughters. Her husband had left her two years ago and had recently remarried. Janet was devastated by the news of her illness, which had been diagnosed quite early. She drank more and more, and her daughters struggled to cope. Janet was terrified, but her daughters were filled with rage. They felt abandoned by both parents. Janet died about six months after her diagnosis. Her daughters were relieved at first but then felt guilty. They had had to grow up quickly and were always trying to hide Janet's alcoholism, never inviting friends home and often going without food. Janet's death brought up new issues, but they felt that they could move on with support.

Beliefs about the cause of the illness which involve shame and blame can be particularly difficult for the family to work through (Rolland, 1991). Smoking-related illnesses might be an example of illness associated with blame, and AIDS often raises many issues about shame.

Assessing the family structure

Most health and social care professionals know the value of using a family tree or genogram to get a picture of the patient's family. Some units have developed tools to assess family functioning (Kissane and Bloch, 2002). However, when people are assessed, it is crucial to develop a relationship first. Empathy, respect and genuineness are essential in order to build trust. They are the core values of social work, counselling and psychotherapy, and encompass the individual's right to self-determination, a non-judgemental attitude towards clients and an understanding of culture and diversity. Why do we need to know? For example, if I was asked about my family I would need to have this explained to me. Making an assessment should involve people and give them a chance to tell their story – it is not something that is done to people.

Alison was a 67-year-old retired businesswoman. She had recently asked for help, by telephone, from a specialist nurse following a cancer diagnosis which had left her acutely anxious and unable to function. Alison became very annoyed when she was asked lots of questions, and she became very suspicious. She asked the nurse why she wanted to know. The nurse became defensive and Alison put the phone down. Later the nurse found out that Alison had made a complaint about her. The nurse contacted Alison again, apologised, and asked whether she would like to see a counselling colleague. Alison agreed to this. In the session with the counsellor the issue of record keeping and confidentiality was addressed, and it was agreed that all records would be written jointly. Alison acknowledged in subsequent meetings that she did lack trust, due to childhood abuse, and told the counsellor that she had been in care as a child. She said that she had spent years trying to escape her childhood experiences, and that she had been thrown back into worries about control and dependence when she became ill. The nurse did not know any of this when she asked her initial questions.

The family tree or genogram shows in a diagrammatic form the construction of the family, usually over three generations. As people engage in building the family tree, they often reflect on how they coped before the patient became ill. The diagram aims to show when losses have occurred. It also identifies the changes in family life, because it provides a record of when people were born and/or died and what the family relationships were.

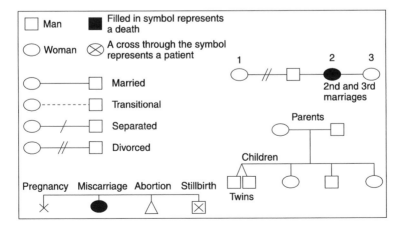

Figure 15.1   Key for drawing a genogram.

The family tree can also show patterns which may sometimes help to explain why the current situation is especially problematic. I have already referred to the work of Byng-Hall (1985, 1988), who introduced the concept of a 'family script' to describe how families seem to repeat behavioural patterns or scenarios when similar contexts are experienced. These family scripts are passed down from generation to generation, and become problematic if they are too rigid and prevent change.

Another very useful tool is an ecomap. This allows people to show who is important to them, and that does not always mean family members, and may include professionals. Sometimes this can be done by using objects to represent people. Children often enjoy using buttons or stones to represent people who are significant in their lives.

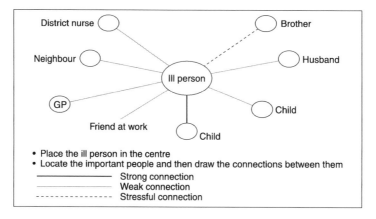

Figure 15.2 Ecomap: identifying networks.

Assessments should always be partnerships and involve a circular process of gathering information, making an informed assessment, agreeing goals or priorities, planning, interventions, review and evaluation (Oliviere *et al.*, 1998). We have already recognised that families develop patterns of doing things, and that these are likely to be repeated when the family members have to adjust to serious illness in the family.

A psychosocial assessment must take into account the stressors of family life. Where service users are consulted, they are keen to emphasise the need for good-quality information and access to services that support their care. Serious illness occurs within a social context – it can lead to lack of money, and concerns about work, school and older members of the family.

The financial hardship caused by serious illness is potentially more severe if it is the breadwinner who is ill. If it is the mother of dependent children who is seriously ill, who will care for the children? Some individuals are disconnected from their family of origin and are reliant on friends and neighbours for help.

> Dawn was dying of breast cancer. She had one daughter aged 13 years. She had left the child's father 10 years ago, and they had never married. There had been some contact between the couple, but it was always acrimonious, and the girl did not really know her father. Dawn was an only child estranged from

her own parents, who lived in Ireland. However, she had some very close friends and she was a very popular member of staff at the care home where she worked as a secretary. Everybody rallied round to take her for her treatments and look after her daughter when she went into hospital. She retained great hope that she would be cured, and she always changed the subject when the Macmillan nurse asked her about the long-term care of her daughter. The school became concerned about the behaviour of her daughter, and asked Dawn to meet with them. As a result, Dawn agreed to meet with the hospice social worker, partly because she acknowledged that she always hated going to meetings at school and she was scared about being criticised. The social worker met Dawn twice at home, and developed enough trust with her to make a family assessment. They agreed that it was important to have hope, and that Dawn had always done the best for her daughter. Dawn contacted her ex-partner and he began to visit the family regularly, eventually coming back to care for Dawn and his daughter during the terminal stage of her illness. The assessment had shown that Dawn and her ex-partner had the capacity to do what was right for their child. Dawn's friends continued to support her child and her ex-partner long after Dawn's death.

Earlier in this chapter, communication issues were raised. The need to talk will vary from one family to another. Some families do not talk about death and dying (Fredman, 1997).

However, the need for information about the illness, treatment and the side-effects of treatment has been shown to be extremely important (Payne *et al.*, 1999), and the issue of communication is linked to problem solving. If a family has very rigid boundaries and finds it difficult to allow outsiders to be involved, they limit the flow of information and therefore their options for resolving issues. Conversely, some families have very weak boundaries, and this can also cause difficulties. One family told their 6-year-old twins absolutely everything about their father's illness. The children were very anxious about going to school, and found it hard to leave their parents. Eventually the parents were able to use the support offered and process information before they talked to the children. Practitioners need opportunities in training and clinical supervision to examine and then discuss their own attitudes to talking about death and dying. A course looking at family and palliative care could include an exercise that allows participants to consider their own views.

This issue of talking to children about the serious illness of a close family member is very important (Christ, 2000). Adults cannot fail to communicate their concerns to children, who sense family tension, notice changes in routine and overhear adult conversations. However, it is necessary to recognise the need to talk to children about what is happening, and some helpful and informative publications are now available (Heegaard, 1991; Stokes, 2000). The professionals, including doctors, nurses, teachers and social workers, need to be taught about the effects of serious illness and bereavement on children. Training courses can make use of a series of new videos in which children talk about having an ill parent, or being bereaved. A recent video, entitled *No – You Don't Know How We Feel!*, has been made by children themselves and facilitated by Chowns *et al.* (2003). The cameraman Nick Lunch helped the children with their filming. The Childhood Bereavement Network

(2003) has also produced a number of new videos about childhood bereavement, including *You'll Always Remember Them ... Even When You're Old*, which shows young people talking about their experiences of bereavement.

A specialist hospice social worker was running a workshop for health and social care workers. She had talked to the group about the sensitivity of the session, and suggested that if anyone did find themselves upset by the material they could either stay or leave the room and make a drink. The session was drawing to a close when she put up a quote from a woman talking about the death of her mother 20 years ago. One of the school nurses ran out of the room. The session ended shortly afterwards, and the teacher was told that the nurse had left alone. Later she was contacted and the teacher and the nurse met with each other. The social worker/teacher gave the nurse information about counselling, which she did access. On reflection, the social worker realised that she should have asked whether anyone had experienced a close family bereavement as a child. Also, the quote had been introduced near the end of the session, when she should have been reducing the emotional content of the session.

Teaching about family care: who knows about families and what training is available to professionals?

Working with families who are facing the loss of a loved one takes great skill. Until recently it was the domain of specialist social workers (Sheldon, 2003)) to work primarily with families. The social work training, with its emphasis on building and sustaining helping relationships, knowledge of family law, sociology, psychology and family and group work, provides the basic training for helping families in situations of loss. Social workers encounter the consequences of loss in a variety of work settings on a daily basis. In the UK, Middlesex University has been unique in providing a specific pathway in palliative care on the basic social work degree course. However, many social workers in Europe and the USA are finding that their roles are changing to include more case management, and that their skills are being undermined and undervalued. The Project on Death in America's Social Work Leadership Development Program has led to the development of programmes and models of education in the USA which have begun to address the educational and knowledge deficit and to increase the valuing of the social work role (Walsh-Burke and Csikai, 2005).

In the UK, the Association of Hospice and Specialist Palliative Care Social Workers, now known as the Association of Palliative Care Social Workers, has provided support, training and advocacy for over 240 members, currently mostly working in hospices. Many members have engaged in counselling and family therapy training to enhance their skills.

Recently, psychologists and counsellors have been employed in cancer care, and this trend will increase following the publication by the UK government of a document entitled *Improving Supportive care for Adults with Cancer* (National Institute for Clinical Excellence, 2004). This document recognises the depth and range of psychological support that is needed by patients with a diagnosis of cancer. In a recent mapping exercise in one Cancer Network area it was very evident that there was a great scarcity of psychological care for cancer patients and their families until they used palliative care facilities such as hospices and specialist palliative care teams. However, it is the family and particularly the family caregiver who may need help after the death. Community bereavement services are often patchy. Cruse Bereavement Care and voluntary bereavement networks do not cover the whole country, and often focus on offering individual support.

There is also a growing need to provide childhood bereavement services, but again service provision is patchy. The Childhood Bereavement Network holds a directory of services, and is seeking to support new services as well as to develop standards and quality measures. A recent educational initiative between Help the Hospices and St Christopher's Hospice, validated by Middlesex University, provided the first undergraduate and postgraduate training in Childhood Bereavement Studies. Students on the first course were from a variety of backgrounds, including nursing, teaching and social work.

The educational needs of members of the multi-disciplinary team in family work can be met in many different ways. One approach is to provide input on Master's courses. The author taught on the excellent Masters in Psychosocial Care at Southampton University for many years. Here students came from a great variety of professional backgrounds. King's College London also provides training in family work as part of their Masters course for palliative care practitioners. St Christopher's Hospice in South London continues to provide a wide range of workshops for people who wish to know more about working with families, and this pattern is repeated throughout the UK, but it is often at a basic level. The Tavistock Clinic in London offered a valuable one-term part-time course entitled *A Psychodynamic Approach to Cancer Care for the Patient and His Family*. The course was structured so that there were lectures from psychologists, psychotherapists, family therapists and psychiatrists, followed by small group work in which there was an opportunity to discuss case material.

It is vital that the training in palliative care in relation to families is undertaken by practitioners who are skilled and have the necessary training in this specialist field.

Hostad (2004) believes that education in palliative care should reflect the principles and practices of palliative care. The multi-disciplinary team approach offered in hospice and palliative care teams also provides a great opportunity for all team members to learn from each other. Sharing rather than disempowering each other can bring great benefits to patients. However, team rivalries and differences can sometimes get in the way. It is easier to identify with one's own professional group, and issues about power and differences in individual professional ethics can prevent workers from listening to each other (Firth, 2003). Clinical supervision which is multi-disciplinary in nature can help, particularly if it is offered by an outside consultant and has a focused teaching and learning component.

Many large hospices have their own education units which offer a wide range of education – a very different model to the small unit that provides local education and is generally run by a nurse lecturer. The larger units are well placed to provide education that is not only multi-professional but also inter-professional (Hostad, 2004). The blurring but respecting of professional boundaries can sometimes be achieved by educational initiatives such as that of Wee *et al.* (2001), who use the carers of cancer patients to provide much needed direct information from their own perspective for students from different professional backgrounds.

Teaching about family care

Teaching about palliative care for families is more demanding on the teacher and student than teaching factual information about diagnosis and treatment. It requires flexibility and concentration to monitor the effects of the material on group members. There is a place for more formal lectures as well as the main teaching models used in this chapter; namely learning by experience and learning from experience. Even a formal lecture can be broken down and facilitated (Faulkner, 1993). It is important to acknowledge that the teacher's approach to teaching can be an example of the way that clinicians need to engage with their clients and patients. An enthusiastic teacher inspires others, and a teacher who talks about family work with sensitivity, humility and genuine concern is modelling how to be with people in distress and crisis.

Hostad (2004) argues that the sensitivity of the teacher is crucial in defining a good teacher in this field. A teacher with good communication skills, such as the ability to pick up subtle and non-verbal clues, can help to assess how students are managing material that is personal and sometimes painful. An educational system is, after all, a form of communication – the teacher and the students communicate meaning and then clarify issues that relate to it. The teacher is responsible for providing a safe learning environment which takes into account the risks in experiential learning. Experiential learning values reflective practice and aims to link theory to practice, which can be demonstrated when students are asked to supply their own case material or to examine case material that has been supplied by the teacher. Burnard and Chapman (1990) has identified five key elements of experiential learning.

1 There is an emphasis on personal learning.
2 It is an active process.
3 Students are expected to reflect on and learn from their own experiences.
4 Experience is valued as a learning episode in itself.
5 The teacher adopts a supportive role in the learning process.

In educational establishments that offer training courses in counselling and psychotherapy, it is common practice for the course to include group or individual support/counselling to provide students with an opportunity to reflect on material that affects them personally and professionally, to make links, and then to bring about change in functioning if appropriate. This opportunity is very rarely offered in the teaching of palliative care. An experiential group in which students would have space to reflect on material and then to make connections could be useful if it was offered regularly, perhaps monthly throughout the course, especially if the learning style is encouraging and promoting self-learning (Firth, 2005).

How to plan a one-day workshop about working with families in cancer care

Size of the group and content

The first consideration is the size of the teaching group. This will determine the content and the style of teaching. A formal lecture can be given, followed by a seminar in which the group is split up into groups of a maximum of 20 students each. When teaching in an interactive style, it is important to begin the day by setting out ground rules that emphasise the responsibilities of students and tutor, as well as the importance of listening to and valuing contributions made by individuals. Students need to be told the content of the course, and the issue of emotional safety must be explained. This should be followed up by a discussion with the group about triggers and how people might manage to cope if they feel upset. If the family content is taught in a large group, it is much more difficult to monitor the effects of the material on the group. It is for this reason that most trainers prefer to use small groups, with a maximum of 20 students led by two trainers, or up to 12 students with one trainer. The smaller groups allow more personal attention to be provided by the teacher, and give more people an opportunity to take part in the discussion. The emotional content can be built up during the day and then reduced towards the end of the workshop.

Exercises

Most teachers are familiar with a range of introductory exercises, some of which, if they are not managed properly, can take up a lot of time. If the topic is about families and the students do not know each other, it can be useful to ask people to introduce themselves by stating their name and what it means to them. This can sometimes produce material which is very pertinent to the session. (e.g. someone might disclose that they were named after a dead sibling, etc.). Another longer exercise that is favoured in family therapy training and is more effective with a large group of 20 or more students is to ask everyone to walk around the room and to look closely at each other. They are asked to choose a partner who either reminds them of someone in their family or who would fit into their family. In discussion, students often find great commonality with their families of origin. When they then choose another couple they can find even more similarities to their personal histories. This is clearly not scientific, but it does demonstrate that we can be drawn to people for a variety of reasons, and family therapists suggest that we try to find people who are in some way familiar. For example, people who were brought up in care often choose other people with similar backgrounds. In one training group the author asked the members of the small group to introduce each other. One group member turned to the person next to her and said 'I sat next to you because I think you are like me and I wanted support.' In fact, both of them had been to special schools for children with unruly behaviour, but they had not known this in advance.

Agenda setting can be useful, so that students take some responsibility for the content. The teacher may give a plan of the session and then offer to negotiate about part of the day. For example, a session on *Difficult Situations* could be added, in which students would be free to raise issues that were troubling them. This also demonstrates to the students that the teacher has to be flexible and may have to face unfamiliar situations, just like the students (Faulkner, 1993).

One way to start the day is to show a clip of video material or audio material and then to follow discussions with the more formal input on a PowerPoint display. The order can be reversed, but the aims are the same, namely to use different media to give the students information. This could be followed by prepared case material that students could work on in small groups. The tutor can then identify links with theory – for example, they could get the group to consider the family script and to identify some family beliefs.

A more emotionally challenging exercise would be to ask the students to draw their own family tree and then to share significant parts of it with a partner, or to ask them to draw a lifeline with dates showing when they experienced episodes of loss and change. This last exercise is useful when beginning to discuss family life cycles.

Burnham (1999) suggests a range of different exercises, focusing around the basic ideas of family therapy, either to be used with a group of students or for individuals to try themselves. McLeod (2004) has written a book about counselling skills, entitled *The Counsellor's Workbook*, and some of his exercises can be extremely useful in helping students to think about the way in which their own life experiences have shaped their lives. This focuses students' thinking on self-knowledge and self-awareness, both of which are crucial for people in helping professions. However, the material is more suitable for use over several sessions.

Role play

Many students are anxious about taking part in role play. Unfortunately, they may have had experiences of role play that was not well managed, and that was short of time and emotionally unsafe. However, role play can be very helpful because it allows students to practise their skills (Faulkner, 1993). This author prefers to get the students to practise in small groups of three. Most people are anxious about being asked to perform in front of the whole class, so this is more acceptable. The importance of feedback can be emphasised by using one member of the small group to act as observer. Many training organisations use this method in skills and competency training (e.g. the Counselling and Psychotherapy Central Awarding Body, which requires students to provide evidence of competency via written feedback from peers in the observer role). In the absence of actual observers in interviews, this can have some value at a basic level.

Sculpting

The use of sculpting can be very helpful when considering a difficult situation that has been brought by a student. The author would not use this method of teaching in a one-day workshop unless the day was part of a training sequence. Sculpts can take time to execute, and they need to be managed carefully by teachers who are competent. Sculpting has some important advantages. It allows someone to get into the skin of another individual for a short time and thus to appreciate that person's feelings. Other members playing a given role in the exercise can give their own perspectives (Faulkner, 1993). Family therapists have used sculpting to help family members by encouraging them to swap roles in an attempt to see the other person's perspective. For example, a teenager might be asked to change roles with a parent.

This way of working needs to be positively presented, and its effects can be powerful (Burnham, 1999). (Role play and sculpting will be considered in more depth in the third book in this series.)

If the day has started with some agenda setting, after two or three hours it is important to revisit the agenda and check it with students. The value of space in the day to reflect and review can slow things down and help the group to think. The remainder of the session can involve some more theory, or it can be focused solely on experiences. Evaluations of a one-day workshop of this nature suggest that focusing on case material and student examples is particularly valued. The tutor/ teacher needs to be careful not to introduce too many emotive ideas towards the end of the day, and to find some way of checking out the group so that students have a chance to express any strong feelings or concerns that they may have. The group may value the opportunity to unwind by playing a game/performing an ending ritual, or simply telling each other about ways in which they unwind. Do check this out with the group first, as some groups hate games. One useful exercise is to give each student a handout entitled *First Aid Kit* (Sunderland and Engleheart, 1993). The students are asked to think about how they manage their professional lives so that they take care of themselves, and what they do that they find helpful. The first-aid kit can provide a pictorial record of how they cope.

Evaluations

Allow time for this if you really value feedback, otherwise the whole exercise is pointless. Evaluations need to address content and level of content. Quite often palliative care education is delivered to groups of people with very varied experience, education and training, so that pitching a session at an acceptable level is quite challenging.

Key points

- Families are all different, and they change as society changes. Teaching about families needs to address the definition of a family.
- Palliative care involves providing care for the patient and their family, yet most healthcare practitioners have little or no training in working with families.
- Interviewing families as a group can be very useful, but practitioners need education to do this competently.
- Assessing families using a genogram is helpful, but needs to be done within the professional relationship, and requires the professionals to have built up a sense of trust.
- All training about working with families assumes that workers have basic communication skills training.
- The role of family carers and the effects on the health of these individuals are becoming a major area of research and concern. Palliative care education can emphasise the need for support and understanding of the carer at a time in society when so much of the burden of caring for sick family members falls on the family in the community.

- The role of children in families with a member who has a life-threatening illness must not be forgotten, and teachers need to emphasise the position of children in families.
- All families live within a social and cultural context and are part of larger systems.

Conclusion

This chapter has explored some current ideas about families and family care when a patient has a life-threatening illness. Most of the ideas come from family therapy and allow the reader to consider the way in which meaning is ascribed to powerful individual/family events. Family organisation and family belief systems can give new insights for the professional involved in providing care. The brief case examples were included to demonstrate the way in which these ideas can help our thinking.

The second part of the chapter focused on teaching ideas and highlighted the need for teaching in this area to be undertaken by teachers who are sensitive and who have good communication skills. The organisation of the teaching needs to acknowledge that students will inevitably look at their own families and their own personal/professional experience, and that this is an essential part of learning, but also requires the teacher to monitor the students for distress. Recognising the effects that working in palliative care can have on us is also an essential part of self-monitoring which teachers need to instil into their students. Practising good self-care is a vital part of good palliative care, and needs to be emphasised by teachers.

The chapter underlines the value of genuine, respectful, caring and sustaining relationships with families and individuals. Families need to adapt and change as the patient's illness progresses. Educators should provide appropriate training to equip the professionals to provide care for patients and their families that is flexible and which can meet their changing needs.

Implications for the reader's own practice

1 How is education about family care delivered in your locality?
2 What sensitive approaches to delivering education in family care do you use?
3 How do you manage family interviews?
4 In what ways has your own family history of loss affected you?
5 Television and radio programmes and novels all include accounts – both fictional and real – of families coping with illness and bereavement. How might these be used to teach about the diversity of family life?
6 Consider how you manage your own family life while working with so much family distress.

References

Altschuler J. Illness and loss within the family. In: Firth PH, Luff G, Oliviere D, editors. *Loss, Change and Bereavement in Palliative Care.* Buckingham: Open University Press; 2005.

Bowen M. Family reaction to death. In: Walsh F, McGoldrick M, editors. *Living Beyond Loss: death in the family*. New York: Norton; 1991.

Bowlby, J. *Attachment and Loss. Volume 3. Loss, sadness and depression*. New York: Basic Books; 1980.

Burnard P, Chapman C. *Nurse Education*. London: Scutari; 1990.

Burnham J. *Family Therapy*. New York: Routledge; 1999.

Byng-Hall J. The family script. A useful bridge between theory and practice. *J Fam Ther*. 1985; **7**: 301–5.

Byng-Hall J. Scripts and legends in families and family therapy. *Fam Process*. 1988; **27**: 167–80.

Carter B, McGoldrick M. *The Changing Family Lifecycle: a framework for family therapy*. 2nd ed. Boston, MA: Allyn & Boston; 1989.

Childhood Bereavement Network. *You'll Always Remember Them ... Even When You're Old* (video). London: Child Bereavement Network; 2003 (available from Childhood Bereavement Network, 8 Wakley Street, London ECIV 7QE).

Chowns G, Bussey S, Jones A. *No – You Don't Know How We Feel!* (video) (further details available from gillian.chowns@berkshire.nhs.uk).

Christ GH. *Healing Children's Grief*. Oxford: Oxford University Press; 2000.

Dallos R, Draper R. *An Introduction to Family Therapy*. Buckingham: Open University Press; 2000.

Faulkner A. *Teaching Interactive Skills in Health Care*. London: Chapman & Hall; 1993.

Firth PH. Multi-professional teamwork. In: Monroe B, Oliviere D, editors. *Patient Participation in Palliative Care. A voice for the voiceless*. Oxford: Oxford University Press; 2003.

Firth PH. Group work in palliative care. In: Firth PH, Luff G, Oliviere D, editors. *Loss, Change and Bereavement in Palliative Care*. Buckingham: Open University Press; 2005.

Fredman G. *Death Talk. Conversations with children and families*. London: Karnac Books; 1997.

Freud S. Mourning and melancholia. In: Strachey J, editor. *The Standard Edition of the Complete Psychological Works of Sigmund Freud. Volume 14*. London: Hogarth; 1957 (original work published in 1914).

Heegaard ME. *When Someone Has a Very Serious Illness: children can learn to cope with loss and change*. Minneapolis, MN; Woodland Press; 1991.

Hostad J. An overview of hospice education. In: Foyle L, Hostad J, editors. *Delivering Cancer and Palliative Care Education*. Oxford: Radcliffe Publishing; 2004.

Hua Ching Ni. *Complete Works of Lao Tzu: Tao Teh Ching and Hua Hu Ching*. Los Angeles, CA: Book World (Seven Star Communication); 1993.

Kissane D, Bloch S. *Family-Focused Grief Therapy*. Buckingham: Open University Press; 2002.

McGoldrick M. The legacy of loss. In: Walsh F, McGoldrick M, editors. *Living Beyond Loss. Death in the Family*. New York: Norton; 1991.

McLeod J. *The Counsellor's Workbook*. Buckingham: Open University Press; 2004.

Machin L. Research in practice. In: Firth PH, Luff G, Oliviere D, editors. *Loss, Change and Bereavement in Palliative Care*. Buckingham: Open University Press; 2005.

National Institute for Clinical Excellence. *Improving Supportive Care for Adults with Cancer*. London: National Institute for Clinical Excellence; 2004.

Oliviere D, Hargreaves R, Monroe B. *Good Practices in Palliative Care*. Aldershot: Arena Ashgate; 1998.

Payne S, Smith P, Dean S. Identifying the concerns of informal carers in palliative care. *Palliat Med*. 1999; **13**: 37–44.

Payne S. Overview. In: Payne S, Seymour J, Ingleton C, editors. *Palliative Care Nursing*. Buckingham: Open University Press; 2004.

Rolland J. Helping families with anticipatory loss. In: Walsh F, McGoldrick M, editors. *Living Beyond Loss. Death in the Family.* New York: Norton; 1991.

Sheldon F. Social impact of advanced metastatic cancer. In: Lloyd-Williams M, editor. *Psychosocial Issues in Palliative Care.* Oxford: Oxford University Press; 2003.

Silverman PR. Mourning: a changing view. In: Firth PH, Luff G, Oliviere D, editors. *Loss, Change and Bereavement in Palliative Care.* Buckingham: Open University Press; 2005.

Smith P. Working with family caregivers. In: Payne S, Seymour J, Ingleton C, editors. *Palliative Care Nursing.* Buckingham: Open University Press; 2004.

Stokes J. *The Secret C.* Gloucester: Winston's Wish; 2000.

Stroebe M, Stroebe W, Hansson R. Bereavement research and theory: an introduction to the handbook. In: Stroebe M, Stroebe W, Hansson R, editors. *Handbook of Bereavement.* Cambridge: Cambridge University Press; 1997.

Sunderland M, Engleheart P. First Aid Kit. In: *Draw on Your Emotions.* Bicester: Winslow Press; 1993.

Tan A, Zimmermann C, Rodin G. Interpersonal processes in palliative care: an attachment perspective on the patient–clinician relationship. *Palliat Med.* 2005; **19:** 143–50.

Walsh-Burke K, Csikai E. Professional social work education in end-of-life care: contributions of the project on death in America's Social Work Leadership Development Program. *J Soc Work End Life Palliat Care.* 2005; **1:** 11–24.

Wee B, Hillier R, Coles C *et al.* Palliative care: a suitable setting for undergraduate inter-professional education. *Palliat Med.* 2001; **15:** 487–92.

Wright LM, Leahey M. *Nurses and Families. A guide to family assessments and intervention.* 3rd ed. Philadelphia, PA: FA Davies Company; 2000.

Chapter 16

Mapping the landscape: spirituality in cancer and palliative care education

Elizabeth Foster

What we call the beginning is often the end
And to make an end is to make a beginning.
The end is where we start from.

We shall not cease from exploration
And the end of all our exploring
Will be to arrive where we started
And know the place for the first time.

TS Eliot

Aim

The aim of this chapter is to explore the issues around spirituality and palliative care education, taking account both of multi-disciplinary working and of the unique contribution of each healthcare professional. The complexity of the subject and the challenges involved are highlighted, and are set alongside creative ideas and approaches to generating engagement and discussion in the teaching environment. The chapter also affirms the importance of each of us recognising our individual potential and learning to define what it is to be fully human.

Learning outcomes

- Recognise the importance of spiritual care and the associated educational responsibilities.
- Be aware of the need to develop creative approaches to the teaching of spirituality.
- Consider the qualities and skills required by those facilitating spiritual care education.
- Appreciate the need for continuity rather than an isolated approach to education.

Introduction

When diagnosed with a life-threatening illness and in a place of transition, patients may find that previously held beliefs and values either sustain them or become an uncomfortable landscape of shifting sand. Significant distress can then be experienced as they are drawn to review and possibly reconstruct their sense of self and the forces that motivate and support them. Palliative care is predicated on its attention to holistic care and the associated humanist values, and aims to prevent and reduce the suffering of vulnerable patients and their families. Importantly, caring for the spirit can enable patients to find meaning and hope in the face of suffering. Therefore spirituality is a vital component of the palliative care agenda (Cobb, 2001).

Acknowledging that patients seek spiritual support from those professionals with whom they have developed a trusting relationship, guidelines indicate that every healthcare practitioner should have an awareness of spirituality and spiritual care (National Institute for Clinical Excellence, 2004).

However, the evidence suggests that healthcare professionals are cautious about engaging with this aspect of care, for the following reasons.

- There is little or no educational preparation for this, the training that is provided often concentrating on dietary requirements and religious customs around the time of death (McSherry, 2000).
- Spiritual care, both clinically and educationally, is usually seen as the responsibility of someone from an established faith tradition. Therefore healthcare professionals may view spirituality as synonymous with religion (Greenstreet, 1999).

For caregivers to become effectively involved, they require opportunities to increase their knowledge and skills, and this also involves exploring personal beliefs and values.

The issue therefore is to determine how educational initiatives respond to this challenge. This chapter provides some signposts to help the reader to negotiate the landscape of spirituality, espousing the idea that this is not just about acquiring theoretical knowledge but also involves the whole presence of the professional carer.

Definition of spirituality

There is no universal definition of spirituality. However, at some point we are all aware of another dimension in our lives that informs the way we live, imbuing our existence with meaning that goes beyond the ordinariness of everyday life and our physical existence. This wider aspect of our personhood includes the need for:

- meaning/purpose
- love/relatedness
- forgiveness
- hope/inspiration.

These are the hallmarks of all humanity, including – but extending considerably wider than – religious affiliation or practice. McSherry and Draper (1998) have integrated these factors along with other qualities into the visual representation of a football (*see* Figure 16.1). With its integrated components, the football (spirituality) is then kicked throughout the game (life). Consequently, through personal experience this vital but intangible life force is uniquely shaped for each one of us. This model elucidates the fact that spirituality is not synonymous with religion, while at the same time capturing the sense of it being unique, in flux and deeply personal.

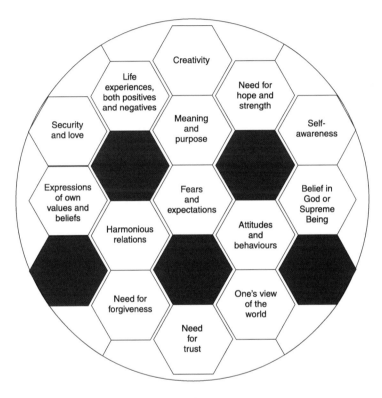

Figure 16.1 Diagrammatic model of spirituality.

The nature and interrelatedness of the core constituents suggest that spiritual need is heightened in the palliative care setting, as these elements suddenly face assault. Patients need to discover a way forward, and to make sense of the experience within the context of their belief system. Facilitating this process constitutes effective spiritual care, which influences the quality of the remaining lifespan, a determinant of skilful palliative care (Cobb, 2001).

The spiritual journey

Because spirituality has a personal meaning to those we care for, we need to attend to their individual stories. There is a wide range of beliefs and rituals among those who do not espouse a particular religion and within each faith tradition. A continuum also exists, extending from those who observe the prescribed rituals to those who take little part in formal practices. Further current issues are the implications of economic migration, asylum arrangements, conversion to new faith practices and changing populations, which mean that both society and the spiritual journey may be becoming increasingly pluralistic.

This diversity of spiritual grounding can have an enormous impact on how patients cope with death and dying from an existential perspective, and on decisions with regard to specific treatment options. We diminish spiritual care if we identify a particular religion, or none, with the aim of completing healthcare records or contacting a faith leader. Truly incorporating this knowledge into supportive, meaningful care demands that we engage in dialogue with patients about their specific wishes and needs.

Patients and carers are clear that they want us to acknowledge and address the spiritual dimension, and our failure to do so actually heightens their distress and affects the way that they perceive the competency of their care (National Council for Hospice and Specialist Palliative Care Services, 2003).

Role of education

Although patients want professionals to engage with the spiritual dimension, and guidelines suggest that everyone requires awareness, it seems unacceptable to expect a level of competence from staff who have received little or no educational preparation. Education has a poor record of preparing professionals, one of the major reasons for this being the focus on information giving. However, education is not just about providing cultural or clinical information, but rather about enabling professionals to have the courage to stay with those who are suffering, and to listen to their fears, hopes and beliefs.

Educationally we need to pay attention to the concepts of both art and science.

We cannot simply rely on analytical techniques and the acquisition of skills. Spiritual care is about developing a certain type of character, where we bring our whole being to the encounter with those who are weak and vulnerable (Byrne, 2002). Consequently, effective teaching and learning can only be accomplished through a range of strategies and approaches, both within and outside the classroom.

Although education can increase competence, it would also help staff to recognise their limitations, and the resources available to support and empower them. Factors to consider include the following:

- who should be included in educational programmes
- the implications for multi-disciplinary working
- the skills required by the professional caregiver
- creative approaches to teaching
- identifying the educator.

The professional caregiver

To determine educational initiatives, one must first identify the caregiver. Recent evidence and guidelines suggest that a multi-professional approach to spiritual care is required. The reasons for this include the following (National Institute for Clinical Excellence, 2004):

- an insufficient range of people to whom patients might turn for help
- insufficient numbers of chaplains within the hospital sector
- faith leaders who are not easily accessible or part of healthcare teams within primary care
- it is impossible for one care setting or professional group to take responsibility, given the definition of spirituality and the fact that spiritual needs change.

Whoever initiates the spiritual dialogue, the patient needs to understand that the subject is a legitimate aspect of care, and to feel affirmed in their spiritual journey (Heaven and Maguire, 1997). Deeply personal questions relating to spirituality may only be raised once, and the professional must be in a position to work with this. In a research study conducted by the author, one participant summed this up as 'seizing the moment' (Foster, 2001). This is analogous to the principles of breaking bad news. Other professionals may subsequently be involved, but it is crucial that the person who is first asked the difficult question responds appropriately.

Addressing spiritual support services for specialist palliative care, Marie Curie Cancer Care (2003) has defined four levels of competency for all staff, including volunteer workers.

- Level 1 – staff who have casual contact with patients to understand that all people have spiritual needs, which can be distinguished from religious needs.
- Level 2 – staff whose duties require contact with patients to understand how spiritual needs might be identified and responded to. This includes the ability to identify personal learning needs.
- Level 3 – members of the multi-disciplinary team are able to assess spiritual and religious need and develop a plan of care, recognising complex needs. This includes issues of confidentiality and documentation.
- Level 4 – professionals are able to manage complex spiritual and religious needs of patients, also acting as a spiritual and educational resource to others. At this level a clear understanding of personal beliefs is required.

This framework can be applied in order to consider educational provision within both specialist and generalist palliative care, recognising that all staff need to be included.

The skills required

For professional caregivers to engage with the spiritual dimension, it is necessary to identify the key skills required and to provide a clear educational emphasis on achieving these.

As well as developing new skills, all professionals need to recognise and celebrate the ways in which they already contribute. Spiritual care can be provided at an unconscious level, and education has a role in bringing this into a more conscious awareness (Milligan, 2004).

Communication skills

The quality and nature of the interpersonal relationship are critical to the delivery of competent spiritual care (Clark and Seymour, 1999). However, the therapeutic relationship requires underpinning skills. These include empathy, unconditional positive regard and genuineness. Importantly, not just the words themselves but also the way in which they are spoken, the pauses in between, and the body language that accompanies them are vital ingredients. Unsurprisingly, patients rate sensitive communication skills and presence higher than either technical or religious knowledge (Cornette, 1997). The question underpinning communication in spiritual care is not 'How are you?' but 'Who are you?' (Clark, 2002).

This defines spiritual work as hard work, and professionals require their own inner resources to stay with situations that potentially expose the vulnerability of both themselves and the patient.

Skilled companionship

Valuing the patient and providing a supportive, trustworthy presence is a way of validating the patient's self-worth. This is demonstrated by respectful attention, gentleness and silence. This is the profound but unspoken language of spirituality (Byrne, 2002). It involves recognising that it is not what we do that helps or heals, but who we are. Our very presence is part of the healing environment. We cannot be 'fixers' who provide the answer, as is so often the case in professional care, but instead we need to be attentively present while the patient explores the questions him- or herself, searching for meaning within the suffering.

This skilled companionship has been variously described as 'journeying together' (Stoter, 1995) and the 'spirituality of presence' (Cassidy, 1988). Although there are assessment tools for spiritual care, it is the self-aware use of presence that allows a real understanding of spirituality (Wright, 2005). We can use rhetoric and clinical models, but this skilled companionship is what people see us do, and through which they understand the genuineness of our concern. We need to learn to value this quality in ourselves and in others.

Self-awareness

Although we claim to be comfortable with notions of death and dying, there is little attention to humanistic principles in education, or emphasis on exploring our own beliefs (Cobb, 2001). However, personal experiences and beliefs affect the way in which we approach and interpret spiritual care (Foster, 2004). Therefore in order to help others we need to explore and understand this dimension for ourselves, reflecting on our motivations, prejudices and wounds, as learning to understand and accept ourselves is the cornerstone of person-centred care.

Healthcare professionals witness suffering on a daily basis, and this provides opportunities for change and growth. Education should help staff to acknowledge this challenge and prepare for it. The concept of burnout is viewed by some as the healthcare professional's own experience of spiritual distress (Wright and Sayre-Adams, 2000). If they are invited to explore spirituality, staff can clarify their individual values and identify their support mechanisms.

Creative approaches to spirituality and education

When considering the skills required for spiritual care, there is a need to think creatively about individual teaching techniques and how we expose professionals to spiritual concepts generally. The aim is to create the maximum potential for self-development and changed behaviour.

Developing workshops that include staff from different clinical settings or groups will enable staff to see how their skills contribute to the whole, enhancing the potential for learning both from and about each other. However, certain teaching approaches may be more familiar to some groups than others, with some participants being more confident about articulating their views and taking part in discussion. Given that all staff have a role to play, it would be equally appropriate to focus on discrete teams, exploring how each staff group can engage with the spiritual dimension.

Art and literature

The humanities offer a balance to the didactic approach, and allow course participants to explore a concrete expression of spiritual distress or harmony. This is working at a human level that we can all recognise, whatever our professional group. In multi-professional groups it can offer a bridge between professionals, helping them to achieve a universal understanding (Johnson and Jackson, 2005).

For example, discussing extracts from prose or poetry which contains examples of loss, suffering or transcendence helps to facilitate the use of language and communication skills that staff can utilise outside the classroom. It allows them to rehearse and prepare for talking with patients in a conscious and articulate way about spirituality.

Considering the way in which we use the words 'spiritual', 'inspiring' and 'dispiriting' in everyday conversation and in literature also helps to tease out the essence of spirituality.

In the USA, a number of medical schools are now teaching concepts of spirituality, using the humanities as a platform to explore this.

Case studies

Aldridge (2000) claims that we dismiss anecdotal material, but apart from the conference podium, this is how we understand the world on a daily basis. Case studies are available in textbooks, or educationalists may wish to develop their own case material.

Case studies are a potent catalyst for reflection and discussion, enabling healthcare professionals to understand how spiritual needs arise, and how reported physical symptoms or behaviour can be an expression of those needs. This includes exploring what constitutes a spiritual question or an instance of spiritual distress.

Combining the use of literature and case studies, the author has used the children's tale of Paddington Bear as an 'anonymous' case study, exploring all of the issues with which Paddington finds himself confronted – geographical dislocation, loss of family identity and support, and abandonment. When Paddington is finally 'revealed', this usually leads to humour, which can ease the tension in such a complex subject. Given the multi-cultural diversity of educational groups, considerable reflection has gone into considering whether this was an appropriate image to use. However, to date the feedback has been positive. Even those who are unfamiliar with this story have been able to recognise both the pathos and humour that it contains.

Spiritual practices

Spiritual practices and ritual give form and guidance at times of great vulnerability. Such practices may include religious observance, meditation, or the development of creative pursuits.

Rather than viewing them as a list of requirements, workshops could include discussion on the spiritual significance and personal meaning of these practices, exploring how we can facilitate time and space for them in the context of home and clinical environments. Workshops could also consider increasing awareness of the daily routines that give our own lives meaning, and our reactions to and feelings about providing this space for others.

Because spirituality is anchored in everyday experiences, the physical environment is important. We therefore need to understand how we can create healing space in the various care settings. This includes, for example, our use of religious symbols, art, music, literature, colour and aroma.

Model of spirituality

Utilising the above-mentioned image of the football to depict spirituality, healthcare professionals could consider how they attend to each of the components in the personal stories that they encounter. They could then reflect on how these factors can affect the needs of a patient, and how they might be aware of and respond to those needs. Different groups could examine the model from different professional perspectives, or use it as a framework to give direction when exploring more focused case studies.

When working with healthcare professional groups or individuals, this model also provides a structure that enables them to begin to map their own support systems.

Journals/supervision

Reflective strategies may be employed throughout a course and beyond it to help to facilitate self-awareness and understanding. They provide rich opportunities to uncover thoughts, feelings and behaviours, enabling the healthcare professional to gain a greater understanding of him- or herself as a result (Schon, 1987). They can be used to clarify responses to art and literature or the model of spirituality, and to reflect on clinical experience, which may be a gateway to the bigger spiritual questions. A structured reflection tool could be used, or in the case of a journal, personal artistic expression could be incorporated. (This type of reflective journal writing will be explored in detail in the third book of this series.)

Another approach would be to explore 'presence' by sitting in stillness for a short period of time as a group, or in pairs, with or without touch. This can allow the participant to understand and process reflectively in journal writing their feelings associated with this, and the possible barriers. The central factor is the healthcare professional's commitment, and the availability of support if and when difficult issues surface.

Identifying the educator

Given the multi-professional nature of spiritual care, this philosophy can be translated into educational provision, recognising that the teaching of spirituality is not the prerogative of one group or setting. Crucially, as with the provision of spiritual care, it is best taught by those who have an awareness and acceptance of their own spirituality (McSherry, 2000). Those with a genuine interest in this aspect of education are already likely to be involved in reflecting on their own life philosophy. Becker (2004) considers that cancer and palliative care education is arguably unique, and that a 'reflective maturity' is required of the educators. This seems particularly appropriate here. Importantly, in teaching the concept sensitively and with empathy, the teacher is role modelling spiritual care.

Delivering spiritual care in a curriculum as an isolated module or workshop appears to be at odds with the very concept. However, because spirituality is a thread running through all aspects of palliative care, we can underpin this by acknowledging spirituality in other topic areas, too – for example, within presentations on the experience of pain, the breaking of bad news, and loss and bereavement. If the educator has a remit to teach other sessions, this will better enable this topic to be integrated. Ideally, for registered professionals it would be appropriate to instigate the topic of spirituality in undergraduate education as a theme, so that students' understanding of the subject develops in line with their experience.

Spirituality requires attention both within and outside the classroom to truly demonstrate its validity and to change practice. Providing support and supervision outside the classroom suggests that clinical and educational areas need to work together in a synergistic manner. This takes us back to the beginning, recognising the importance of increasing the awareness of all staff. It also suggests that the educator could be someone who has both educational and clinical responsibility, in order to maximise this collaboration.

The individual who takes an educational lead, with its challenges and responsibilities, requires commitment to ongoing study and supervision. This could range across focused study days, conferences, theology degrees, courses related to interfaith perspectives and mentoring relationships. We must honour opportunities for personal development as educators, and be committed to enhancing the very same skills as those required for spiritual care.

Key points

- Spirituality is a universal dimension.
- As effective spiritual care requires a multi-professional approach, all staff must have an awareness of spirituality. However, certain professionals need to develop further expertise.
- Education has a role in effectively preparing staff to address spiritual care. This is wider than information giving, and includes an emphasis on exploring personal experience and developing self-awareness.

- Education needs to take the long view, recognising that encouraging staff to reflect on their own spirituality requires time and ongoing support.
- Spirituality needs to be acknowledged and addressed in other areas of palliative and cancer care education, which includes working collaboratively with clinical environments.
- The educator should have an awareness of their own spirituality and be committed to self-development, interfaith dialogue and respect for humanistic values.

Conclusion

While recognising that spirituality is important and profound, we should not over-complicate it to a point where we become incapacitated. Like many changes in practice, it can begin with small incremental changes. By improving our communication skills and valuing ourselves as part of the therapeutic environment, we must have the courage to take the first steps. We should ask patients what lifts their spirits and what dispirits them, what gives them strength and hope, and how we as professionals are able to support them. With the patient's permission we could include this information in our documentation, rather than restricting the patient experience to sterile descriptions of practical care. Similarly, in multi-professional settings we should aspire to be advocates, recognising that if we do not acknowledge the spiritual dimension we cannot hope to provide holistic care. We ought to review and refresh our surroundings.

Education has enormous potential to facilitate these changes, but we need to take the 'long view', recognising that changes in practice take place over time as self-awareness, knowledge and appropriate confidence develop. Both the educator and the clinician have the capacity to act as pebbles in a pool, initiating new ways of thinking and being.

The beginning of spiritual care in part involves reflecting on what we already do and who we are, and recognising the significance of this, perhaps for the first time. It is also about enhancing the humanistic and pastoral aspects of our work, which can then be a stimulus for our own spiritual journey. Again we are back at the beginning, as this exposes our vulnerability alongside our expertise. It is a paradox, because the experience of vulnerability is the place from which we develop our reflective maturity and insights about what it is to be human, so that we may stand alongside those who are suffering, and listen to the full depth of their experience.

> *No man can reveal to you aught but that which already lies half asleep in the dawning of your knowledge. The teacher ... if he is indeed wise ... does not bid you enter the house of his wisdom, but rather leads you to the threshold of your own mind.*
>
> *Kahil Gibran*

Implications for the reader's own practice

1 What examples of art/literature/music might you use in a teaching session to generate discussion on the issues of suffering and loss?
2 What innovative ways can you think of to develop multi-faith and multi-cultural understanding in your educational and/or clinical setting?
3 What could you do to ensure that students who are exploring spirituality are adequately supported while considering their own values and beliefs?
4 How do you reflect on your own spiritual values and remain committed to self-development?
5 How would you motivate other healthcare professionals to include spiritual awareness in their educational and/or clinical area?

References

Aldridge D. *Spirituality, Healing and Medicine. Return to the silence*. London: Jessica Kingsley Publishers; 2000.

Becker R. Education in cancer and palliative care: an international perspective. In: Foyle L, Hostad J, editors. *Delivering Cancer and Palliative Care Education*. Oxford: Radcliffe Publishing; 2004.

Byrne M. Spirituality in palliative care: what language do we need? *Int J Palliat Nurs*. 2002; **8**: 67–74.

Cassidy S. *Sharing the Darkness. The spirituality of caring*. London: Darton Longman and Todd; 1988.

Clark D, Seymour J. *Reflections on Palliative Care*. Buckingham: Open University Press; 1999.

Clark B. Spirituality and ethnicity. In: Charlton R, editor. *Primary Palliative Care. Dying, death and bereavement in the community*. Oxford: Radcliffe Medical Press; 2002.

Cobb M. *The Dying Soul. Spiritual care at the end of life*. Buckingham: Open University Press; 2001.

Cornette K. For whenever I am weak, I am strong ... *Int J Palliat Nurs*. 1997; **3**: 6–13.

Foster E. *A study of the qualified nurse's perception of spirituality and spiritual care in the palliative care settings of a hospice and a nursing home*. Unpublished MSc dissertation, University of Hull, 2001.

Foster E. Exploring the territory: nurses' perceptions of spirituality and the implications for nursing care and education. In: Foyle L, Hostad J, editors. *Delivering Cancer and Palliative Care Education*. Oxford: Radcliffe Publishing; 2004.

Greenstreet W. Teaching spirituality in nursing: a literature review. *Nurse Educ Today*. 1999; **19**: 649–58.

Heaven CM, Maguire P. Disclosure of concerns by hospice patients and their identification by nurses. *Palliat Med*. 1997; **11**: 283–90.

Johnson A, Jackson D. Using the arts and humanities to support learning about loss, suffering and death. *Int J Palliat Nurs*. 2005; **11**: 438–43.

McSherry W. *Making Sense of Spirituality in Nursing Practice. An interactive approach*. London: Churchill Livingstone; 2000.

McSherry W, Draper P. The debates emerging from the literature surrounding the concept of spirituality as applied to nursing. *J Adv Nurs*. 1998; **27**: 683–91.

Marie Curie Cancer Care. *Spiritual and Religious Care Competencies for Specialist Palliative Care*. London: Marie Curie Cancer Care; 2003.

Milligan S. Perceptions of spiritual care among nurses undertaking post-registration education. *Int J Palliat Nurs*. 2004; **10**: 162–71.

National Council for Hospice and Specialist Palliative Care Services (NCHSPCS). *Care of the Dying and the NHS: some carers' views*. London: NCHSPCS; 2003.

National Institute for Clinical Excellence. *Guidance on Cancer Services. Improving supportive and palliative care for adults with cancer.* London: National Institute for Clinical Excellence; 2004.

Schon DA. *Educating the Reflective Practitioner.* San Francisco, CA: Jossey Bass; 1987.

Stoter D. *Spiritual Aspects of Health Care.* London: Mosby; 1995.

Wright S. *Reflections on Spirituality and Health.* London: Whurr Publishers; 2005.

Wright S, Sayre-Adams J. *Sacred Space. Right relationship and spirituality in health care.* Edinburgh: Churchill Livingstone; 2000.

Chapter 17

'Let's talk about it – we never do.' Sexual health in cancer and palliative care: an educational dilemma?

Janis Hostad

> *If we fail to assess each patient's sexuality, we are denying them of their fundamental human right.*
>
> *Parke (1991)*

Aim

One of the aims of this chapter is to provide an overview of the complexity, diversity and sensitivity of issues related to sexual health affecting cancer and palliative care patients and their families.

However, the primary and most vital aim is to examine the difficulties involved in teaching such a challenging subject, which not only has many dimensions but also, due to its sensitivity, remains shrouded in taboos and myths. This involves finding successful ways of teaching the topic to ultimately improve this specific aspect of care for the patient, with the minimum of embarrassment and the maximum dignity and respect.

Learning outcomes

- Understand the importance of this subject in relation to cancer and palliative care.
- Reflect on the complexity and elusive nature of sexuality, and consequently the difficulties involved in teaching this topic.
- Appreciate the need to balance the challenging of students' beliefs and attitudes, while at the same time role modelling the sensitivity that they will require when dealing with patients.
- Consider different approaches to achieving success in teaching the topic, so that students may meet each patient's individual requirements with skill, tact, diplomacy and confidentiality.

Introduction

This chapter encourages the reader not only to challenge their approaches to teaching this topic, but also, as a result, to re-examine their own beliefs, attitudes and vulnerability, and to question whether such issues and views could impact on their teaching. It is intended that the content will be both thought provoking and challenging.

> *Trying to achieve sexual rehabilitation is a mission that could well fit into our own idealistic perception of our profession. Let us strive to make it a standard aspect of nursing care all over the world.*
>
> Yaniv (1992)

It may not be possible for us all to be evangelists like Yaniv. However, if everyone tries to improve this standard aspect of holistic palliative care in their own area (across all disciplines, not just nursing), then perhaps one day a global improvement may be accomplished. To this end, it is anticipated that this chapter will work in some small way to achieve this aim. The problems related to teaching this topic, and integrating this learning back into practice, are due to four main factors.

- Sexuality is not easy to define.
- Sexuality includes aspects of people's lives that usually remain private.
- Only limited research has been undertaken in this field.
- There is a lack of training and education available in this field.

All of these issues will be discussed and debated, and some thoughts, ideas and solutions will be offered. Other questions are left for the reader to ponder and to find their own solutions that are unique to their own specific patient groups, their students and their locality.

Over the years, little attention has been paid to this topic, even though it continues to be clear that these patients' needs are not being dealt with (Gamlin, 2005). Equally, the topic has not been addressed in the classroom (Grigg, 1997). It seems a great shame that so little effort has been activated in teaching and learning about sexuality in cancer and palliative care, especially in view of the fact that when workshops have been conducted where healthcare professionals have the opportunity to explore issues related to sexuality, a more positive approach has been adopted (Frazer *et al.*, 1982; Kautz *et al.*, 1990; Matocha and Waterhouse, 1993; Hostad, 1999). A number of publications have highlighted this lack of specific training available for healthcare professionals in relation to sexual health issues (Purdie, 1996; Waterhouse, 1996; Crouch, 1999).

The content of this chapter is the result of this author's experience of having run many workshops over a number of years. These have included different groups, course durations and venues. Each session has generated new ideas, challenges and discoveries, which have then been incorporated into subsequent workshops, resulting in useful strategies and approaches.

Based on the above, the contents of this chapter are often a personal view, underpinned where possible with appropriate theory. One of the vital features of the training and education described here is that it is experiential in nature. Not only is it a way to provide specific facts and to focus on the wider aspects of sexuality, but it also raises issues relating to belief systems, prejudices and comfort zones. This allows attitudes and personal values to be gently challenged in a safe environment.

As the chapter develops, possible teaching approaches, activities and methods will be suggested for consideration by the reader. However, in order to discuss various aspects of teaching this subject, the difficulties and complexity of defining the topic need to be demonstrated in the first instance. This is one of the main problem areas with regard to education in this topic, as already mentioned.

The difficulties of definition

Sexuality means different things to different people, and there are a myriad definitions – some very similar, some very different. There is a school of thought which suggests that many of these definitions are too complex, and therefore somewhat elusive (Fonseca, 1970; Rafferty, 1995).

Indeed, Rafferty proposes that finding an effective, short, simple definition is fraught with difficulties, due among other things to the powerful and emotive nature of the topic.

While some authors limit their definition of sexuality to the sexual act (Hohman, 1972), others provide a much broader definition, taking into account the holistic nature of sexuality, and the fact that the identity of an individual cannot be separated from their sexuality (Stuart and Sundeen, 1979; Hogan, 1980; Savage, 1987).

Stuart and Sundeen (1979) reinforce the notion of the uniqueness of every person. However, Hogan (1980) chooses to underline the diversity of ways in which sexuality may be expressed, including perceptions of male and female roles, and interpersonal expressions of affection. These latter definitions refer to the whole person, including his or her thoughts, experiences, learning, ideas, values, fantasies and emotions, and to being male or female. The World Health Organization (1986) has published a description of what they describe as the three elements of sexual health:

1 a capacity to enjoy and control sexual and reproductive behaviour in accordance with a social and personal ethic
2 freedom from fear, shame, guilt, false beliefs and other psychological factors which inhibit sexual response and impair sexual relationships
3 freedom from organic disorders, diseases and deficiencies which interfere with sexual and reproductive functions.

An earlier definition of sexual health, also published by the World Health Organization (1975), was as follows:

> The integration of the social, emotional, intellectual and social aspects of sexual being in ways which are positively enriching, and which enhance personality, communications and love.

The concern is that this holistic multi-dimensional complex phenomenon may be confusing, and that it may be considered to be related solely to sexual intercourse rather than to who the person is, from birth to death. Girts (1990) separates the two succinctly, defining sex as something that we do, and sexuality as something that we are. Poorman (1988) reinforces this by suggesting that sexuality is interwoven with every aspect of human existence, and is expressed and lived in our daily lives, and in how we relate to our friends, family and work.

The healthcare professionals and educators working in cancer and palliative care need to be able to define sexuality, as they have a vital role to play in the promotion of the importance of sexual health, and its future dynamic progress.

Providing an exact scientific definition of sexuality is somewhat like trying to catch a shooting star, as sexuality is a dynamic, multi-faceted, lifelong process. However, trying to capture the essence of this in a classroom is essential. Rather than showing a series of PowerPoint slides detailing the many available definitions, it is useful to let the students do the work themselves. To gain a clearer perception of the difficulties related to definition, and to act as a catalyst for wider debate, educators might use the following activity.

Exercise 1(a)

Divide the students into small groups, with flipchart and pens.
Ask the groups to:

1 brainstorm and list all of the elements which are important and relevant to our sexuality
2 on a separate sheet, decide on a composite definition of sexuality (one which all members of the group can agree upon).

Discuss within the full group the different elements that they have documented, and the reasons why they have done so.

This exercise is more difficult if only a definition is requested, especially if the students have never considered the topic before. However, by asking them to first consider all of the different elements, this allows 'thinking outside the box.' Much more lateral thinking seems to provide a wider definition, and allows students to discuss elements of sexuality which they might not otherwise have considered.

The second part of the exercise can then match the theory to the practice.

Exercise 1(b)

Ask the students to comment on a number of the definitions (perhaps on PowerPoint).

What are the differences and similarities to their own definition?

Are there any different implications as a result of using any of these in practice?

This seems to be a very good way of starting a session. However, prior to this, much thought needs to go into the setting and observance of ground rules. This must be the precursor to any such session.

Ground rules

Ground rules are always important, especially when teaching with an experiential workshop-type approach (Faulkner, 1993). They are also important when role modelling different approaches with the participants, which you would in turn expect them to utilise with patients. Having ground rules can add to participants' comfort, as they have been involved, and have agreed to the rules for the session. These rules often include such aspects as being punctual, switching off mobile phones, respecting others and their point of view, the option to opt in or opt out, and treating all comments as confidential.

As a facilitator, confidentiality needs to be a priority and must be handled carefully. Often facilitators remind participants about their code of conduct (e.g. do not mention patients by name, or say anything which might identify them). The facilitators may also inform the participants that this confidentiality does not prevent them from cascading the session's general information, and its application, to others on return to their own clinical setting. However, what often fails to be mentioned is that confidentiality agreements at the beginning of a course are not legally binding! This is particularly relevant in this field, as it is not uncommon for participants to share sensitive personal details.

The author is aware of a number of occasions when sharing within the group was encouraged by facilitators (after confidentiality had been agreed as part of the ground rules), to the detriment of the participants. On one occasion, these self-revelations, which were intended to increase self-awareness, included one individual stating (for the first time) that she was gay. Subsequently, she was seen by the manager of the gynaecological department where she worked, and was asked whether she considered it appropriate for her to work in this specialty, given her sexual orientation. While the manager's approach was totally unacceptable, the fact was that confidentiality had been breached, which is vitally important in this context.

How can you be expected to trust implicitly fellow participants whom you have never met previously? The author always reiterates the above example (or a similar one, of which there are many), suggesting that participants should only share information which they would be comfortable about being public knowledge.

This usually leads to discussions about the confidential nature of intimate conversations with patients, and these being shared with other colleagues. It may not always be necessary to share all information with the entire team (Becker and Gamlin, 2004). It is useful to explore with the group when it is appropriate to share such information, and when it is not.

Within any teaching session, the aims of the session need to be ascertained. This is particularly important in view of the sensitive nature of the topic, and relating this to the time available and the number of participants in the group. What you could accomplish in an informal setting with 8 or 10 students is going to be very different to what could be achieved with 80 to 100 students in a lecture theatre.

Versatility of teaching style and methods is of paramount importance, in order not only to engage the students, but also to enable them to learn, and to examine and challenge their own practice.

The methods might include carefully thought out self-awareness exercises, case studies, reflective accounts, critical incidents, discussions that relate to specific problems, role play, use of actors, patient involvement, questionnaires, action learning, problem solving, group work, goldfish-bowl exercises, and many more.

There are in fact some reports and studies which state that students prefer group work, and that it is the most useful way of learning about issues related to sexuality (Dow and Schlone, 1982; Hostad, 1999).

If the aim is to raise awareness, the activity will be somewhat different to that which would be used if the aim was to change attitudes. It has to be acknowledged that it is difficult for clinicians to address this potentially very embarrassing topic with patients (Booth, 1990; Kautz *et al.*, 1990; Bor and Watts, 1993; Lewis and Bor, 1994; Clifford, 2000). However, if we accept this, then we need to realise that it might also be difficult to address the topic in the classroom.

This point can be very effectively illustrated to the class by asking them to consider how many people they would confide in about problems and issues of an intimate nature related to sexuality. Very few would talk to anyone other than their partner, a close friend, or both.

It can be very useful in a short awareness-raising session to invite the students to think about how they would react to and feel about their own sexuality, relating this to different aspects of the topic. They should then collectively brainstorm all the different possible answers, most importantly considering the implications and possible consequences of each answer. This exercise aims to increase self-awareness, which is vitally important, but because the students don't need to have personal owner-ship of their contributions it is not too threatening.

> *Education and training in sexual health have to take into account that within this area of care there is a delicate interface between 'professional' and 'per-sonal.'*
>
> *English National Board (1994)*

One effective way to engender student participation would be to provide the group with literature which illustrates that patients, although they may feel embarrassed, still wish the professional to start the conversation (Kreuger *et al.*, 1979; Baggs and Karch, 1987; Jenkins, 1988; Young *et al.*, 1989, Waterhouse and Metcalfe, 1991). Dividing students into groups and asking them to talk about how best to broach the topic, and how to tackle such problems in their own area, prompts much debate and discussion. It also encourages those who perhaps were not too sure about the importance of the topic to begin to increase their awareness of it.

Teaching about sexuality in the context of illness and treatment related to cancer and palliative care

> *Almost all patients with advanced cancer and non-malignant disease experience debilitating fatigue at some time during their illness.*
>
> *Gamlin (2005, p. 204)*

Accepting that this axiom is true, all healthcare professionals should have a good working knowledge of how their particular patient group is affected. This includes situations involving fatigue, surgery, wounds, breathlessness, syringe drivers, cath-eters, pain, weight gain, weight loss, nausea, constipation, effects or side-effects of drugs, depression and anxiety.

Some of the above may be applicable to all patients, while others may have specific implications for certain diseases and treatments.

Little has been written on the above issues in relation to sexuality, and it has been reported that some staff suggest that if a person is dying, such matters are considered irrelevant (Hostad, 1999; Searle, 2005).

One way to get students to focus on this aspect is described below.

Exercise 2

Ask the students in the group to list all of the different ways in which patients' sexuality is affected by their illness and treatment.

Report back and discuss the group's findings.

Develop this further by giving each student a card with one of the above-mentioned problems written on it.

Ask each student to suggest how this problem might affect their patient group and, if they wish to do so, how it would affect them.

Then ask all members of the group to contribute their suggestions about each problem.

This exercise is designed to increase awareness of the extent to which patients' sexuality is affected, and to increase students' empathy.

Another way to increase students' awareness is by the use of case studies. Gamlin (2005) provides a poignant extract from *Cancer Ward* by Solzhenitsyn (1968) to make his point most incisively. This extract transfers most effectively to the learning environment (*see* Further reading section at the end of this chapter).

The author has a colleague who is a cancer patient (and who was formerly a Macmillan nurse). She not only shares her experiences with various groups for teaching purposes, but her moving account is contextualised and conceptualised particularly effectively due to her background.

Exercise 3 (The Patient's Account)

A moving, eloquent and emotional account by a patient, whether written or verbally presented, always has a strong effect on the group.

It is usually accompanied by questions which the facilitator asks the group, such as the following.

- What do you think was good about the care that was provided?
- What do you think led to the negative aspects of the care?
- What do you think could have been done to improve the care?

The exercise is completed by asking the patient how they feel that the various aspects of their treatment and care could have been improved.

This type of exercise always generates much useful dialogue between students and patient.

The author has a number of patients who are willing to tell their personal story in this way. The preparation, training, utilisation and support of these individuals as trainers is beyond the scope of this chapter. However, it will be discussed in detail in the third book of this series.

The following activity is less emotive and emotional, but nevertheless very useful.

If the students are on a longer course, they can be asked to report back on the care related to sexuality in their areas for the next session. This should include both positive and negative aspects. How did they achieve success with the good practice? What are they doing to improve the bad practice?

In another similar homework-type exercise, the students are asked to return and share information on how medications specific to their specialty affect their patients' sexuality. When they present this research to the group, everyone benefits from the knowledge and ideas of their fellow students.

Body image

Body image is sometimes taught separately, as if it were a different topic. However, the author would suggest that 'sexuality' is the umbrella term, and 'body image' is one aspect of this, although nevertheless a very axiomatic element of the overall topic. This aspect is often very distressing, disturbing and damaging to this client group. Much has been written about this specific aspect of sexuality (Piff, 1985; Anderson and Wolf, 1986; Dewing, 1989; MacGregor, 1989, 1990; Price, 1990; Burbie and Polinsky, 1992; Salter, 1997; Newell, 1998). In the field of cancer and palliative care, the literature suggests that body image problems tend to be addressed when they relate to a specific body part.

> *Perhaps in such circumstances, sexual implications are more overt, and clinicians can be confident that sexuality is a legitimate focus of care.*
>
> *Cort et al. (2004)*

There are a number of models related to body image which might be useful (Price, 1990; Salter, 1997; Newell, 1999). However, Newell (1999) recognises the inherent danger of following one specific model. He examines the over-emphasis of certain aspects by some of the models. Although there have been some criticisms of Bob Price's model, it has much to offer in a classroom situation. In particular, his book entitled *Body Image* has useful exercises at the end of each chapter, which could be utilised to very good effect.

So far, the author has considered the main issues with regard to the wider aspects of body image and sexuality. However, it has to be borne in mind that even a dying patient with low libido may still wish to engage in the sexual act from time to time. Education about how this might be achieved should be included when teaching students how to talk to patients and how to assess their patients' needs (*see* below).

Relationships, love and intimacy

In most cases, a couple's sexual relationship will remain deeply private. When a patient is diagnosed with cancer or some other life-threatening illness, their relationship will be affected. This may affect their usual levels of intimacy, and their ways of giving and receiving love. Patients often question whether they can still be found attractive when they are thin and emaciated, or disfigured, or have a catheter, a colostomy, bad odour, no hair, or any of many other problems. In fact, some relationships continue to thrive and the couple remain close, whereas other relationships fail because one or the other partner cannot see beyond (or cope with) the presenting problem. An excellent list of the fears of such patients has been presented by Gamlin (2005, p. 209). For most couples, the desire is not for sexual intercourse, but for closeness and intimacy. They need their partners to touch them, hold them and talk to them. Coping with cancer and dying can be very lonely without the closeness of loved ones to share the journey.

Helping patients and their relatives to come to terms with their problems can be very rewarding. However, as a teacher, one should explain that outcomes are not always successful. Indeed, many participants talk of couples whom they have nursed, and whose relationship was never the same again, the illness acting as the catalyst for its subsequent failure.

Within most healthcare settings, some information (albeit minimal) is available. However, ongoing support for patients and their partners is limited. This is a crucial area, which therefore needs to be reiterated in the classroom! It is important to emphasise to students how painful and daunting it must be to cope with the feelings of loss that both partners can experience when faced with a life-threatening illness which may ultimately lead to the death of one of them (Searle, 2002; Cort *et al.*, 2004).

The author remembers a bereaved husband who never hugged, loved or touched his wife after she was diagnosed, because he was fearful that he might hurt her. Subsequently he felt that he had been denied his right to comfort her, to say goodbye to her properly, and to be at one with her before she died.

It is easy to see how his wife might have felt, suddenly bereft of all the normal intimacy that they had shared. It is very saddening to know that a simple conversation with them both would have remedied the issue at the time, and prevented the husband's subsequent problems during his bereavement.

Different scenarios like this could be presented to the group for discussion. Actors can be very useful here, both to allow the student to practise in safety, and also when teaching very large groups, to allow the student to participate at a more 'feeling' level. (This will be discussed in greater depth in the third book in this series.)

Searle (2005) has presented a very workable model, adapted from Sternberg's theory of love, which may be utilised to teach some of these intimate aspects of care (*see* Figure 17.1).

Whilst Searle substitutes the central theme of love with sexuality, perhaps both should be emphasised, each one being equally important in different ways. As a result, this model has been further adapted to include love and sexuality.

The uniqueness of the triangle is defined by the individual. Sternberg states that there should be a close match between our own triangle and that of our partner when they are placed together. Further details can be found in a chapter in which Searle (2005, p. 130) illustrates clearly how useful these diagrams can be.

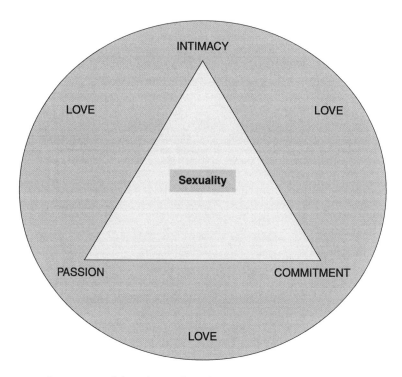

Figure 17.1 The concept of the relationship (the rudiments of a model). Based on the work of Searle.

Exercise 4

An exercise which has worked well with groups involves teaching them about Sternberg's theory, and then giving them one or two detailed case histories of different relationships between couples.

The students then discuss in groups what type of relationship it is (well matched, closely matched or mismatched).

(This exercise can be extended by looking at each case history and asking the group 'What would happen if ...?', posing different hypothetical situations which might affect the dynamics of the relationship.)

The students then discuss the possible implications of using such a model in practice.

Finally, they may consider formulating a different model of their own.

It is important to acknowledge that, for most individuals, having and maintaining a close relationship is of paramount importance during such life crises. Expressing and receiving love are among life's most rewarding and treasured experiences. The more help that is given to the practitioner by the teacher, the more acceptable the patient's journey may be, and the more cherished the memories for the bereaved.

Teaching about sexual orientation: can it work in the classroom?

The previous section discussed relationships, and this aspect could undoubtedly be incorporated within it. However, this topic was considered too important by the author not to have a separate section devoted to it. Literature in this area continues to indicate that lesbians and gay men are discriminated against in all areas of their lives, and this attitude is pervasive throughout society (Deaney, 1989; Plummer, 1992; Rose, 1993; Wilton, 2000).

> *Until relatively recently, the argument shaping homosexuality in Euro-American societies was so deeply rooted that it was not thought necessary to explain why being homosexual disqualified one from basic human and civil rights.*
>
> Wilton (2000, p. 136)

There often seems to be a misconception that lesbians, gay men and bisexuals are campaigning for 'special treatment', when all that they are requesting is to share other users' fundamental human rights and needs, and to be dealt with in an appropriate way. This misconception is perpetuated by cultures, society, religions and the communication media's beliefs about what is 'normal.'

Sadly, the view that heterosexuality is 'normal' and homosexuality is 'abnormal' pervades the thinking of most countries worldwide. Although there have been some changes, most recently in the West, in many countries around the world homosexuality remains illegal and very much a taboo subject.

Lesbian and gay subcultures continue to grow slowly and thrive, giving much needed support to one another. However, when an individual from the gay population requires healthcare, it can be a very lonely place.

Social exclusion has diminished over the last few decades in most Western societies, and tolerance has increased. However, it is still far from being an accepting, equal society, and as Wilton (2000, p. 1) says, 'tolerance exists side by side with the extremes of prejudices.'

Most healthcare services are no exception to this, and literature paints a rather depressing picture of discrimination against these minority groups being rife. Platzer (1993) supports this view, commenting that as a result of being subject to bias and prejudices, lesbians and gay men can be marginalised within all healthcare settings.

Corr (1991) suggests that nurses have a poor knowledge of homosexuality, and this in turn results in their responding inadequately to the needs of homosexual patients. Irwin (1997) postulates that gay patients are often avoided, ridiculed and exposed to a range of negative behaviours. Homophobic nurses have reported high levels of apprehension about caring for people who have a diagnosis of AIDS (Taylor and Robertson, 1994).

Research conducted by the author contained vignettes in which a dying female patient asks if her partner can sleep with her at the hospice, because she is feeling lonely and frightened.

Most of the respondents said that they would cope with the situation, but felt uncomfortable, shocked and awkward. One respondent actually wrote 'totally disgusted!' It is interesting that only in this vignette (relating to homosexuality) did the responses refer to the patient's needs as a 'problem.'

The respondents were also given a separate long list of factors that might improve or inhibit their ability to discuss issues of sexuality with patients. By far the greatest inhibiting factor was the patient being gay, with 88% of the participants highlighting this as a major inhibiting factor.

These factors were measured again at the end of the sexuality workshop. Although the overall learning was significant, the area with the lowest shift as a result of learning was this topic.

It is a great challenge for all educators to incorporate this topic into their teaching. It breaks all the taboos of cancer, death, dying and homosexuality. Given the level of growing evidence of poor practice, both research based and anecdotal, it really is time to act!

Take care when choosing which exercises to use, as some do not always have positive effects. Some of the negative personal experiences of attending previous workshops will deter participants from revisiting the topic. These experiences include being asked to share their first sexual encounter with the group, or to place themselves on an imaginary 'sexual orientation' continuum that runs across the classroom (like the continuum described by Kinsey *et al.*, 1948). The latter exercise is supposedly designed to illustrate how heterosexual or gay the participants are! Educationalists should think carefully about the implications and consequences of such activities. They have a very responsible role which cannot be compromised, and the learning outcomes for the student should always aim to be positive, as this will ultimately benefit their patients.

The following exercises may be useful ways of introducing the topic gently.

Exercise 5 (the Facilitator)

Collect a number of mainstream magazines, as well as a number of specifically lesbian and gay magazines.

Divide the students into groups, with some participants looking at heterosexual magazines, and some looking at the lesbian and gay magazines.

Mainstream magazines:

- Are there any articles related to gay issues?
- How are couples depicted?
- How could they be different?
- How would you feel if they depicted same-sex couples embracing?

Gay and lesbian magazines:

- Are they what you expected?
- How did you think they might be different?
- How do they make you feel?
- How could they be different?

The groups should then exchange magazines and give feedback collectively.

They can then discuss what is similar, and what is different.

Adapted from Wilton (2000)

Some of the underpinning theory and relevant information could be taught at this point. However, a word of warning – even the above seemingly innocuous exercise may cause much heated discussion and emotional distress. If you are new to teaching this topic, it is wise to initially teach as part of a team if possible. This is particularly useful if the person who teaches with you is already experienced, so that you can learn from their responses, sensitive interactions and gentle challenges.

The following exercise also proves useful.

Exercise 6

Present a number of cancer and palliative care scenarios and vignettes that include sexual orientation-specific elements.

Then ask the students individually to state what they would expect, like, dislike and feel if they were the patient.

Brainstorm all four of these categories (expectations, likes, dislikes and feelings) as lists and discuss them. This exercise is more effective if it is completed individually in a small group. However, it can be useful when teaching a larger audience, if it is conducted in smaller groups.

Finally, ask the group to state what the implications of this exercise are for their practice.

Often discussions include patient documentation, such as admission questions, which assumes heterosexual orientation. For example, the question 'Are you married?' should be changed to 'Do you have a partner?'. Caulfield and Platzer (1998) suggest that 'next of kin' in care plans should be replaced with 'contact person.' Fortunately, this admission information is improving.

Other discussion revolves around partners being excluded from the care of their loved one, because they have not 'come out.' Sadly, it is a common experience for a gay partner to be excluded from the funeral of their loved one.

The Royal College of Nursing (1994) has recognised the discrimination and prejudices faced by lesbian and gay patients. Their document entitled *The Nursing Care of Lesbians and Gay Men* outlines their commitment to developing and promoting good nursing practice for this minority group, and all educators would do well to familiarise themselves with this document.

An excellent book by Wilton (2000), entitled *Sexualities in Health and Social Care: a textbook*, addresses these issues eloquently and provides excellent exercises which could be adapted by a skilful teacher to reflect issues related to cancer and palliative care.

'Let's talk about it' – assessing and supporting patients' sexual needs: educational underpinnings

This chapter has already discussed how to deal with some specific aspects of sexuality. However, a simple assessment model (PLISSIT) has been effectively utilised across not only different healthcare settings but also different social settings, by Relate counsellors and social workers, among others (Annon, 1976).

This model may be successfully used to benefit cancer and palliative care patients who need help, support and information with regard to sexual matters.

Permission

The healthcare professional sets the scene, and either initiates the discussion or gives the patient permission to do so by raising the topic, and ensures that the patient understands how and when they are personally available should they wish to discuss matters further.

Limited information

If the patient does not wish to talk, they may want to have written information to take away and read. This may involve specific facts (e.g. 'It is not possible to pass the cancer on by having sexual intercourse because ...').

Specific suggestions

This involves providing both simple and complex advice. These types of suggestions will mainly be generated by the patient's (and their partner's) questions. Having knowledge of the professional's own expertise (e.g. the effects of treatment) will help to provide more accurate answers, along with good communication skills.

Intensive therapy

As some problems are sometimes much more complex than was initially realised, the patient and/or their partner may benefit from being referred to a sexual counsellor, a therapist or a clinical psychologist.

This model is illustrated in Figure 17.2 and highlights levels of intervention.

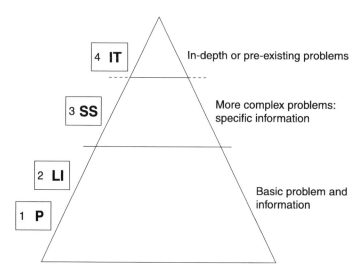

Figure 17.2 The PLISSIT model. Adapted from Annon (1976).

With the help of education, training and good clinical supervision, the healthcare professional should be able to increase their knowledge and skill in order to be able to support their patients up to the dotted line shown in Figure 17.2. It has been suggested that healthcare professionals can support the patient at the first two levels, and can be trained up to the third level (Schover, 1993; Zarwid, 1994).

Exercise 7

The case studies or scenarios that the students have already worked on could be returned to at this point.

Ask the groups to determine how much of this model they have already used, and what else they would need to do in order to achieve the outcomes up to the dotted line in Figure 17.2.

In order to move up this triangle, it is imperative that the healthcare professional continues to improve their communications skills. Egan (2002) has provided a useful model which intertwines effectively with the PLISSIT model. An understanding of transactional analysis is also beneficial (Berne, 1964). Being au fait with the ego states can enhance empathy with the changes in relationships, and how they might affect the patient and their partner. We all conduct our lives in our different ego states of parent, adult and child, with a propensity to fulfil different roles depending on where we are, what we are doing, who we are with, the way that we have been brought up, life crises, and so on. When someone is ill, a partner who has had a tendency to adopt their child ego state may take on the parent role instead, in order to support their partner. The patient who has had parent ego state tendencies may now have to take on more of the child role because they are ill. Helping them to come to terms with some of their problems with regard to adult ego states can be very effective.

Searle discusses the usefulness of transactional analysis, and how a clearer understanding of this process and its dynamics 'may be a route to a more fulfilling relationship' (Searle, 2005, p. 137). She also illustrates her point succinctly by utilising the well-accepted social dictum that 'One does not have sex with one's child.'

More in-depth training could be offered where necessary for healthcare professionals working in specialist areas. The author regularly runs three-day workshops, with follow-up days to increase the skills of those who work regularly with individuals with sexuality-related problems.

Learning how to formulate, implement and monitor sexual strategies, protocols, standards and policies

As this is such a neglected area of care, it is fairly safe to say that very few organisations possess adequate relevant documentation with regard to sexual health. For instance, the care plan is often inadequate in relation to this area of care, and this leads to poor documentation by the various healthcare professionals involved. However, when participants on courses are asked what documentation in their area relates to sexuality, few of them have such documentation, and very few indeed have any idea what they do have! The teacher could get the group to identify what different documentation needs to be put in place in order to assist the implementation and monitoring of this specific aspect of care. Small groups could each consider an aspect of a strategy as course work, or as homework for the next session. Questions for the group might include the following.

- What is the aim of the strategy?
- What is the scope of the strategy, including all parameters and boundaries?
- What problems does the strategy seek to address?
- What background information can the group collect?
- What is the national perspective?
- What are the main objectives?
- Are there any valuable findings?
- How will the group produce a detailed action plan with specific targets and timescales?

A collectively produced strategy could then be taken away and adapted for the student's own clinical setting.

One of the activities in Chapter 21 could be adapted to help students to relate to the importance of policy and its development regarding sexuality. At the Marie Curie Centre in Liverpool, the multi-disciplinary healthcare professionals have a very proactive group which formulates and implements standards (after much consultation). The Liverpool group evaluates and adapts this excellent document according to the feedback that they receive.

At a macro- and micro-level, educators would do well to influence practice and policy in this and other ways.

Clinical supervision

This is particularly important here, where issues might relate not only to lack of knowledge and skills, but also to attitudinal issues concerning assumptions, judgements and prejudices about the patient (Palmer and Samociuk, 2000). It is obvious that clinical supervision provides great potential for the practitioner's continuing development. Sexual health presents many challenges, and will continue to raise issues which the practitioner may find difficult. Much has been written over the years on the topic of supervision, providing many useful models to follow (Faugier, 1992; Butterworth, 1994; Heaven *et al.*, 2006), but a discussion of these is beyond the scope of this chapter. It is vital that educators espouse the advantages of clinical supervision. It is often the process of supervision that individuals are unsure about.

Palmer and Samociuk (2000) suggest that the model of Page and Woskett (1994) is used. This provides five stages which are easy to understand and utilise in practice (*see* Figure 17.3).

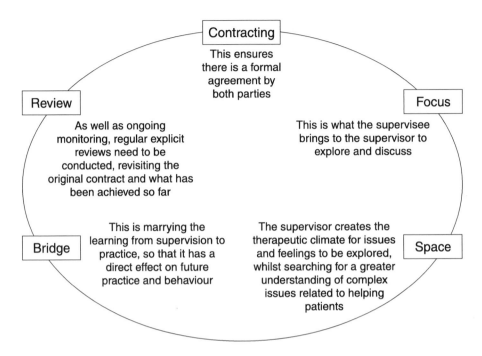

Figure 17.3 Cyclical model of counselling supervision. Adapted from Page and Woskett (1994).

In relation to sexuality, the issues that may arise during clinical supervision can be quite diverse. A few examples are listed below.

- The patient wanted to know if she and her partner could still have sex ... I didn't know the answer. I felt embarrassed.
- The patient is having an affair, and wants us to arrange for her lover to visit.
- I don't like the fact that they are always kissing, and on the bed together when I visit.
- The patient said that he would like me to hold him.
- This patient is the same sex as myself, and I feel strongly attracted. This has never happened before.
- My long-term bereavement client seems to be making comments which are over-familiar.

These are just a few of the many issues that healthcare professionals have brought to the author's supervision sessions. All of them need to be dealt with using the utmost sensitivity.

The educational implications of clinical supervision are far reaching, and some of the more salient points to consider are listed below.

- The importance of supervision needs to be expounded when teaching both formally and informally.
- Exercises to illustrate its importance could be incorporated into the session.
- Students need to be aware that they should choose someone whom they completely trust, and with whom they feel comfortable.

- Staff/students/participants need to be aware that it is important to choose someone who is also skilled at providing clinical supervision, and who has highly developed communication skills and counselling expertise.
- In-depth knowledge of the topic is not necessary, but it does help.

Thus the educator needs to ensure that adequate training is provided in clinical supervision, communications, counselling, and knowledge of relevant sexual health issues, or alternatively they need to ensure that members of the group know where such training is available.

The following exercise has been found to be useful with different groups of students.

Exercise 8

Ask each of the students to think of a sexuality-related problem in the clinical setting.

Then ask them to think about what they could have discussed during supervision.

List the group's ideas on a flipchart.

Choose one problem, and ask the student to share this with the group.

The group should act as a 'collective' supervisor.

The facilitator should stop and start the discussion, providing constructive feedback and role modelling good techniques.

Note: This exercise requires prior discussion with the proposed supervisee, to ensure that he or she is comfortable to do this, and to agree to post-session debriefing.

Many individuals will not have utilised a number of the above-mentioned approaches to sexual health before. Getting it right requires more than just the theory that is taught in the classroom. Even for those who have a good knowledge base and practical skills, supervision allows them to reflect, and to continually learn and improve within the clinical setting.

Key points

- The topic of sexual health is hard to define, and consequently difficult to teach.
- Sexuality is as much a private and sensitive topic for students as it is for patients.
- Students do not always admit their personal biases, beliefs and attitudes.
- If we accept the notion that self-awareness is fundamental to working with patients, and to teaching the topic of sexual health, how might this be realistically and successfully achieved with regard to sexuality?
- There is only very limited education available on sexuality in healthcare. There is even less training available for the trainer in this area.

- Many students who have had training recall poor practice in teaching methodology.
- Sexual health is not often considered to be an essential element of healthcare training either pre- or post-registration/qualification.
- Oncology and palliative care courses (accredited and non-accredited) and other study days could serve as useful forums at which to introduce members of the multi-disciplinary team to the potential benefits of teaching this topic.
- Always remember the student and their own vulnerability.

Summary and conclusion

This chapter has considered the importance, complexity and elusive nature of sexuality. It has also discussed the difficulties and possible solutions involved in teaching about sexuality in relation to cancer and palliative care. It has highlighted a number of different approaches, but further elaboration of these ideas is beyond the scope of this book. It is hoped that the above account goes at least some way towards ensuring that this topic does not remain a hidden aspect of cancer and palliative care in future years.

Guilfoyle (1990) has suggested 'the importance of how sexuality theory can be combined with practice, to promote better education of nurses, and move towards a more holistic approach to patient care, which is often ignored.' Searle (2005) argues that it is a hidden area of palliative care, and that the evidence is demanding. In addition, she suggests anecdotally that the experience of various groups which have studied cancer and palliative care reveals that little or no thought is given to addressing this area of practice. This author's experience has been the same.

Searle also states most succinctly that 'if dying is part of life and sexuality a part of adulthood, and experiences constitute quality of life, hidden sexuality can no longer remain.'

Back in 1980, Macleod-Clark informed the workforce that there was evidence that general nurses were not equipped by their training with either the knowledge or the skills to meet patients' needs. What has changed?

Most of the studies conducted to date have confirmed that the more knowledge nurses have about sexuality, the more positive their attitude is, and the more comfortable they are in dealing with patients' concerns appropriately (Page and Woskett, 1994; Webb, 1988; Lewis and Bor, 1994).

It is time for an attitude change, and in order to provide high-quality holistic care for this patient group and their families, practitioners and educators must rise to the challenge of teaching this topic more effectively.

This chapter demonstrates that although there remains a scarcity of research and publications on this subject, it is still possible to teach students the fundamentals. These elements, when taught in an interesting and sensitive manner, can still challenge attitudes and beliefs, yet remain supportive of the students' inherent vulnerabilities.

Implications for the reader's own practice

1 In what ways might you adapt your role as a result of reading this chapter?
2 Do you teach the subject as a stand-alone topic, or integrated into other subjects? What are the implications of each approach?
3 How might you be even more challenging, yet remain sensitive and respectful?
4 Consider and explore how you might utilise patients and/or their loved ones as part of the learning event. What are the limitations and benefits of this approach?
5 How do you think you could realistically measure your success?
6 What new creative approaches could you develop to teach this topic?

References

Anderson B, Wolf F. Chronic physical illness and sexual behaviour: psychological issues. *J Consult Clin Psychol.* 1986; **54:** 168–75.

Annon J. The PLISSIT model: a proposed conceptual scheme for the behavioural treatment of sexual problems. *J Sex Educ Ther.* 1976; **2:** 1–15.

Baggs JG, Karch AM. Sexual counselling of women with coronary heart disease. *Heart Lung.* 1987; **16:** 154–9.

Becker R, Gamlin R. *Fundamentals of Palliative Care Nursing.* London: Quay Books; 2004.

Berne E. *Games People Play.* Harmondsworth: Penguin; 1964.

Booth B. Does it really? *Nurs Times.* 1990; **86:** 50–52.

Bor R, Watts M. Talking to patients about sexual matters. *Br J Nurs.* 1993; **2:** 657–61.

Burbie GE, Polinsky ML. Intimacy and sexuality after cancer treatment: restoring a sense of wholeness. *J Psychosoc Oncol.* 1992; **10:** 19–33.

Butterworth CA. Preparing to take on clinical supervision. *Nurs Stand.* 1994; **8(52):** 32–4.

Caulfield H, Platzer H. Next of kin. *Nurs Stand.* 1998; **15(7):** 47–9.

Clifford D. Professional awareness in health care. In: Wells D, editor. *Caring for Sexuality in Health and Illness.* Edinburgh: Churchill Livingstone; 2000. pp. 11–18.

Corr G. Sexuality: a topical issue for nursing. *Nurs Standard.* 1991; **6:** 52–5.

Cort E, Munroe D, Oliviere D. Couples in palliative care. *Sex Relationship Ther.* 2004; **19:** 2004–19.

Crouch S. Sexual health. 1. Sexuality and nurses' role in sexual health. *Br J Nurs.* 1999; **8:** 601–6.

Deaney S. When Mom or Dad come out: helping adolescents cope with homophobia. *J Psychol Nurs.* 1989; **27:** 33–6.

Dewing J. Altered body image. *Surg Nurs.* 1989; **2:** 17–20.

Dow MGT, Schlone AP. Teaching medical undergraduates about psychosexual problems. *Br J Sex Med.* 1982; **8:** 24–9.

Egan G. *The Skilled Helper: problem management and opportunity development approach to helping.* Florence, KY: Wadsworth; 2002.

English National Board. *Sexual Health Education and Training.* London: English National Board; 1994.

Faugier J (1992) *The Supervision Relation: clinical supervision and mentorship in nursing.* London: Stanley Thomas; 1992.

Faulkner A. *Teaching Interactive Skills in Health Care.* Kingston upon Thames: Nelson Thornes Ltd; 1993.

Fonseca JD. Sexuality – a quality of being human. *Nurs Outlook.* 1970; **18:** 25.

Frazer J, Albert M, Smith J *et al*. Impact of a human sexuality workshop on the sexual attitudes and knowledge of nursing students. *J Nurs Educ*. 1982; **21**: 6–13.

Gamlin R. Sexuality and palliative care. In: Lugton J, McIntyre R, editors. *Palliative Care: the nursing role*. London: Elsevier; 2005.

Girts C. Nursing attitudes about sexuality needs of spinal cord injury patients. *Rehabil Nurs*. 1990; **15**: 205–6.

Grigg E. Guidelines for teaching about sexuality. *Nurse Educ Today*. 1997; **17**: 62–6.

Guilfoyle JF. Responding to a human need. *Prof Nurse*. 1990; **6(1)**: 33–6.

Heaven C, Clegg J, Maguire P. Transfer of communications training from the workshop to the workplace: the impact of clinical supervision. *Patient Educ Counsel*. 2006; **60**: 311–25.

Hogan R. *Human Sexuality: a nursing perspective*. New York: Appleton Century Crofts; 1980.

Hohman GW. Consideration in management of psychosexual readjustment in the injured male. *Rehabil Psychol*. 1972; **19**: 50–58.

Hostad J. *A sensitive question? Impact of sexuality study day on the sexual knowledge and attitude of nurses on a palliative care course*. Unpublished MSc dissertation, University of Southampton, 1999.

Irwin R. Sexual health promotion and nursing. *J Adv Nurs*. 1997; **25**: 170–77.

Jenkins BJ. Patients' reports of sexual changes after treatment for gynaecological cancer. *Oncol Nurs Forum*. 1988; **15**: 349–54.

Kautz DD, Dickey CA, Stevens MN. Using research to identify why nurses do not meet established sexuality nursing care standards. *J Nurs Qual Assurance*. 1990; **4**: 69–78.

Kinsey AC, Pomeroy WB, Marks CE. *Sexual Behaviour in the Human Male*. Philadelphia, PA: WB Saunders; 1948.

Kreuger JC, Hassell J, Goggins DB *et al*. Relationship between counselling and sexual readjustment after hysterectomy. *Nurs Res*. 1979; **28**: 145–50.

Lewis S, Bor R. Nurses' knowledge of and attitudes towards sexuality and the relationship of these with nursing practice. *J Adv Nurs*. 1994; **20**: 251–9.

MacGregor FC. Social, psychological and cultural dimensions of cosmetic and reconstructive plastic surgery. *Aesthetic Plast Surg*. 1989; **14**: 249–57.

MacGregor FC. Facial disfigurement: problems and management of social interaction and implications for mental health. *Aesthetic Plast Surg*. 1990; **14**: 249–57.

Macleod-Clark J. Communications with cancer patients: communications or evasion? In: Tiffany R, editor. *Cancer Nursing Update*. London: Bailliere Tindall; 1980.

Matocha LK, Waterhouse JK. Current nursing practice related to sexuality. *Res Nurs Health*. 1993; **16**: 371–8.

Newell R. Altered body image: a fear-avoidance model of psychosocial difficulties following disfigurement. *J Adv Nurs*. 1999; **30**: 1230–38.

Page S, Woskett V. *Supervising the Counsellor: a cyclical model*. Routledge: London; 1994.

Palmer H, Samociuk S. Sexual health: support and supervision. In: Wilson H, McAndrew S, editors. *Sexual Health: foundation for practice*. London: Harcourt Publishers; 2000.

Parke F. Sexuality in later life. *Nursing Times*. 1991; **87**: 40–2.

Piff C. *Let's Face It*. London: Victor Gollancz; 1985.

Platzer H. Nursing care for gay and lesbian patients. *Nurs Standard*. 1993; **7**: 34–7.

Plummer K. *Modern Homosexualities: fragments of lesbian and gay experience*. Routledge: London; 1992.

Poorman SG. *Human Sexuality and the Nursing Process*. Norwalk, CT: Appleton and Lang; 1988.

Price B. *Body Image: nursing concepts and care*. New York: Prentice Hall; 1990.

Purdie H. Management of sexuality in a mental health setting. *Nurs Standard*. 1996; **11(12)**: 47–50.

Rafferty D. Putting sexuality on the agenda. *Nurs Times.* 1995; **91:** 28–31.

Rose P. Out in the open? How do nurses treat their patients and colleagues who are lesbian? *Nurs Times.* 1993; **89:** 50–52.

Royal College of Nursing. *The Nursing Care of Lesbians and Gay Men.* London: Royal College of Nursing; 1994.

Salter M. *Altered Body Images: the nurse's role.* 2nd ed. London: Bailliere Tindall; 1997.

Savage J. *Nursing Today. Nurses' Gender and Sexuality.* London: Heinemann Nursing; 1987.

Schover LR. Sexual rehabilitation after treatment for prostate cancer. *Cancer.* 1993; **71:** 1024–30.

Searle E. Sexuality and people who are dying. In: Heath H, White I, editors. *The Challenge of Sexuality in Health Care.* Oxford: Blackwell Science; 2002. pp. 153–60.

Searle L. Sexuality and palliative care: a journey of discovery and understanding. In: Nyatanga B, Astley-Pepper M, editors. *Hidden Aspects of Palliative Care.* London: Quay Books; 2005.

Solzhenitsyn A. *Cancer Ward.* Harmondsworth: Penguin Books; 1968.

Stuart GW, Sundeen SJ. *Principles and Practice of Psychiatric Nursing.* St Louis, MO: CV Mosby; 1979.

Taylor I, Robertson A. A sensitive question. *Nurs Times.* 1994; **90:** 31–2.

Waterhouse J. Nursing practice related to sexuality: a review and recommendations. *Nurs Times Res.* 1996; **1:** 412–18.

Waterhouse J, Metcalfe M. Attitudes towards nurses discussing sexual concerns with patients. *J Adv Nurs.* 1991; **16:** 1048–54.

Webb C. A study of nurses' knowledge and attitudes about sexuality in health care. *Int J Nurs Stud.* 1988. **25(3):** 235–44.

Wilton T. *Sexualities in Health and Social Care: a textbook.* Buckingham: Open University Press; 2000.

World Health Organization. *Education and Treatment in Human Sexuality: the training of health professionals.* Technical Report Series 572. Geneva: World Health Organization; 1975.

World Health Organization. *Concepts of Sexual Health.* Copenhagen: World Health Organization; 1986.

Yaniv H. Sexuality of cancer patients: a palliative care approach. *Eur J Palliat Med.* 1992; **2:** 69–72.

Young EW, Knoch PB, Preston DB. AIDS and homosexuality: a longitudinal study of knowledge and attitude changes among rural nurses. *Public Health Nurs.* 1989; **6:** 189–96.

Zarwid CS. *Sexual Health: a nurses' guide.* Real Nursing Series. Amsterdam: Delmor Hamilton Hill; 1994.

Further reading

The following websites, books and booklets, although few in number, offer further ideas to extend and develop the reader's practice. Much of this information can be adapted for use as teaching material with little effort.

Useful websites

- www.cancerbacup.org.uk
- www.cancerbacup.org.uk/info/sex/sex_9.htm
- www.mautnerproject.org-lesbians with cancer
- Gay and Lesbian Medical Association; www.glma.org/policy/hp2010/pdf/cancer.pdf

Books

- Gamlin R. Sexuality and palliative care. In: Lugton J, Miltye R, editors. *Palliative Care: the nursing role*. London: Churchill Livingstone; 2005. This text provides an excellent accompaniment to this chapter. The author has tried as far as possible not to overlap too much with this text (in particular by utilising different exercises). Most of Gamlin's reflective points and learning exercises may be used by the educator in different settings. It is hoped that the use of both texts will provide the reader with a rich supply of resources which could not have been presented in one short chapter.
- Wilton T. *Sexualities in Health and Social Care: a textbook*. Buckingham: Open University Press; 2000. This book takes a different focus to most of those written for healthcare professionals on sexuality. The primary aim is to support improvements in service delivery to lesbians, gay men and bisexuals by offering a foundation of sound information to be laid down during training. The book is designed to be appropriate for use in both basic and post-basic training, and to be used either as a classroom text or by the individual reader. All educationalists ought to have a copy of this on their bookshelves.
- Becker R, Gamlin R. *Fundamentals of Palliative Nursing*. London: Quay Books; 2004. The chapter on sexuality in this book is short but succinct, providing an excellent foundation for those who have never focused on this subject, whether they are students or qualified nurses. Again, there are useful exercises which can easily be adapted by the teacher.

Other books which contain useful chapters are listed below.

- Nyatanga B, Astley Pepper M. *Hidden Aspects of Palliative Care*. London: Quay Books; 2005. The reader is recommended to consult the chapter entitled 'Sexuality and palliative care: a journey of discovery and understanding' by E Searle. However, there are also many useful educational resources in other chapters, relating to psychosocial care.
- Heath H, White I, editors. *The Challenge of Sexuality in Health Care*. Oxford: Blackwell Science; 2002. This book contains much useful information, but the chapter entitled 'Sexuality and the dying patient', again written by E Searle, is particularly relevant.

Useful booklets

- CancerLink. *Body Image: sexuality and cancer*. 4th ed. London: CancerLink; 1995.
- CancerLink. *Close Relationships and Cancer*. London: CancerLink; 1998.
- Cancer BACUP. *Sexuality and Cancer: a guide for people with cancer and their partners*. London: Cancer BACUP; 1995.

Chapter 18

Complementary therapies: progressing from knowledge to wisdom

Ruth Sewell

> *The test of a system of medicine should be its adequacy in the face of suffering.*
> *Cassell (1991, p. vii)*

Aim

The popularity of complementary therapies is increasing worldwide, with substantial evidence of growth in the use of such therapies among people at all stages of their cancer journey. The aim of this chapter is to explore the important, unique and crucial contribution that complementary therapies can make within a healthcare approach that genuinely seeks to provide holistic and integrative care for the patient, and those who are supporting them, particularly during the palliative phase of illness. An integrative approach also emphasises the importance of education for all professionals, whether they are representing mainstream or complementary therapies within palliative healthcare.

Learning outcomes

- Reconsider the importance of holistic approaches to care.
- Appreciate that complementary therapies (usually) arise from different models, philosophies and paradigms of healthcare practice, which may not appear to be concordant with current practice within mainstream palliative care.
- Consider key issues in the creation of educational opportunities which can effectively guide healthcare professionals and complementary therapy practitioners to form an effective integrative model of palliative care.
- Consider how education enables the integration of complementary therapies within mainstream palliative care practices.
- Consider key issues when creating training and continuing professional development courses for complementary therapists who are seeking to work within mainstream palliative care.
- Reflect on the role of education in identifying and encouraging appropriate methods of research that are sensitive to the different paradigms, particularly in broadening world views of healthcare.

Introduction

Individuals need to retain as much control over their lives as possible, and this is also true at times of illness, and in the presence of advancing disease. One of the most encouraging trends in healthcare lies in patient-led incentives concerning disease management information, along with greater involvement of patients in their own care at all stages of their illness experience (Thomas, 2001). Concurrently, there is wider access to information about, exposure to and access to other forms of healing and healthcare, particularly in the form of complementary and alternative medicine (CAM) and complementary therapies. With regard to complementary therapies (CTs), it is evident that they are therapeutically significant for individuals affected by long-term or chronic conditions (Partnership on Long-Term Conditions, 2005). In the UK, a survey by Thomas and Coleman (2004) found that 1 in 10 of the population actively sought to incorporate some form of complementary therapy within their conventional healthcare. Furthermore, surveys of the NHS affirm greater progress towards the integration of complementary therapies within mainstream healthcare, with 50% of GPs and over 43% of primary healthcare trusts providing access to complementary therapies for patients/service users (Wilkinson *et al.*, 2004).

In relation to cancer, surveys have identified a global trend in the application and integration of complementary therapies among patients during and after treatment for cancer (Ernst and Cassileth, 1998; Scott *et al.*, 2005). Whatever the circumstances of the use of complementary therapies, the underpinning principles are concerned with helping the individual to maximise their quality of life. They are also concerned with preparing and educating practitioners and professionals alike to provide the highest possible quality of care. The importance of this cannot be overstated, and it emerges as a significant feature of *The NHS Cancer Plan* (Department of Health, 2000), through the provision of 'supportive care.' Supportive care is defined as approaches to care that are intended to empower and help patients to cope during their experience of cancer and its treatment. It is concerned with helping each individual to maximise the benefits of treatment, while living as well as possible. The National Institute for Clinical Excellence (2002) emphasises that supportive care should be considered to have equal priority with disease management, and it is designed around the provision of nine services, complementary therapies being one of these.

Definitions

Complementary medicine/therapies, alternative medicine/therapies, integrated medicine and holistic medicine are all terms that regularly appear within the literature, or as part of health awareness publicity. It is not uncommon for the differences and similarities to appear indistinguishable, and the terms are often used interchangeably, which can be confusing for all concerned. However, what is more frequently seen, particularly within professional publications, is the abbreviated term 'CAM.' The terms 'CAM' or 'CAMs' denote therapies and approaches that are used within complementary medicine and alternative medicine. In its broadest sense, CAM involves approaches to diagnosis, treatment or prevention that complement mainstream (conventional) medicine by contributing to a common whole, by satisfying a demand that is not met by conventional medicine, or by diversifying the conceptual framework of medicine (Ernst *et al.*, 1995). At the present time there is little consensus concerning the difference between the terms 'complementary medicine' and 'complementary therapies.' One of the clearest definitions of CAM is the following:

> *A broad domain of healing resources that encompasses all health systems, modalities and practices and their accompanying theories and beliefs, other than those intrinsic to the politically dominant health systems of a particular society or culture in a given historical period.*
>
> *Cochrane Collaboration (1996)*

This definition serves to simplify and demystify complementary approaches, and at the same time discourages the dominance of prevailing social or political trends. It also encourages the fostering of acceptance of therapies and approaches to health that are not seeking to contradict or compete with those that are established, or which are considered to have become historically 'the norm.' Perhaps what is most significant in terms of educational objectives is the observation by Rankin Box (2006) that rather than debating the therapies, there is more of a need and desire for educators and clinicians/practitioners to understand which therapies are actually capable of making a clinical difference. Once this happens there can be better outcomes for all concerned, not least the patient or client. For them, there should be every encouragement and education to expect holistic care along with the best of unbiased palliative care, including the appropriate integration of complementary therapies.

A wider selection of definitions has been provided by Zollman and Vickers (1999). For the purpose of this chapter, the term 'complementary therapies' will be used to refer to complementary therapies that seek to support and complement conventional/mainstream healthcare practices. In contrast, 'alternative medicine/therapies' are usually considered to be used in place of mainstream healthcare. Although there is always a potential role for alternative therapies, it is beyond the scope of this chapter to explore the indications for alternative treatment within mainstream palliative healthcare services.

Complementary therapies: the link back to holism and healing practices

> *Healing is a process of integrating and balancing the parts of oneself at a deep level of inner knowledge that gives each part equal importance and value.*
>
> *Sandor (2005)*

Complementary therapies are generally considered to be based within a philosophical model of holistic or whole-person healthcare. This proposes that each person is viewed as an organic intact whole, composed of inseparable dimensions identified as those related to the physical, intellectual, psychological, emotional (feeling), social and spiritual dimensions (Benor and Benor, 1997). It is therefore suggested that the individual's development, which must include their responses to illness and health, is a function of all of these dimensions (Bolletino Cohn, 2002). Unlike the biomedical approach, the holistic approach does not limit itself to signs and symptoms, functions, body chemistry, mood and emotions, the presence or absence of religious belief or spiritual alliance. Instead, as Fulder (2005, p. 775) suggests, holism requires the practitioner to delve more deeply into the overall life and situation of the client, even 'digging below the obvious symptoms.' From this perspective it is clear that if a holistic approach to care is to be pursued, there is a need to keep educating and re-educating healthcare professionals and practitioners about holism, and furthering the attitude of always approaching each individual in their entirety. However, Fulder (2005) makes the significant point that holism is at risk of being swept up in the new terminology of integration, or integrative care, which has come to mean the blending of mainstream (conventional) healthcare approaches with complementary medicine/therapies. While integration is moving practice forward for the benefit of both patient and practitioners, it may well be at the risk of overshadowing the importance of holism by losing the patient in a sea of over-blended treatments and therapies which may not even be arising from a complete holistic assessment.

Holism is not about which treatment approach should be taken, but rather it is concerned with a view of reality – it is more to do with the 'how' than the 'what' of it. Holism offers the potential for the practitioner, in accordance with the needs, desires and expectations of the patient, to apply sound informed clinical logic and judgment, capable of intelligent selection of treatment. Fulder (2005) considers that it is essential to think both logically and impressionistically in order to help the patient towards greater life awareness and health. In other words, education needs to support the practitioner – whether mainstream or complementary – in thinking holistically even in the presence of increasing pressures over resources and a mainstream healthcare culture that is moving towards increasing governance and control. It can be difficult to sustain a humanistic holistic approach when environments of care are, for whatever reason, unable to commit totally to the practitioner in their ambitions for their patients/clients.

However, it is worth remembering that there is a temptation to assume that if complementary therapies are embraced, such therapies will be holistic. This may not necessarily be the case, as therapies that are applied without taking into consideration the whole person simply lead to a reduction of therapeutic effects. Furthermore, holistic assessment will vary according to the tradition in which it is found. For instance, the merging of westernised medicine and eastern medicine demands cooperation, education and a willingness among practitioners to respect different traditions that together integrate what might appear to be disparate paradigms of health (Thomson, 2005).

The earliest dialogues in both holism and complementary therapies were championed by nurses and also within the hospice and palliative care movement in the 1980s (Benor, 1996). Since that time, the term has enabled practitioners to engage with patients 'outside the box' of the biomedical model. Wilber (2005) suggests that it is not so much about the contents in the 'bag of medicine' that is carried, as it is about the person who is carrying the bag. At a time when increased efforts are being made to render healthcare more humane at the least and more inclusive and whole person centred at best, there continue to be challenges to the practice and delivery of holistic care. In addition, it is important to recognise the constraints on both healthcare professionals and the system of westernised healthcare which regularly encounters times of crisis, the cost of care being exacerbated by dwindling resources which not only interrupt the continuity of care, but also undermine the confidence of care providers. These constraints are occurring at a time when healthcare is actually seeking to be more effective in enabling patients to be actively involved in their treatment. Furthermore, there are concerns about the growing trend towards medicalisation within palliative care provision (Corner and Dunlop, 1999). If this is the case, then the more important implications include the risk of a biomedical model dominating and narrowing the healing environment of care, with the further risk of ultimately directing care away from a holistic and integrative approach. Wilber (2005) suggests that this process may not only limit healing practices, but can also be a painful undertaking for those professionals who are attracted to approaches in healthcare that are concerned with the whole person rather than merely focusing on an aspect of a disease or somatic/mental functioning. Here Wilber is referring to the importance of recognising that holistic practice is applicable not only to the patient, but also equally to the practitioner.

Even though resources are limited and modern healthcare seems to be completely subsumed in meeting targets, Morrison (2004) suggests that returning to the real meaning of holistic practice may well serve to renew the vision of what health and healing are all about. It is also the case that education can help all practitioners to re-evaluate their personal and professional values, and specifically to see themselves within a holistic paradigm through working effectively as a whole team.

Education that serves to prepare the patient for complementary therapies

The existential plight that arises is a larger picture and produces its own set of problems and issues to be resolved or not. However, when the larger issues are distilled by the day-to-day reality of coping, dealing with pain and other symptoms, and living with uncertainty, the most important matters for the individual are how they can function well and not be overcome or compromised in their ability to function, to make decisions, and to concentrate on what they need to do for themselves or how they will respond to the uncertainty that frequently accompanies their illness. However, Bolletino Cohn (2002) suggests that despite these very human experiences and all that they have to deal with, the fact is that each individual is quite capable of making choices, particularly inner choices and changes in the way in which they view and live their life and continue to grow. The vehicle for this may well be the use of complementary therapies that enable the individual to be more involved in, responsible for and responsive to the healing process that they seek to find, whether that healing involves living to the full until they die, improving their quality of life, or contributing to a 'healing unto death' (Benor, 1993, 2001). Mackereth (2006, p. 25), illustrating his considerable experience of providing touch therapies in palliative care, finds that 'massage and reflexology' can provide a nurturing source of support and comfort for patients in advanced stages of disease. He adds that so long as touch is welcomed, it can lead to a deeply relaxing response that imbues comfort and the feeling of being cared for. When describing his experience of offering touch therapies, he points out that some patients may initially be rather hesitant about accepting the treatment. However, he describes how change take place through the 'domino' effect, which can happen once a patient observes the positive, relaxing and comforting effects of treatments on fellow patients. Then even the most hesitant patient wants to experience such effects for him- or herself. The role of educating the patient's partner/carers about the benefits of receiving complementary therapy is a vital one. It is important to acknowledge the potentially demanding situation and not infrequent exhaustion that can arise for the carer(s) of a person with advanced cancer (Turner *et al.*, 2005). Carers may also be reluctant to take time out for themselves, or they may underestimate their own need for care and comfort (Veach *et al.*, 2002). Mackereth (2006) further illustrates the positive role modelling and 'domino' effect for carers by providing chair massage by a patient's bedside, which can in turn encourage other carers to receive the same relaxing treatment themselves.

The role of supportive literature

Science is the tool of the western mind, and with it more doors can be opened than with bare hands. It is part and parcel of our knowledge, and only obscures our insight when it holds that the understanding given by it is the only kind that exists.

Developing knowledge into wisdom is concerned with knowing the obvious, and not being seduced into believing that (and behaving as if) knowledge is fixed. Complementary therapies are no longer a novelty, or merely an option to be used if all else fails. The House of Lords Select Committee Report (2000) found 15 million users of complementary and alternative medicine/therapies nationwide. It is evident that many individuals at all stages of the disease process are using some form of complementary therapy, and many are using alternative approaches (Yates *et al.*, 2005). Therapies are used by patients to enhance their quality of life (Rees *et al.*, 2000), and to help to reduce the side-effects of cancer treatment (Walker *et al.*, 1997, 1999; Lee and Jang, 2005) and the symptoms related to increasing disease progression, particularly within palliative care (Lewith, 2002).

Criticism of complementary medicine and therapies is often levelled at the lack of substantial research and evidence-based practice. However, Molassitotis *et al.* (2005) suggest that patient satisfaction can be an appropriate end-point outcome for evaluation of such therapies, rather than relying exclusively on clinical outcome studies. Furthermore, the problem of insufficient evidence/information has been highlighted by Shekelle *et al.* (2005) specifically with regard to the inconsistencies and biases in publication and indexing of complementary therapies/medicine research. They point out the tendency of complementary and alternative medicine journals to highlight the positive results of studies, while the negative or inconclusive results are more likely to appear in mainstream medical journals. Language is also found to compound the problem, with a tendency towards the exclusion of non-English-language reports, which may result in lower estimates of intervention effects.

Palliative care education about complementary therapies has a crucial role to play in highlighting such constraints. Difficulties in understanding who might benefit from complementary therapies are complex, and usually arise from lack of research within the evidence-based literature (e.g. gender-specific research). Complementary therapies are used more widely by women during all phases of cancer (Rees *et al.*, 2000). In contrast, men with cancer have been reported to use them less (Sparber *et al.*, 2000; Smith, 2004). Complementary therapies have a potentially important role in supporting men with cancer, particularly in providing them with an opportunity to talk, encouraging them to communicate their needs with regard to comfort, and enabling them to receive emotional and psychological support. Moynihan (2002) warns that men who are not encouraged to communicate may become depressed or anxious, and these conditions may persist long after treatment ends.

A study of note of respondents receiving palliative care was conducted by Molassiotis *et al.* (2005). This descriptive survey was designed to explore the use of complementary and alternative medicine/therapies in cancer patients from 14 European countries, with data collected from 956 respondents. It was found that over 35% of cancer patients were using some form of CAM, with 58 therapies identified, the most popular ones being herbal medicines/teas, relaxation techniques, homoeopathy, dietary supplements/minerals/vitamins and spiritual therapies. Information on complementary approaches was provided by friends, family and the media, but only limited information was provided by the patients' doctors and nurses. The main reasons cited for using complementary therapies were to help the body to fight the cancer, and to improve physical and emotional well-being. Most of the respondents reported beneficial effects, and a few had experienced transient side-effects. A later study by Molassiotis *et al.* (2006) reported a positive correlation between improved quality of life in people with lung cancer and use of complementary therapies across eight European countries. With the increasing use of complementary therapies by cancer patients, Molassiotis *et al.* (2005, 2006) emphasise the importance of education for both patient and professional on the appropriate use of complementary therapies and the level of effectiveness that can potentially be expected from such therapies, while encouraging both practitioners and educators towards supportive integration of complementary therapies into mainstream practice.

Research: a changing world view

MacNish (2001) makes the valid point that some of the primary philosophical differences between complementary therapies and mainstream medicine are a result of the biomedical model's separation of body, mind, spirit and the environment in seeking to come to a diagnosis, finding treatment which is underpinned by research initiatives that are designed to reflect only one aspect of the individual. There are also discrepancies in the evidence base for complementary therapies when research methods are inappropriately applied. However, this problem can be resolved when research initiatives are allowed to reinstate subjectivity and consciousness into both research and scientific debate. Andrews (2006) suggests that there is a unique opportunity not only to educate about the importance of studies on complementary therapies, but also to encourage the building up of capacity to make such research possible for professionals who may not have considered its relevance within their own clinical or research field.

There is patchy research evidence in palliative care in general, but particularly with regard to the effectiveness of complementary therapies in palliative care. Palliative care education can serve to stimulate questioning around research at the most simplistic level by bringing healthcare teams together. Questioning results, thoroughness in recording observations and particularly patient satisfaction are all valid end points for research, and can serve as building blocks to increase research

capacity among dedicated professionals who might not otherwise consider themselves adept, familiar or confident enough with research methodologies.

Education serving to help the patient

One of the most important contributions that complementary therapies can make is
to help the individual to find hope and to live as full a life as possible, which after all
is the tenet on which all palliative care is based. An increase in hope and a decrease
in despair and hopelessness are all functions of the mind, and may be critically
important factors in determining how we live our life and deal with distress, pain,
dying and death (Ray, 2004).

The selection of therapies needs to be based on the level of need and the perceived
level of independence sought by the patient. Like any mainstream treatment,
therapies can be 'done to' the patient (e.g. acupuncture, massage, aromatherapy,
shiatsu), or they may be prescribed (e.g. homoeopathy, herbal medicine, flower
essence therapies). A qualitative study by Chessman *et al.* (2001) of shiatsu for
patients in a hospice found an improvement in the patients' quality of life, including
a reduction in pain and nausea, relief of constipation, a reduction in swelling and
oedema, and an improvement in mobility and flexibility. The deeper relaxation
effect following the shiatsu treatment produced other important changes, including
a reduction in the preoccupation and feelings of forboding resulting from a poor
prognosis, a sense of mental and emotional calmness, and alleviation of the physical
depletion and exhaustion caused by the advanced disease process.

Other therapies are more amenable to self-help. These include relaxation exercises, visualisation, meditation, the use of simple remedies (e.g. ginger extract to
relieve nausea, or flower essence remedies to ease emotional stress), and appropriately prescribed vitamin and dietary supplements. A study by Walker *et al.*
(1999) of women undergoing chemotherapy reported a reduction in nausea and
vomiting, but also found that these women reported a lower level of anxiety, with
less inclination to suppress their emotions, as a result of learning to use the self-help
therapies of relaxation and guided imagery. Walker *et al.* (1997) also found in an
earlier study that women with advanced breast cancer who used relaxation and
guided imagery were able to cope better, were less anxious, and had a more positive
mood and improved levels of concentration.

Palliative care is an elastic term, with many people living far beyond their original
prognosis. It is therefore important to consider that while complementary therapies
are used to help to relieve symptoms, or to improve well-being in general, use of the
same therapies can be appropriately encouraged at other times, in order to maintain
a person's level of health or quality of life. Adopting a variety of approaches to
complementary therapy encourages the patient and their carers to be independent
and empowered again. At stressful times, when worries and concerns arise, or
when the symptoms are overbearing, it is enormously helpful for patients to have
something they can do for themselves. As healthcare professionals we cannot be
there in the middle of the night when they wake with pain or distress. We cannot
provide a soothing massage at these times, but with some training and support
either the patient him- or herself or a carer can improve the patient's well-being. It is
well worth investing time in educating the patient about such approaches.

Although a detailed discussion of key educational incentives with regard to suitable therapies in palliative care is beyond the scope of this chapter, it is possible to highlight those therapies that are available for use in supervised practice, or which are now increasingly being used within palliative care settings. These include aromatherapy, massage, reflexology, relaxation exercises and guided imagery. All of them produce in the patient a 'relaxation response', with physiological changes associated with decreased arousal of the sympathetic nervous system (lowered heart rate, blood pressure and breathing rate). The obvious benefit of complementary therapy is that these treatments have the potential to induce rest, relaxation and a sense of being cared for, while at the same time helping to reduce the patient's actual (physiological) and perceived (psycho-emotional and social) levels of stress and distress. This is also consistent with the growing literature on the integral connection and bidirectional flow of information and responses between the mind, body, emotions and spirit. The importance of acknowledging this connection and its relationship to the integration of complementary therapies is increasingly reported in the research literature on psychoneuroimmunology (PNI) (Spiegel and Septon, 2001; Cunningham and Watson, 2004). A detailed discussion of PNI has been provided by Spencer-Grey (2004).

Key issues and considerations when designing education programmes for the successful integration of complementary therapies in palliative care settings

It is important to remember that cancer and other life-threatening diseases are complex, experiential events that have a life-altering effect. Therefore a range of therapeutic options that acknowledge the ongoing process of change for the cancer patient and their family is required. Education has a crucial role in guiding and designing programmes to reflect this process.

Educational considerations

The delivery of healthcare is no longer considered to be static, but rather to respond dynamically to change and progress. Education needs to influence and guide the design of educational programmes that are capable of modelling a holistic approach for the successful integration of complementary therapies into all services and settings that provide palliative care.

When considering the course content, it is important to focus on the potential benefits of complementary therapies, which include the following.

- Patients report an overall improvement in quality of life (Rees *et al.*, 2000; Lewith, 2002; Cunningham and Watson, 2004).
- While undergoing treatment, the patient can usefully apply self-help approaches (e.g. breathing exercises, simple relaxation exercises, using the power of the imagination to distract them). These practices can also help to give the patient a greater sense of active participation in disease management and any associated side-effects of treatment (Luebbert *et al.*, 2001). Comfort can be gained from

receiving touch therapies (Post-White *et al.*, 2003; Fellowes *et al.*, 2004; Soden *et al.*, 2004).

- Complementary therapies can help to promote hope, and may help to strengthen coping skills and rebuild confidence and a sense of personal control (Walker *et al.*, 1997, 1999).
- These therapies help to reduce the effects of current and future stress (Cunningham and Watson, 2004).
- They can foster a more tolerable dying process when death is inevitable (Barnet, 2001).

It is important to anticipate potential barriers within the programme for integration of complementary therapies, which may include any of the following:

- financial cost
- time
- access
- cultural and religious considerations
- sensitivities within the family/community
- healthcare professionals' reactions/responses.

There are several core components that are essential to consider in the delivery of programmes that can directly guide clinicians/practitioners towards an effective integrative service. These include the following.

- Education should be given on the importance of careful assessment of complementary therapies, guided by the stage of disease and the treatment.
- Tools need to be developed which can enable all practitioners to identify their 'gaps' in knowledge of complementary therapies, and how they might 'fill the gaps.' Design creative learning opportunities to attract mixed group participation (i.e. mainstream healthcare professionals and complementary therapy practitioners).
- Education programmes should guide practitioners on when and when not to refer patients for complementary therapies (National Council for Hospice and Specialist Palliative Care Services and the Prince of Wales Foundation for Integrated Health, 2003).
- Practitioners should be educated in the use of effective communication skills in relation to complementary therapies, in order to prevent unrealistic expectations about outcome and/or the raising of false hope (National Council for Hospice and Specialist Palliative Care Services and the Prince of Wales Foundation for Integrated Health, 2003, p. 32).
- Education on effective communication should be provided to help all practitioners to support the individual patient in choosing complementary therapies based on what they have feel they want to achieve. For example, some individuals may not feel well enough or motivated enough to take on self-help exercises such as relaxation or guided imagery, and would prefer to receive massage or other touch therapies (Taylor, 2002, 2003).
- Education needs to be geared towards the development of appropriately pitched policies, protocols and standards of practice that include both healthcare professionals and complementary therapies. Standards of working collaboratively should include education on safe practice, which requires the design of reliable audit and evaluation tools to ensure demonstration of work-based practice that is

informed by the most recent research findings in integrative and complementary therapy practices (Tavares, 2004).

- Education provides the opportunity to encourage and support the high degree of inter-disciplinary collaboration, respect and trust that is required in order to achieve the best outcomes for the patient and their family.
- Education helps to raise awareness and increase understanding that an integrated approach utilising complementary therapies is about enhancing quality of life for the patient and their family, or supporting a 'healing unto death' (Benor, 1993, 2001).

The role of education in guiding the healthcare professional and complementary practitioner

Courses should be based on sound educational principals to better prepare complementary therapy practitioners for working in mainstream palliative care environments and services. It is essential that reliable peer-reviewed and evidence-based journals on the application of complementary therapies are available for course participants, and that healthcare professionals are educated to read around the subjects.

Educationalists need to be aware of those therapies that may be available within their own healthcare service provision. However, the patient who reports an improvement may be the best end point of research.

In addition, palliative care education should seek to support practitioners and service providers by training them to be resourceful and to look for funding to provide therapies within clinical areas. This should include the recruitment of appropriately qualified complementary therapists, who are offered terms and conditions based on a salaried position. Educationally driven incentives that are capable of supporting commissioners in determining future funding of complementary therapies and the recruitment of complementary therapy practitioners should not be overlooked.

Guidance on how to prepare both local and national information for patients about how to obtain reliable information on safe, competent complementary practitioners within their own communities is pivotal in palliative care education.

Similarly, educationalists and practitioners should participate in the building of information and educational resources for patients and their carers on the role of the complementary therapies in palliative care.

There are numerous courses on complementary and integrative therapies in the UK, one of which provides PhD level training. Furthermore, with growing incentives for complementary therapies to strive for regulation of training and the pursuit of continuing professional development, there is increasing access to reliable and well-designed courses of training.

Key points

- Despite the current debate about holism, it remains fundamental to healthcare professionals' approach to and delivery of complementary therapies.
- Education should serve patients and professionals equally.
- Research has a part to play in strengthening the evidence base for complementary therapies, but patients' reports of the effects of these therapies should remain of paramount importance.
- The patient/client should be involved and at the forefront of considerations before courses are devised for healthcare professionals and therapists.
- There are numerous therapy practitioners, but awareness of local resources and constraints is essential for service integration and educational developments.

Conclusion

It is evident that complementary therapies are increasingly being incorporated into palliative care settings, and greater opportunities are being offered for those in the palliative and terminal phases of illness to receive quality of care, to be comforted and to be relieved of their suffering. Even though there is in general a greater need to encourage demonstration of the effect of work-based practices on effective integration, along with the need to guide practice through research evidence, there is no question that complementary therapies have an invaluable contribution to make to holistic practice. Therefore, in order to take our current knowledge and move it towards a deeper understanding, it is important to recognise that holistic and integrative care is as much about the practitioner as it is about the patient. This means that interest in complementary therapies is a marker for other factors, such as healing, health and care, rather than merely a means of symptom control. Wisdom is about knowing and understanding how to translate approaches to healing and care which essentially come from different traditions and paradigms, which may at first appear too different to each other, but which in fact – with a willingness to be open-minded and a commitment to looking for how the best of one can be blended with the best of the other – can produce a satisfying outcome for the patient, their family and the healthcare practitioners and professionals involved. At a practical level this can be fostered through education that responds by supporting, coaching and training, and which realistically reflects resources at a local level. It is equally important to encourage research initiatives and methodologies that are sensitively and appropriately designed to take in the subtle differences in healing modalities. Education is needed on methods that can reflect the holistic approach in order to more fully explain and expand on the experience of both patient and practitioner when an integrated model of palliative care is sought.

Implications for the reader's own practice

1 How would you map the types of training in complementary therapy that are available in your area for healthcare professionals?
2 What teaching strategies would you employ to ensure that apparently different paradigms and values and underlying differences in philosophical approaches to healthcare can work and be translated into practice?
3 How would you set about developing training programmes that provide opportunities for gradual attainment of knowledge and skills?
4 What training could you initiate for complementary practitioners to empower them to make a significant contribution during clinical management team meetings?
5 What type of course could you design to include creative workshops on shared cases and highlight the differences in assessment models, in order to find a shared language and make the clinical intention clear to all?
6 Who else do you need to involve in teaching in order to ensure that quality standards are set and audited in clinical areas and that research initiatives achieve academic rigor?

References

Andrews G. Encouraging additional research capacity as an intellectual enterprise: extending Ernst's engagement. *Complement Ther Clin Pract.* 2006; **12**: 13–17.

Barnett M. Overview of complementary therapies in cancer care. In: Barraclough J, editor. *Integrated Cancer Care: holistic, complementary and creative approaches.* Oxford: Oxford University Press; 2001.

Benor R. Healing unto death. *Doctor Healer Network Newsletter.* 1993; **4**: 19–21.

Benor R. A holistic view to managing stress. In: McDaid P, Fisher R, editors. *Palliative Day Care.* London: Edward Arnold; 1996. pp. 126–38.

Benor R. Healing unto death. In: Benor DJ, editor. *Healing Research. Volume 1. Spiritual healing: scientific validation of a healing revolution.* Southfield, MI: Vision Publications; 2001.

Benor R, Benor D. The missing 'w' in wholistic, whole person care. *Complement Ther Nurs Midwifery.* 1997; **3**: 1–3.

Bolletino Cohn R. Responses to 'attachment and cancer: a conceptual integration.' A reality check. *Integr Cancer Ther.* 2002; **1**: 382–6.

Cassell E.J. *The Nature of Suffering and the Goals of Medicine.* New York: Oxford University Press; 1991.

Chessman S, Christian R, Cresswell J. Exploring the value of shiatsu in palliative care day services. *Int J Palliat Nurs.* 2001; **7**: 234–9.

Cochrane Collaboration Complementary Medicine Field (1996) *The Cochrane Library.* Oxford: Update Software Ltd; 1996.

Corner J, Dunlop R. New approaches to care. In: Clark D, Hockley J, Ahmedzai S, editors. *New Themes in Palliative Care.* Buckingham: Open University Press; 1999.

Cunningham AJ, Watson K. How psychological therapy may prolong survival in cancer: new evidence and a simple theory. *Integr Cancer Ther.* 2004; **3**: 214–29.

Department of Health. *The NHS Cancer Plan: a plan for investment, a plan for reform.* London: Department of Health; 2000.

Ernst E, Cassileth BR. The prevalence of complementary and alternative medicine in cancer. *Cancer*. 1998; **83**: 777–82.

Ernst E, Resch KL, Mills S *et al*. Complementary medicine: a definition. *Br J Gen Pract*. 1995; **45**: 506.

Fellowes D, Barnes K, Wilkinson S. Aromatherapy and massage for symptom relief in patients with cancer (Cochrane Review). In: *The Cochrane Library. Issue 3*. Oxford: Update Software; 2004.

Fulder S. Remembering the holistic view. *J Alt Complement Med*. 2005; **11**: 775–6.

House of Lords Science and Technology Committee. *Complementary and Alternative Medicine, HL Paper 123*. London: TSO; 2000. www.publications.parliament.uk/pa/ld/ldsctech.htm

Lee MS, Jang HS. Two case reports of the acute affects of Qi therapy (external Qigong) on symptoms of cancer: short report. *Complement Ther Clin Pract*. 2005; **11**: 211–13.

Lewith G. Complementary cancer care in Southampton: survey of staff and patients. *Complement Ther Med*. 2002; **10**: 100–6.

Luebbert K, Dahme B, Hasenbring M. A review of the impact of hypnosis, relaxation, guided imagery and individual differences on aspects of immunity and health. *Stress*. 2001; **5**: 147–63.

Mackereth P. Nurturing resilience: touch therapies in palliative care. *Holistic Healthcare*. 2006; **3**: 24–9.

MacNish S. Complementary therapies. In: Kinghorn S, Gamblin R, editors. *Palliative Nursing: bringing comfort and hope*. London: Royal College of Nursing and Bailliere Tindall; 2001.

Molassiotis A, Fernandez-Ortega P, Pud D *et al*. Use of complementary and alternative medicine in cancer patients: a European survey. *Ann Oncol*. 2005; **16**: 655–63.

Molassiotis A, Panteli V, Patiraki E *et al*. Complementary and alternative medicine use in lung cancer patients in eight European countries. *Complement Ther Clin Pract*. 2006; **12**: 34–9.

Morrison S. Holism and interprofessional learning: from the whole person to the whole team. *J Holistic Healthcare*. 2004; **1**: 15–18.

Moynihan C. Psychosocial aspects of men and cancer. *Cancer Topics*. 2002; **11**: 8–11.

National Council for Hospice and Specialist Palliative Care Services and the Prince of Wales Foundation for Integrated Health. *National Guidelines for the Use of Complementary Therapies in Supportive and Palliative Care*. London: Prince of Wales Foundation for Integrated Health; 2003.

National Institute for Clinical Excellence. *Guidance on Cancer Services: improving supportive and palliative care for adults with cancer. Second consultation document*. London: National Institute for Clinical Excellence; 2002.

Partnership of Long-Term Conditions. *17 Million Reasons: improving the lives of people with long-term conditions*; www.17millionreasons.org

Post-White J, Kinney ME, Savik K *et al*. Therapeutic massage and healing touch improve symptoms in cancer. *Integr Cancer Ther*. 2003; **2**: 332–44.

Rankin Box D. Shaping medical knowledge. *Complement Ther Clin Pract*. 2006; **12**: 1–2.

Ray O. How the mind hurts and heals the body. *Am Psychol*. 2004; **59**: 29–40.

Rees RW, Feigel I, Vickers A *et al*. Prevalence of complementary therapy use by women with breast cancer: a population-based survey. *Eur J Cancer*. 2000; **36**: 1359–64.

Sandor MK. The Labyrinth: a walking meditation for healing and self-care. *Focus*. 2005; **1**: 480–83.

Scott JA, Kearney N, Hummerston S *et al*. Use of complementary and alternative medicine in patients with cancer: a UK survey. *Eur J Oncol Nurs*. 2005; **9**: 131–7.

Shekelle PG, Morton SC, Suttorp MJ *et al*. Agency for Healthcare Research and Quality: challenges in systematic reviews of complementary and alternative medicine topics. *Ann Intern Med*. 2005; **142**: 1042–7.

Smith SS. Who uses complementary therapies? *Holistic Nurs Pract*. 2004; **18**: 176.

Soden K, Vincent K, Craske S *et al*. A randomised controlled trial of aromatherapy massage in a hospice setting. *Palliat Med*. 2004; **18**: 87–92.

Sparber A, Bauer L, Curt G *et al.* Use of complementary medicine by adult patients participating in cancer clinical trials. *Oncol Nurs Forum.* 2000; **27:** 623–30.

Spencer-Grey SA. The role of psychoneuroimmunology in oncology and palliative care. In: Foyle L, Hostad J, editors. *Delivering Cancer and Pallliative Care Education.* Oxford: Radcliffe Publishing; 2004.

Spiegel D, Septon SE. Psychoneuroimmunology and endocrine pathways in cancer: effects of stress and support. *Semin Clin Neuropsychiatry.* 2001; **6:** 252–65.

Tavares M. *Guide for Writing Policies, Procedures and Protocols: complementary therapies in supportive and palliative care.* London: Help the Hospices; 2004.

Taylor EJ. Transformation of tragedy among women surviving breast cancer. *Oncol Nurs Forum.* 2002; **27:** 781–8.

Taylor E.J. Spiritual needs of patients with cancer and family caregivers. *Cancer Nurs.* 2003; **26:** 260–66.

Thomas H. Complementary care in oncology: a patient-led revolution. In: Barraclough J, editor. *Integrated Cancer Care: holistic, complementary and creative approaches.* Oxford: Oxford University Press; 2001.

Thomas K, Coleman P. Use of complementary or alternative medicine in a general population in Great Britain. Results from the National Omnibus Survey. *J Public Health.* 2004; **26:** 152–7.

Thomson A. *A Healthy Partnership: integrating complementary healthcare into primary care.* London: Prince of Wales Foundation for Integrated Health; 2005.

Turner J, Kelly B, Swanson C *et al.* Psychosocial impact of newly diagnosed advanced breast cancer. *Psycho-Oncology.* 2005; **14:** 396–407.

Veach TA, Nicholas D, Barton M. *Cancer and the Family Cycle: a practitioner's guide.* New York: Routledge; 2002.

Walker LG, Walker MB, Simpson E *et al.* Guided imagery and relaxation therapy can modify host defences in women receiving treatment for locally advanced breast cancer. *Br J Surg.* 1997; **84** (**Suppl. 1):** 31.

Walker LG, Walker MB, Ogston K *et al.* Psychological, clinical and pathological effects of relaxation training and guided imagery during primary chemotherapy. *Br J Cancer.* 1999; **80:** 262–8.

Wilber K. Foreword. In: Schlitz M, Amorak T, Micozzi M, editors. *Consciousness and Healing: integral approaches to mind–body medicine.* St Louis, MO: Elsevier Churchill Livingstone; 2005.

Wilkinson J, Peters D, Donaldson J. *Clinical Governance for Complementary and Alternative Medicine in Primary Care.* London: University of Westminster; 2004.

Yates JS, Mustian KM, Gillies LJ *et al.* Prevalence of complementary and alternative medicine use in cancer patients during treatment. *Support Care Cancer.* 2005; **13:** 806–11.

Zollman C, Vickers A. ABC of complementary medicine. What is complementary medicine? *BMJ.* 1999; **319:** 693–6.

Resources for training in complementary medicine and therapies

There are a number of accredited postgraduate academic courses in complementary medicine and therapies throughout the UK, details of most of which can be found at www.scit.wlv.ac.uk/ukinfo/uk.map.html

Examples of higher degree courses on complementary medicine/therapies (e.g. acupuncture, aromatherapy, body therapies, reflexology, healing, homeopathy), with open access for healthcare professionals and other practitioners, involving part-time, full-time and distance learning, are listed below.

- University of Westminster, School of Integrated Health; www.wmin.ac.uk/sih
- University of Exeter, Peninsula Medical School; www.ex.ac.uk, www.pms. ac.uk
- Liverpool John Moores University; www.livjm.ac.uk/default.asp
- Queen Margaret University College, Edinburgh; www.qmuc.ac.uk
- Oxford Brookes University; www.brookes.ac.uk
- University of Greenwich; www.gre.ac.uk

The *Certificate of Working with People with Cancer for Complementary Therapists*, run by the Bristol Cancer Help Centre, is a course for complementary therapists on the integration of complementary therapies for people affected by cancer. This course leads to a certificate of attendance, the *Working with People with Cancer Certificate*, and can be taken at an advanced level as an Evidencing Work-Based Learning module accredited by the University of the West of England. Further details can be found at www.bristolcancerhelp.org or by emailing education@bristolcancerhelp.org.

The Prince of Wales Foundation for Integrated Health seeks to promote better understanding of and wider access to integrated healthcare, along with education on and development of confidence in integration of complementary medicine as part of an integrated healthcare approach. Further details can be found at www. fih.org/resources

The National Association of Complementary Therapists in Hospice and Palliative Care (NACTHPC) is a relevant organisation for any complementary therapist who is seeking to work or already working within palliative and terminal care. Further details can be found at www.helpthehospices.org.uk/NPA/complementarytherapists/ index.asp or by emailing nacthpc@hotmail.com

The Royal College of Nursing Forum on Complementary Therapies is a useful resource for nurses who are interested in the integration of complementary therapies into healthcare settings. Further details can be found at www.rcn.org.uk

Information about the American Holistic Nurse Association (AHNA) can be found at www.ahna.org

Organisations that hold information on current research into complementary medicine and therapies are listed below.

- Bristol Cancer Help Centre; www.bristolcancerhelp.org
- British National Health Service; www.library.nhs.uk/cam and www.cancer.gov
- Research Council for Complementary Medicine; www.rccm.org.uk, www.rccm. org.uk/cameol/include/login.aspx?ReturnUrl=%2fDefault.aspx
- National Institutes of Health, USA; http://nccam.nih.gov/health/whatiscam

Useful journals

- *Journal of Holistic Health Care: Developing Whole Person Approaches.* The official journal of the British Holistic Medical Association; www.bhma.org
- *Complementary Therapies in Clinical Practice and Complementary Medicine*; www.elsevierhealth.com/journals
- *Spirituality and Health International*; www.interscience.wiley.com/jounal/shi
- *Alternative Therapies in Health and Medicine*; www.Alternative-Therapies.com
- *Integrative Cancer Therapies*; www.sagepub.com

Help with appraising a website can be found at www.discern.org.uk

Chapter 19

Rehabilitation: imperatives in cancer and palliative care education

Kim Platt-Johnson

> *You matter because you are you. You matter to the last moment of your life, and we will do all we can not only to help you die peacefully but to live until you die.*
> Dame Cicely Saunders

Aim

The aim of this chapter is to explore the process of rehabilitation for cancer and palliative care patients, and to identify teaching strategies that will enhance the learning of those clinicians delivering rehabilitative care.

Learning outcomes

- Have a greater understanding of the concept of rehabilitation and its relationship to cancer and palliative care education.
- Demonstrate increased awareness of the importance of a multi-disciplinary rehabilitation approach in cancer and palliative care education.
- Demonstrate an increased awareness of the implications of integrating the concept of rehabilitation into practice via education.
- Have a greater knowledge of the role that the educator can play in supporting the development of rehabilitative cancer and palliative care education.

Introduction

A diagnosis of cancer can affect any aspect of our lives, and may lead to physical, psychological, spiritual and social distress. Supportive care is now seen as integral to any treatment plan for those with cancer and palliative care needs. In order to improve the illness experience, services are increasingly integrating rehabilitative interventions into their supportive care provision.

The first part of this chapter will look at rehabilitation in the context of cancer and palliative care services. The second half will look at the key issues in the provision of rehabilitative education and the teaching strategies that will assist in the delivery of that education.

The National Institute for Clinical Excellence (NICE) (2004) recommendation entitled *Improving Supportive and Palliative Care for Adults with Cancer* includes *Key Recommendation 16*, which promotes the formation of systems to enable cancer rehabilitation services to develop.

> Commissioners and providers, working through Cancer Networks, should insti-
> tute mechanisms to ensure that patients' needs for rehabilitation are recognised
> and that comprehensive rehabilitation services and suitable equipment are
> available to patients in all care locations.
> National Institute for Clinical Excellence (2004, p. 12)

A rehabilitative approach to care integrates strategies that are aimed at reducing the impact which the disease, the illness experience and the ensuing treatments can have on the quality of life. The key focus throughout the journey is on supporting patients and their carers in regaining control, maintaining realistic hope, and understanding and making choices that lead to adaptation and empowerment in the changing situation.

Much has been written about the elements necessary for effective rehabilitation. The following essential components have been identified by Habeck *et al.* (1984).

- Comprehensive input is needed to address the needs of the whole person, recognising that each person's life involves a unique blend of psychological, social, vocational, economic and physical factors.
- A team approach is required to achieve coordinated inter-disciplinary care.
- Goals for rehabilitation are derived from the effects of medical problems in accordance with prognostic expectations.
- Education is a major component of the rehabilitation process.
- Intervention occurs as soon as likelihood of disability is anticipated.
- The unit of care includes both the patient and their family.
- Rehabilitation needs must be reassessed on a continuing basis and met through-out all phases of care.

The principles outlined above do not appear to be at odds with agreed best practice in cancer and palliative care. Therefore it could be expected that there would be few obstacles to the combining of philosophies. Certainly, in recent years, cancer and palliative care services have seen a more widespread acceptance of a more patient-focused, rehabilitative approach. Rehabilitation needs are no longer regarded as the 'Cinderella area' of care (Traynor, 1995), as they once were in cancer and palliative care service provision.

Despite this, active rehabilitation for some groups of cancer and palliative care patients has been slower to gain acceptance than that for others. For patients who anticipate long years of remission or even cure, the idea of active rehabilitation in order to promote maximum independence raises few concerns for healthcare professionals. It is accepted that there may be a need for rehabilitative support aimed at enabling cancer survivors to rebuild a life that has been altered by the intrusion of the illness.

As well as those patients who can expect to be cured of the disease, there are those who can expect a long and active life with cancer. Cancer treatments are now becoming more effective at controlling disease. Many patients and their families may find themselves facing repeated adaptation and re-evaluation of their lives, while coping with ongoing treatments and their unwanted side-effects. The patient and their family may grieve over repeated physical, psychological, emotional and spiritual losses, and may have to cope with permanent disability and stigma. The more chronic nature of many cancers forces on many a life that includes a need for ongoing adaptation to change and disability. As Watson *et al.* (2005) state:

> *the length of survival for most patients with cancer and other chronic progressive cardiac, respiratory and neurological illnesses has increased over the past 25 years. In some patients this is associated with prolonged disability due to the disease itself and/or the side-effects of treatment.*

The need for support to adjust to such changes may begin at the point of diagnosis and can be required throughout the illness experience, with increased need for input at various points of concern or crisis.

Living in the face of ongoing life-threatening disease places demands on both personal and professional resources. Support is sometimes required not only to manage the physical repercussions but also to actively take control of the emotional, psychosocial and spiritual dimensions of the illness experience.

Belief in the importance of maintaining hope and supporting adaptation, regardless of the anticipated prognosis, or time, creates an environment within which individual flourishing and growth can continue even when some aspects of life have to be relinquished, albeit reluctantly.

> *The patient may be faced with constructing a new 'self' linking his/her present experience to his/her former life, before diagnosis, and linking into the future through aims and goals. The skills of the entire multidisciplinary team may be involved in this reconstruction.*
>
> *Hopkins and Tookman, 2000, p. 126*

For those patients whose illness is considered to be advanced at diagnosis, for the elderly who often have a number of coexisting problems, and for those perceived to be close to death, the idea of active rehabilitation has been slower to gain acceptance than in other areas, sometimes being seen as unnecessary, inappropriate or even unduly interventional in certain circumstances.

For patients with complex and advancing care needs, the offering of appropriate rehabilitative support in the face of physical deterioration can be demanding. As evidence (to be discussed later in the chapter) suggests, motivation, teamwork, support from the specialists in this area, and knowledge of the patient's fears, concerns and desires can bring worthwhile, if subtle benefits for the patient in terms of reducing disability and increasing individual independence and control.

The educator has an important role to play in encouraging the wider use of rehabilitation techniques for all who require cancer and palliative support. As rehabilitation services in this area develop, and such services refine and evaluate their skills, the education process offers an opportunity to disseminate information about such development and facilitate the transfer of such skills into practice. Greater understanding of the benefits, and wider application of rehabilitation principles, will help to ensure that evolving services include appropriate rehabilitative interventions, equipment and resources.

Objections to active rehabilitation, particularly for patients with advanced disease, often stem from confusion about the application of its principles. Common misconceptions include the belief that the desired result of rehabilitation should be a measurable improvement or restoration of function (National Council for Hospice and Specialist Palliative Care Services, 2000, p. 2). The concept of rehabilitation is also more generally associated with disability linked to chronic benign disease (Watson *et al.*, 2005).

As many cancer and palliative care patients are seen as having ongoing disease, with deficits that can be progressive, and with an illness that is often perceived as being terminal (Sliwa and Marciniak, 1999), there may be a perception that the patient may be 'beyond' rehabilitative support. This belief, coupled with a poor knowledge of cancer and rehabilitation and inadequate detection of rehabilitation problems (Fulton, 1994), could lead to appropriate rehabilitative services not being available to those who are sometimes in greatest need of them.

The appropriate use of rehabilitation must be addressed educationally both in the classroom and in the clinical setting. Although rehabilitation can, and often does, offer a mechanism whereby one can overcome disability and restore a high level of function, its philosophy can be used effectively to allow us to offer a way of supporting individuals with a far wider range of problems than those we expect will make a significant 'recovery.' Rehabilitative interventions for those experiencing advanced life-threatening disease may be more subtle in their goals, but are no less valuable because of this. Reluctance of healthcare professionals to consider that active rehabilitation can be appropriate for a wide range of patients, regardless of the stage of their illness, may lead to patients with advanced disease experiencing a poorer quality of life. Priorities may shift and goals may change, but the need for hope, regardless of time, requires an active process that is relevant to every minute of a patient's life.

Cancer and palliative care education is necessarily concerned with the quality of a person's experiences of dying. Through incorporation of the rehabilitative approach in education, it is possible to maximise the quality of an individual's life in the face of death.

The next section of the chapter will look at the role that education can play in promoting and supporting rehabilitation-focused cancer and palliative care services.

Education: a forum for discussion of the evidence base

Because interventions have been used less readily for patients with advanced disease, there has been a paucity of evidence available to support the argument for more widespread use of rehabilitation services in cancer and palliative care. Although evidence of the effectiveness of rehabilitative interventions is sparse, it is growing. As Scialla *et al.* (2000, p. 122) state:

> *relatively few studies have examined the effects of cancer rehabilitation. An early study by Dietz qualitatively examined functional improvement in 1019 patients and observed at least moderate functional recovery in 68% of those patients.*

This lack of evidence has led some to question whether rehabilitation is considered a waste of resources for people with life-threatening illnesses (National Council for Hospice and Specialist Palliative Care Services, 2000, p. 2).

Fortunately, in many areas, innovative interventions are being developed and evaluated, and their encouraging results are demonstrating how rehabilitative support can be offered sensitively and appropriately for all patients and their carers.

Skills developed by those trained in rehabilitative techniques are being adapted and integrated into specialist and general palliative care provision. Expertise in cancer and palliative care rehabilitation is developing and expanding. Many professions, such as physiotherapy, occupational therapy, speech therapy and dietetics, are developing expertise in cancer and palliative care. Such expertise is seen as a sub-specialty within their own paramedical field.

If used sensitively, and recognising the limitations relevant to patients with ongoing, sometimes terminal disease, a rehabilitative approach can enhance high-quality supportive care. Those developing rehabilitative interventions have demonstrated improvements in areas where patients express dissatisfaction.

> *Recent studies have highlighted some elements of dissatisfaction with oncology services which include: poor communication (Wilkinson, 1990; Barley et al., 1999); lack of information (Feber, 1998; McNamara, 1999); inadequate psychosocial support and lack of advice about supportive and complementary therapies (Barley et al.,1999).*
>
> Hopkins and Tookman, 2000, p. 123

The interventions are also aimed at addressing patient and carer concerns regarding autonomy and independence. Such concerns are frequently cited by patients and their carers as causing great distress and hopelessness. (This issue is discussed in more detail in the third book of this series.)

Filiberti *et al.* (2001) looked at the characteristics of five cancer patients who found the illness experience so distressing that they eventually took their own lives. The researchers identified that these patients showed great concern about the lack of autonomy and independence, refused to be dependent on others, and feared and worried about losing their autonomy. Four patients presented with functional and physical impairments, uncontrolled pain, awareness of being in the terminal stage of the disease, and mild to moderate depression. They had feelings of hopelessness as a result of their clinical condition. Feelings that were emphasised were fear of suffering, and feeling that they were being a burden to others. Cheville (2000) also noted that the prospect of uncontrolled pain, isolation and crumbling autonomy was reported by patients as one of their most disturbing fears, sometimes more distressing than the fear of ultimately dying. These examples demonstrate the adverse impact of hopelessness and feelings of dependency – issues that may be improved by rehabilitative interventions.

This places a responsibility on the educator to provide opportunities for those involved in cancer and palliative care to explore the relevance and the application of developing rehabilitation interventions in practice.

There are promising research findings about the role that rehabilitative interventions can play in reducing disability and distress in cancer and palliative care. There is also increasing evidence demonstrating how such techniques can be integrated into the practice of a range of disciplines.

Ongoing research into the effectiveness of rehabilitation for cancer and palliative care patients is also offering increasing insights into the beneficial effects that can be achieved for a wide range of cancer and palliative care patients, even for frail elderly patients and those with deteriorating physical functioning and advanced disease.

Scialla *et al.* (2000) studied the effectiveness of an intervention for cancer asthenia (fatigue) in the elderly. An identified group of elderly, fatigued patients was offered a comprehensive individualised inpatient rehabilitation programme in which:

> each patient received psychological counselling, therapeutic exercises, recreational therapy, mobility and self-care training. ... The rehabilitation goal for all patients was to maximise their functional status to a level allowed by their impairments.
>
> Scialla et al. (2000, p. 123)

The results were encouraging, leading the researchers to conclude that regardless of the cancer diagnosis, elderly cancer patients with asthenia did show increases in physical and cognitive function after multi-disciplinary rehabilitation.

Such research is important because it highlights individualised, sensitive adaptation of the principles, taking into account the patient's physical condition, and can benefit even the most elderly patient groups while respecting their limitations. Such improvement appeared measurable and had a positive impact on patients' quality of life. Therefore educationalists need to focus on all phases of the patient journey and all types of patient. Through education, opportunities can be explored which promote the development of rehabilitative, creative and caring strategies that can be adapted and applied in difficult or challenging circumstances.

The multi-centre breathlessness management study (Corner *et al.*, 1996) evaluated the effectiveness of education and support for patients experiencing breathlessness secondary to lung cancer. Those who suffered from this distressing and difficult to manage symptom were offered the opportunity to explore the impact and meaning of their breathlessness, to learn practical interventions for pacing and prioritising their activity, and to integrate helpful breathing and anxiety management techniques into their daily lives. The intervention built on the experiences and expertise of the disciplines of physiotherapy and occupational therapy, and offered those experiencing breathlessness the opportunity to take control of their breathing and also to manage the anxiety often linked to their breathlessness. The positive results which are now being integrated into palliative care professional practice across disciplines demonstrate that patients with lung cancer who suffer from breathlessness can experience improved function, reduced distress and a greater sense of control over an often progressively debilitating symptom.

There is also growing evidence in support of the benefits of physical exercise for improving quality of life for patients undergoing treatment for cancer.

> Early results have so far have been positive, demonstrating that the study participants are showing increased activity, fitness levels, muscle tone and weight, which has led to a more positive outlook.
>
> Cancer Research UK (2004)

Specialists in this area are seeking to demonstrate the importance of integrating exercise into support programmes for patients. Many believe that this is an area that has not received enough attention. The researchers noted that the potential of exercise was to identify the impact on the physical/functional problems of patients, as well as their psychosocial problems. This suggests that it could make a valuable contribution to patient care along with other existing quality-of-life interventions, such as psychological support and complementary therapies (Stevinson and Fox, 2005, p. 68).

Other research is demonstrating the effectiveness of using the principles of rehabilitation in areas such as the following:

- fatigue management
- psychological symptom management
- lymphoedema management
- breathlessness management
- stress management
- grief interventions
- anxiety and depression management.

The previously mentioned research and the above work demonstrate how different professions are using rehabilitation in busy clinical practice areas. Providing a forum for discussion of and reflection upon the use of rehabilitation in a variety of settings is an important responsibility of the educator.

Busy practice areas may offer the practitioner a snapshot of rehabilitative techniques that may be useful to their client group. The educator can provide an opportunity to review the research looking at the entire cancer journey, offering the student an opportunity to analyse the implications for different interventions useful in the different phases of the rehabilitation process.

Useful teaching strategies

Healthcare professionals who have little understanding of the concept of rehabilitation in palliative care should, through a variety of learning strategies, be given the opportunity to question and challenge the strengths and weaknesses of the approach. A change in practice will not come about by transfer of knowledge alone, as change may involve challenging or changing beliefs and behaviours that have previously led to the rejection of rehabilitation for cancer/palliative care patients, particularly those with advanced disease. Having the opportunity to explore this with those colleagues who are actively involved in rehabilitative support can help to break down the barriers that arise from the belief that an active rehabilitative approach is not appropriate for many cancer and palliative care patients.

The educator plays a vital role as the catalyst to encourage closer working with the client, ignoring the professional agenda. This may involve refocusing goals around the patient, working in the best interests of the service user, developing skills of proactive and anticipatory planning, recognising the qualities and skills of other team members, being open to the scrutiny of other professions/patients, and a desire to fulfil the obligation to communicate to the highest possible standard. Development of these qualities will assist greatly in the endeavour to offer effective cancer and palliative care rehabilitation, sometimes in the most distressing and challenging of circumstances.

The aims of the educational input should be as follows:

- to encourage a desire to consider the issues generated by integrating a rehabilitative philosophy into their care
- to facilitate sharing of the lived experience of those actively involved in cancer rehabilitation

- to create innovative opportunities for those offering care to hear first-hand accounts of the benefits to be gained from those who may have accessed such services
- to motivate the student to approach their care from a new perspective.

Getting the environment right

Ensuring that the experience is meaningful and relevant involves providing a learning environment that is conducive to adult learning.

Keogh *et al.* (1999) identified factors which can be seen as stimulating for adult learners. These factors include encouraging the learners' involvement in curriculum planning, identification of the specific needs of the group, and defining objectives and resources, leading to implementation and self-evaluation of learning.

Working together as a team focusing on rehabilitation issues applied to practical scenarios/challenges gives students the opportunity to identify concerns, plan their strategies, and evaluate and review implementation in a neutral setting. Shared problem-based learning (*see* Chapter 3) gives students the opportunity to experience for themselves the benefits of active participation, taking control and active shared decision making without the added clinical and time pressures.

Seeking opportunities for multi-disciplinary learning

It is important that the educator seeks out opportunities for multi-disciplinary education. Rehabilitation requires effective communication across teams. Identification of concerns often involves referral to or consultation with other agencies, as potential needs can be diverse. Busy clinical practice often provides little opportunity to stop and reflect upon the skills and benefits that other team members can bring. The educationalist has an opportunity to support team members in reflecting on practice. Through such reflection the educator has an opportunity to harness a rich diversity of knowledge and stimulate discussion about different approaches to care.

This is an opportunity that is welcomed by professionals. Jeffrey (2004) states that 'A study of educational needs of general practitioners and community nurses concluded that 90% of GPs and 95% of community nurses thought that multi-disciplinary teaching sessions would be helpful.'

Multi-professional communication and teamwork offer a number of opportunities for all involved to develop relationships with other members of the team, allowing clarification of different roles and appropriate referral. Although this can be a mostly positive experience, it could involve unsettling challenge, so it is important that facilitators encourage active dialogue in the classroom and feel confident about managing debate and conflict which will result in a useful outcome.

Blurring of boundaries is to be expected. The impact of this can be explored and an increased inter-disciplinary understanding can be developed in a more objective classroom setting.

> *Given the inter-professional nature of rehabilitation, some skills/roles will be common across the oncology team e.g. communication, a whole person approach.*

> *Although there would be some blurring, many paramedical specialists recognise*
> *that there needs to be recognition of the unique contribution of each member of*
> *the team.*
>
> Chartered Society of Physiotherapy (2003)

Alerting healthcare professionals to blind spots and areas where care could have
been enhanced by multi-disciplinary input is an important role for the facilitator.
The practitioner may be the gatekeeper to other useful services for the patient, but
this can only be utilised if the gatekeeper recognises, and integrates into their
practice, an understanding of the value of others in the team who may offer help. It
is not enough to 'accept' passively the involvement of others, or to expect that other
professionals will be involved without proactive anticipatory planning.

Maintaining realistic hope about the integration of services

Palliative care both nationally and locally emphasises the importance of a rehabilitative approach to care. Once they have reviewed examples of effective use of
rehabilitation in cancer and palliative care, students may continue their journey by
exploring why locally and nationally there are still barriers to such support at all
stages of illness, and why many patients are not appropriately referred to other
services or given social support. For the educator, this is a time to promote the
exploration of reactions to change and loss linked to cancer and palliative care.
Rehabilitative care involves the maintenance or encouragement of realistic hope.
This is a challenge when one is faced with the many fears that surround the disease –
fears that do not escape healthcare professionals. Armstrong-Coster (2004) discusses the reflections of Susan Sontag on attitudes to cancer and the cancer patient.
Sontag discusses how:

> *since cancer is, in the public perception, a disease that causes terror and the cause*
> *of it remains unknown, it is felt ... to be morally if not literally contagious. Thus a*
> *surprisingly large number of people with cancer find themselves being shunned*
> *by relatives and friends.*

Reflections of this kind would make a good discussion point in small group work.
Such small group exploration could involve debate, small group tutorials and role
play to encourage the airing of barriers, misconceptions and prejudice, and an
emphasis on the pivotal role of dialogue. The educator has an important role in
breaking down barriers that would prevent honest and realistic communication.
There is a responsibility to re-emphasise the practical importance of dialogue,
which leads to accurate assessment (the key to successful goal setting) and review of
the situation. The power of the patient's story needs to be heard, and the educator
has a responsibility to incorporate this. Goldie (2005), reflecting on his role as a
psychotherapist working with cancer patients, identifies the following concern:

> *My armentarium of 'just words' was unimpressive in comparison to the*
> *resources of a physician or anaesthetist for treating pain and the high-tech world*
> *of a modern hospital with its 'scans', magnetic resonance imaging, computer*
> *tomography. ... But this leaves out of the account the healing properties of talking*
> *and listening, and the untapped power of the mind for denying or modifying the*
> *effects of sensory input to the body.*

Critical incident and case study discussion enables healthcare professionals to explore patient/carer scenarios and the benefit that could be achieved by offering rehabilitative services focused on improving activity, control, hope and independence. Armstrong-Coster (2004) emphasises the value of exposure to personal testimony:

> *Doing so enables the storyteller to re-order their individual life story. It can also function as a learning aid to carers, helping them to develop their own knowledge of the illness experience, and a telling personal cancer story can serve as an example to others who might, one day, experience the same problem.*

These useful concepts related to storytelling will be explored further in the third book of this series. Such powerful emotional as well as practical learning places on the educator a responsibility to develop skills of personal and group facilitation. The educator needs to develop a learning environment that is able to manage positively difficult personal and professional issues that may arise, maintaining a feeling of safety for the student.

Such difficulties may include the following:

- feeling uncomfortable acknowledging one's lack of knowledge about other roles
- sharing of feelings of negativity toward other healthcare professionals, interventions or groups
- concerns about the realities of individualised care in busy practice
- a challenge to professional boundaries
- personal and professional incidents triggered by discussion in the group.

This is a challenge for rehabilitative education, as rehabilitative multi-disciplinary learning will include development of skills, beliefs and attitudes.

Facilitating the identification of priorities and encouragement of creative solutions

Having encouraged a climate of mutual respect and collaboration, there are a number of strategies available to the palliative care educator to encourage a creative and dynamic learning environment. A range of active learning techniques have been suggested to encourage debate, exploration and reflection on practice, stimulating creative problem solving (Cheville, 2000).

Jeffrey (2004) identifies a number of techniques that are useful for stimulating reflection and discussion. Rather than the more formal lecture format, Jeffrey suggests considering the use of pictures, music, literature and imaginative games. Such group work is aimed at encouraging the practitioner to look at situations from a range of different viewpoints, affirming the fundamental principle that patients are individuals with different ways of coping with, expressing and perceiving concerns. Such differences are sometimes difficult for others to understand. Despite this, it is necessary to use such creative methods of exploration with the patient/carer in order to gain a better understanding of what may help them.

Patients and carers have been sharing their emotions and insights with healthcare professionals in a variety of ways for years.

Alan Bennett, the playwright, shocked the literary world when he revealed his private battle with colon cancer. Rather than being a deterrent, the experience spurred him on to write about personal and private issues. Bennett dealt with his distress privately, recording incidents and feelings, and published them when he was ready to share the experiences with others.

Many people have seen the paintings by the artist Michele Petrone, defining important stages of his cancer journey. In an interview with BBC News, Petrone (cited by Elliott, 2003) reflected on the powerful way in which his art was able to facilitate expression. He stated that 'Painting definitely helped me. I had never been through anything like this before, and I found it very difficult to articulate.' Through his painting he has offered support to others, as many have identified similar feelings themselves and found his art stimulating and uplifting. Despite being in isolation, he identified a need to decorate the door of his hospital room, which became a catalyst for his future paintings about his cancer journey. Through his physical losses he acknowledges having gained so much:

> My cancer journey has taught me so much, about myself and about the world around me. But mainly about the things that most of us are never taught about, and don't feel we can talk about openly.
>
> *Petrone (2006)*

The uncertainty envelope

An example of a creative reflective exercise that could be particularly relevant to exploring attitudes to the use of rehabilitation in a cancer and palliative care setting is the use of the uncertainty envelope (Jeffrey, 2004).

In this exercise, which is aimed at exploring attitudes toward death and dying, each of the group members is given a sealed envelope which contains a fictitious date and time of their own death. After considering the envelope, they are offered the choice of whether to open it or not. Jeffrey (2004) has observed that few students want to open the envelope, but that the exercise leads to discussion around the question 'How long have I got?' Our beliefs concerning death and active intervention for those who are close to death are pivotal to acceptance of rehabilitation for patients with advanced disease, and such an exercise triggers debate around this difficult subject. This exercise could be altered to make it more specific to rehabilitative education. Each envelope could contain the statement 'You will be offered a range of rehabilitative services' or 'You will not be offered rehabilitative services.' The subsequent discussions, whether among individuals or groups, can focus on the implications of either scenario. This should also include eliciting student attitudes and feelings depending upon the group to which they are allocated. Sensitive facilitation is crucial to the success of this teaching strategy. The facilitator needs to be alert to emotional issues for the student that may be triggered by this reflective exercise, and should provide appropriate support when debriefing the students.

Practical solutions

Pragmatic solutions discussed within the group can be applied to clinical practice between sessions, and the outcomes reviewed within the group. Practical integration of rehabilitative strategies/skills is recorded utilising reflective models, and time is allocated within subsequent teaching sessions for the student to share with the group the scenario, ensuing reactions, responses and action planning.

A typical scenario is outlined below.

James is 78 years old and has been living alone since the death of his wife 2 years ago. He has one son who lives 2 hours' drive away and visits at the weekend. James has chronic obstructive airways disease and has been diagnosed with an advanced lung tumour for which he has received radiotherapy to help to improve the symptoms. His GP is working with James to monitor his illness. His ongoing concerns include breathlessness, loss of appetite and low mood, due to his illness and social isolation.

You have been visiting on request as his district nurse. He has a supportive neighbour, but she has been away on holiday for the last week. You have been contacted by his son, as James has fallen and appears to be getting weaker. His son is concerned that James may not cope at home, and is asking for him to be assessed for placement in a nursing home, although James has always resisted this idea, saying that he wants to die at home surrounded by his memories.

Questions to consider could include the following.

- How can James be enabled to live and die in the place of his choice?
- Is this patient being supported as fully as possible?
- Are all steps being taken to maximise his potential?
- Could any other members of the team/other services be of help?
- What went well?
- What could be done differently?
- How will this experience shape your practice in the future?

Existing models for reflection on practice may be used, or the individual or group may prefer to devise their own reflective questions.

Reflection with others could serve as a very useful learning tool, as often the pooling of insights may lead to the selection of solutions previously unknown to or not considered by the practitioner.

> *When a surprise occurs, a learner is caused to pause and reflect on what has happened and on their previous actions. The process of reflection may lead to the selection of a solution.*
>
> *(Macleod, 2004, p. 119)*

Key points

- Integrating the principle of rehabilitation into our practice requires the conviction that active holistic and multi-dimensional support with a focus on independence and autonomy is not an optional extra but a basic right for all, regardless of diagnosis, and clinicians should be educated to integrate this in their delivery of care.
- As hope is fundamental to our existence, it is never absent and therefore always available to be nurtured. The presence of hope, whatever this hope may be for, provides us with the opportunity to integrate the rehabilitative philosophy. This needs to be captured and taught in the classroom.
- Appropriateness depends upon how sensitively rehabilitative support is offered. Key to this is the effective education of those who deliver rehabilitative care. Through educational initiatives, teams have the opportunity to review the impact that rehabilitation is having on patients in cancer and palliative care.

Conclusion

Reflection is a fundamental tool for enhancing and assisting both students and educators in the development of their learning strategies. As clinicians and educators develop their skills through the reflective process, it is essential that they take into account where patients who are being rehabilitated are in their reflective journey. They may be at a pivotal point of reflection in their cancer and palliative care experience. As patients and carers oscillate from one experience to another, they need clinicians who have been educated to ascertain and fulfil their needs in all dimensions, including physical and psychosocial domains. This chapter has outlined definitions of and available research on rehabilitation for patients with a cancer and/or palliative care diagnosis. Teaching rehabilitation in cancer and palliative care may pose challenges, as it is an aspect of care that is gaining a higher profile. This chapter has suggested a range of teaching strategies that may assist those educators who are embarking on the teaching of rehabilitative care in cancer and palliative care.

Implications for the reader's own practice

The National Council for Hospice and Specialist Palliative Care Services (2000) identified questions for services to consider when integrating a rehabilitative approach into their practice. These questions are relevant to both individuals and teams, and are worthy of consideration in relation to education. When reflecting on whether the rehabilitation philosophy is alive in your practice, consider the following questions which are adapted from the National Council document (National Council for Hospice and Specialist Palliative Care Services. 2000, p. 12).

1 Is rehabilitation prioritised as an important part of cancer and palliative care education in your locality?

2 How do you encourage clinicians to address the rehabilitative needs of their patients?

3 What agencies and units are currently providing rehabilitation services/education in the area?

4 What teaching strategies do you employ to teach cancer and palliative rehabilitative care?

5 How might you develop and expand these in the future?

6 Who could you work in partnership with to provide rehabilitation education?

7 Are you aware of what other agencies and units are currently providing rehabilitation services in the area?

8 Do you make the best use of the services and skills available in primary care?

9 Could you work in partnership with others to provide rehabilitation?

References

Armstrong-Coster A. *Living and Dying with Cancer*. Cambridge: Cambridge University Press; 2004.

Barley V, Tritter J, Daniel R *et al*. Meeting the needs of people with cancer for support and self management. A collaborative project between Bristol Oncology Centre; Department of Sociology, University of Warwick; Bristol Cancer Help Centre. 1999; Unpublished.

Cancer Research UK. *Exercise boosts recovery from breast cancer* (press release); www.cancer researchuk.org/news/pressreleases/exercise_breastcancer_8oct04 (accessed 7 October 2005).

Chartered Society of Physiotherapy. *The Role of Physiotherapy for People with Cancer. CSP Position Statement*. London: Chartered Society of Physiotherapy; 2003.

Cheville AL. *Cancer Rehabilitation and Palliative Care. Why does rehabilitation matter in the cancer patient with advanced disease?*; www.findarticles.com/p/articles/mi_qa3946/is_200001/ai_n8878654 (accessed 23 June 2005).

Corner J, Plant H, Ahern R *et al*. Non-pharmacological intervention for breathlessness in lung cancer. *Palliat Med*. 1996; **10**: 299–305.

Elliott J. *Battling Cancer Through Art*. BBC Health Online, 2003; http://news.bbc.co.uk/1/hi/health/2340613.stm (accessed 24 June 2006).

Feber T. Design and evaluation of a strategy to provide support and information for people with cancer of the larynx. *Euro J Oncol Nurs*. 1998; **2(2)**: 106–14.

Filiberti A, Ripamonti C, Totis A *et al*. Characteristics of terminal cancer patients who committed suicide during a home palliative care program. *J Pain Symptom Manage*. 2001; **22**: 544–53.

Fulton CL. Physiotherapists in cancer care: a framework for rehabilitation of patients. *Physiotherapy*. 1994; **80**: 830–34.

Goldie L. *Psychotherapy and Treatment of Cancer Patients*. London: Routledge; 2005.

Habeck RV *et al*. Cancer rehabilitation and continuing care: a case study. *Cancer Nurs*. 1984. **7**: 315–19.

Hopkins KF, Tookman AJ. Rehabilitation and specialist palliative care. *Int J Palliat Nurs*. 2000; **6**: 123–30.

Jeffrey D, editor. *Teaching Palliative Care: a practical guide*. Oxford: Radcliffe Publishing; 2004.

Keogh K, Jeffrey D, Flanagan S. The Palliative Care Education Group for Gloucestershire (PEGG). *Eur J Cancer Care*. 1999; **8**: 44–7.

Macleod R. Challenges for education in palliative care. *Prog Palliat Care*. 2004; **12**: 117–21.

McNamara S. Information and support: a descriptive study of the needs of patients with cancer before their first experience of XRT. *Euro J Oncol Nurs*. 1999; **3(1)**: 31–7.

National Council for Hospice and Specialist Palliative Care Services (NCHSPCS). *Fulfilling Lives: rehabilitation in palliative care,* London: NCHSPCS; 2000.

National Institute for Clinical Excellence. *Improving Supportive and Palliative Care for Adults with Cancer.* London: National Institute for Clinical Excellence; 2004.

Petrone M. *Rapport. Newsletter from St John's Hospice Lancaster;* www.sjhospice.org.uk/mich.htm (accessed 24 June 2006).

Scialla S, Cole R, Scialla T *et al.* Rehabilitation for elderly patients with cancer asthenia: making a transition to palliative care. *Palliat Med.* 2000; **14:** 121–7.

Sliwa JA, Marciniak C. Physical rehabilitation of the cancer patient. *Cancer Treat Res.* 1999; **100:** 75–89.

Stevinson C, Fox KR. The role of exercise for cancer rehabilitation in UK hospitals: a survey of oncology nurses. *Eur J Cancer Care.* 2005; **14:** 63–9.

Traynor BE. A nursing assessment of rehabilitation needs following treatment for cancer. *Eur J Cancer.* 1995; **31:** 294.

Watson M, Lucas C, Hoy A *et al. Oxford Handbook of Palliative Care.* Oxford: Oxford University Press; 2005.

Wilkinson S. Factors which influence how nurses communicate with cancer patients. *J Adv Nurs.* 1990; **16:** 677–88.

Chapter 20

Teaching approaches to survivorship issues in cancer care

Candy Cooley

> *Being a cancer survivor is at the forefront of my self-awareness. It enters into conversations that I have with myself about what I want to do, how I want to spend money, how I want to spend time, my energy, all of that. Being a cancer survivor has added another dimension to my identity. I am a cancer survivor.*
>
> Mortimer Brown, aged 80 years

Aim

This chapter will consider how the educator and the learner can develop their understanding of this new topic of survivorship within the context of cancer care and academic rigour.

Learning outcomes

- Appreciate what survivorship means in cancer care.
- Understand the relationship between length of survival and quality of life.
- Consider a range of teaching options for delivering this topic within a classroom setting.

Introduction

Including a session on 'issues of survivorship' within the curriculum of adult cancer education programmes is a fairly new idea. However, within the field of paediatrics this topic has been included in the curriculum for some time. Advances in cancer treatments and supportive care have led to a situation in which survivorship issues now need to be considered within all cancer courses to ensure that healthcare professionals are aware of this aspect of the patient's cancer journey.

It is well recognised that students are individuals, and in order to sustain meaningful learning that will result in a long-term change in understanding rather than short-term involvement, individual learning preferences need to be considered. The goal for educators is to engage the student in a way that ensures their ability to develop based on this learning and, more importantly, to change and challenge practice.

What is survival?

Survival has been defined as 'how long patients with a given type of cancer live on average after diagnosis – the proportion alive after five years is the standard measure' (National Audit Office, 2004, p. 2).

Worldwide, cancer develops in an estimated 1 in 200 children each year (National Audit Office, 2004). In the UK in 1999, a total of 1,470 children were diagnosed with cancer. Among adults, one in three people in England will develop cancer, and one in four will die from it. In 2003 there were over 220,000 new cases of adult cancer in England, with over 128,000 deaths (National Audit Office, 2004). Survival rates for cancer vary enormously, but it is important to consider that in some cancers the likelihood of survival exceeds 80%, and in others, such as lung cancer, the survival statistics remain poor (6% for lung cancer within the UK).

For the majority of cancers, a higher proportion of women than men survive for at least 5 years after diagnosis (this is known as the 5-year survival rate). The 5-year survival rate for all cancers diagnosed in the early 1990s was 36% for men and 49% for women. Age is also an important factor. Among adults, the younger the age at diagnosis, the higher the survival rate for almost every cancer. In men, the highest 5-year survival rate is for testicular cancer (97% for those diagnosed during the 1990s). For women, the highest 5-year survival rate is for malignant melanoma of the skin (88%).

For paediatric cancers, the early successes seen in survival rates since the 1960s followed the widespread introduction of chemotherapy. In the 1970s, the development of a multi-disciplinary approach to the treatment of childhood cancers enabled more improvements in the 5-year survival rates for both the leukaemias and solid tumours (Meadows *et al.*, 1993). For adult cancers, the first major changes that occurred in the development of cancer services followed the publication of the *Policy Framework for Commissioning Cancer Services* (Department of Health, 1995). This was followed by *The NHS Cancer Plan* (Department of Health, 2000), which set out a national framework for the development and delivery of cancer services.

Now, in the early twenty-first century, advances in treatments, the use of a coordinated approach to surgery, radiotherapy and combination chemotherapy, and service approaches within the field of adult cancer have ensured that we are beginning to see a steady increase in both length of survival and cure rates (National Audit Office, 2004).

Quality of life

Although from a statistical viewpoint it is easy to see that individuals with cancer are surviving for longer, and 5-year 'cure' rates are rising, this gives no picture of the consequences for an individual of being a survivor. We are aware that the three modalities in current regular use all have physical and psychological costs (Souhami and Tobias, 1995).

Surgery may be disfiguring, mutilating or require the removal of an organ or a limb. Chemotherapy has a systemic effect and is known not only to have carcinogenic tendencies but also to cause specific damage to various physiological processes. Radiotherapy is known to indiscriminately damage healthy growing tissue, with possible DNA damage – an oncogenic effect – having the possible major consequence of development of secondary tumours.

> *During my treatment and for several years after ... my primary concern was recurrence and, although I haven't had any, I would be lying if I say I don't think about it all the time. [Now] I worry about secondary cancers.*
>
> Karen Dyer, 24 years old

Quality of life is always a fairly contentious area. Some would say that you can only consider quality of life when there is life. Therefore there is an argument that the experiences and treatments associated with cancer only have long-term sequelae if the patient survives. Ottery (2004) suggests that the quality of the survivorship should be as important as the length of survival. She states that managing the symptoms associated with the long-term chronic sequelae, such as fatigue, not only makes survival a chore but also reduces the willingness of the individual to receive further treatment if the disease does reoccur.

Quality of life is a generalistic concept that encompasses not only physical and psychological function, but also the broader issues of education, job capabilities, and social and family life. The World Health Organization (WHO) defines health as 'a state of complete physical, mental and social well-being and not merely the absence of disease or disability' (World Health Organization, 2004).

This definition is important for the survivor of cancer, as it identifies the emotional and social dimensions as well as the physical ones. Jenny *et al.* (1995) considered the challenges facing medical, nursing and health carers in identifying and minimising the long-term sequelae in order to ensure maximum quality of life. They stated that identifying the health-related quality of life of an individual who has survived cancer is the first step in assessing the impact that the disease and its treatment will have on long-term quality of life for that person.

The price of cure varies according to diagnosis and treatment. However, debates regarding the need for long-term follow-up arise in connection to them all. Long-term follow-up has shown that although many patients survive their disease, they are left with significant long-term sequelae. Therefore when assessing the success or failure of cure, the effect on the patient and their family must be part of the equation (Wen and Gustafson, 2004).

Assessment of quality of life, and for the purpose of this learning quality of survivorship, requires some type of quality-of-life (QOL) tool. However, it has long been acknowledged that such tools can be subjective, and their reliability is often questionable within health/ill health situations (Montazeri *et al.*, 1996). According to the WHO's research in 1994, quality of life is determined by a number of factors which are perceived by an individual within the context of their life, culture and value system (World Health Organization, 2004). This might be the starting point for the students' learning. Do QOL tools easily identify issues for survivors of cancer?

Late effects

Late effects can appear months or years after the patient has completed their cancer treatments. At this stage the patient may be biologically 'cured', in that they show no evidence of biological disease, have the same life expectancy as any other individual, and may die of old age or illness unrelated to cancer.

Late effects can be either physiological or psychological, or a combination of both. These may lead to a chronic impact on the individual's ability to function both physically and socially.

The common physiological effects are often determined by the age of the patient at the onset of treatment and the toxicity of the treatment protocol. Younger patients are usually more able to deal with the toxicity of the initial treatment, and may make an almost total recovery, the only permanent damage being to reproductive function (Byrne *et al.*, 1987).

As might be expected, late effects are influenced by the treatment area. For example, children who receive cranial radiation and/or intrathecal chemotherapy may have cognitive dysfunction (Peck, 1979). Adults with head and neck cancers that have been treated with radiotherapy may present with thyroid function problems, or with salivary gland damage that leads to long-term dental and swallowing problems associated with a totally or partially dry mouth. Post-surgery radiotherapy in breast cancer can lead to lymphoedema or osteoporosis. Chemotherapy is associated with a range of potential systemic long-term problems (Pendersen-Bjergaard, 1995).

Many of the treatments that are used to cure cancer are themselves carcinogenic. Therefore the possibility of secondary cancers being caused by the treatment is a real threat as survival times lengthen (Brada, 1995).

> *Death is not the enemy; living in constant fear of it is.*
>
> *Norman Cousins*

The psychological implications of diagnosis and treatment of cancer are well documented. Anxiety associated with the fear of recurrence, loss of regular contact with the healthcare team, isolation from social groups and fatigue are commonly described (Stark *et al.*, 2002).

Ensuring that the patient has access to resources and follow-up is imperative (Tesauro *et al.*, 2002). It is important that services are initiated to enable follow-up of cancer patients following 'cure' (James *et al.*, 1994). Assessment of the risk of long-term sequelae may enable the healthcare professional to identify and initiate interventions earlier, thereby reducing the impact on the patient's quality of life (Wen and Gustafson, 2004). However, these interventions will only be available if the healthcare professional has considered the important implications of survivorship within cancer care.

Teaching strategies

In 1999, Langton undertook a literature review and documentary analysis of cancer nursing education within England. This identified 'rehabilitation and survivorship' as one of the key significant themes, although this tended to be related to psychological issues. Concerns may not only relate to psychological emotions. Some patients will have to deal with physical changes due to treatments. It is these aspects of survivorship that have until recently received minimal consideration within adult cancer care in general. They have received almost no attention within the curriculum programmes of cancer courses, which will tend to make those involved with the cancer patient think of just two outcomes – the 'good death' and the 'happy cure.'

It is tempting to dismiss survivorship issues as being of minimal importance. Many of us would feel that, looking at the overall survival statistics, anyone should be delighted to survive cancer. However, the small amount of research that has been undertaken with adult survivors would seem to demonstrate that the initial euphoria of completing treatment and follow-up is replaced by feelings of vulnerability and fear. Work with older patients also seems to show that their stoical approach to life may mean that they do not express their concerns (Cooley and Coventry, 2003).

There are a number of teaching strategies which can be implemented for this topic area. It is a subject that lends itself to a range of opportunities for interactive student involvement, the inclusion of the personal experience, reflection and biological exploration. It is tempting to consider that this subject is predominantly about the patient's psychological experience of cancer and the impact on their view of life now that they are a survivor. However, this does not allow the healthcare professional to investigate their own thoughts on cancer survival, possibly at a physical cost, or the impact on the family.

One suggested way of introducing this topic to students is to undertake an exercise based on personal values and health beliefs, asking the question 'Is being alive enough? What would you not be prepared to live with?' If the students are able to work in smaller groups, this usually allows a range of debate around what individuals would be prepared to cope with and what they could not tolerate. There is a tendency to get a range of views, from those who would find any impact on their quality of life untenable to those who would be prepared to put up with many long-term sequelae so long as they survived. Exploring the value statements surrounding these views enables the students to understand the cultural and lifestyle impact on quality of life.

One of the key areas within healthcare at present is that of involving 'users' of the service to support developments. There are two ways in which the involvement of patients and clients can be utilised within the topic of survivorship. The first option involves enabling the students to attend a follow-up clinic and, utilising a critical incident framework, asking a 'survivor' a series of appropriate questions. The findings can then be utilised in the classroom by adopting a case study approach, or simply used as reflective practice.

The other option which may be used is the involvement of the 'survivor' in the classroom setting. This approach has its own potential problems with regard to creating a safe environment for both the 'survivor' and the students, but it has been used in a number of establishments as a key learning tool. People are often concerned that the 'survivor' may feel threatened. However, there is research which demonstrates that people welcome the opportunity to teach the healthcare professionals and to tell their story. Patients are a valuable resource at all stages of healthcare education (Wykurz and Kelly, 2002). It is important to have clear ground rules, an opportunity for debriefing both for the 'survivor' and for the students, and for the educator to have a clear idea of how they will utilise this experience to support the students' learning. If patients are given appropriate support, training and remuneration, the evidence shows that they offer qualities which uniquely enhance the skills of the healthcare professional, specifically with regard to history taking, physical examination and communication (Department of Health, 2000).

Chipas (1995) clearly demonstrated that if students were empowered to be true participants in the learning experience, they became more analytical and better prepared for the future. Enabling students to share their personal reflections and debate the basis of another individual's attitudes ensures that they have a greater breadth as well as depth of understanding of their patients' experiences.

By utilising the 10 'Cs' of reflection suggested by Johns (2000) (*see* Box 20.1), students can move from simple observation and discussion of an experience towards critical analysis and evaluation for future practice.

Box 20.1   The 10 'Cs' of reflection as the basis for learning (Johns, 2000, p. 36)

Commitment – believing that self and practice matters; curiosity and willingness to challenge norms; accepting responsibility for self and practice.

Contradiction – exposing and understanding the reality between desirable and actual practice.

Conflict – using the energy generated to support changing practice.

Challenge and support – empowering others to question and challenge their practice.

Catharsis – dealing with negative feelings, and learning to live with them.

Creation – moving beyond self to see new ways of knowing and doing.

Connection – connecting new knowledge with the reality of practice; realising that experience will alter within time constraints.

Caring – realising desirable practice as everyday reality.

Congruence – reflection being suitable to challenge practice.

Constructing personal knowing in practice – linking experience and theoretical paradigms to develop learning in self.

Johns (2000, p. 36)

Having understood the patient's view of being a survivor, the student needs to consider a number of issues.

- Could the long-term sequelae have been reduced?
- How do we evaluate the impact of these symptoms on the patient's quality of life?
- What systems are in place to support the cancer survivor?
- Do we have an ethical and moral obligation to be responsible for the long-term problems associated with cure?
- What is the impact on family and friends of living with the survivor?

The first two issues relate to understanding the biological impact of cancer treatments on the healthy individual. These could therefore easily be taught in a medical model or using a practical pathology approach. If time is limited, there are a number of online physiology courses that would enable the student to identify any gaps in their knowledge of how the disease or a treatment may impact on the physiology of a patient.

As previously mentioned, discussion could then be focused around considering the QOL tools currently in use in the field of cancer, such as EORTC QLQ or FACT-L (Cella and Tulsky, 1990; Cella, 1995). There are a number of excellent literature reviews that consider QOL tools and their ability to provide a picture of the patient's experience (e.g. Selby, 1993; Jenkinson, 1994).

Then, utilising the critical questioning approach in either the clinical area or the classroom, ensure that the student has the opportunity to link the theory to the personal experiences of a cancer survivor. Encourage debate about the impact on the family and also the social and financial implications, including job prospects, insurance problems and future health problems.

Key points

- It is important to ensure that the student considers the wider implications of being a cancer survivor.
- Encourage the student to consider the physiological impact of survivorship, not simply the psychological impact.
- Empower the student to investigate the patient's experience within a safe environment for both the patient and the students.
- Through the use of critical reflection, enable the student to consider how this new knowledge should impact on their practice, in relation to reducing the risks of long-term sequelae, early identification of problems, and the availability of a service to support these patients in their long-term future.

Conclusion

As an educator, you will be used to the rapid changes within healthcare and the needs of your students. Because this is a fairly new trend for cancer patients and services within the UK, it is a subject which students often do not consider to be particularly relevant to them. However, this topic is having and will continue to have a major impact on treatment decisions and service developments. As a stage is reached where decisions can be made based not just on how *long* the patient will survive, but on how *well* the patient survives, these decisions present a different set of ethical considerations. The students need to be prepared to act on the patient's wishes, based on informed decision making. To do this, they need to have considered the knowledge, skills and expertise that they will require in order to act in the patient's best interest.

For you as the educator it is about mixing the solid medical evidence of the physiological implications of surviving with the philosophical arguments surrounding supportive care and consent. To do this, you need to feel confident of your own knowledge of the long-term sequelae and the problems that may be associated with being a cancer survivor.

And in the end, it's not the years in your life that count. It's the life in your years.

Abraham Lincoln

Implications for the reader's own practice

1 How integrated is the teaching of survivorship in your curriculum?
2 How could you develop learning opportunities to consider the issue of survivorship in the classroom?
3 How will you link this teaching into the practical experiences when students may not meet 'survivors'?
4 How can you raise the importance of this topic in a programme that is often already full of 'active' or intensive-care subjects?
5 Would there be benefits or problems associated with inviting a survivor to the classroom?

References

Brada M. Is there a need to follow up cancer patients? *Eur J Cancer.* 1995; **31**: 655–7.

Byrne J, Mulvihill JJ *et al.* Effects of treatment on fertility in long-term survivors of childhood or adolescent cancer. *NEJM.* 1987; **317**: 1315–21.

Cella DF. Methods and problems in measuring quality of life. *Support Care Cancer.* 1995; **3(1)**: 11–22.

Cella DF, Tulsky DS. Measuring quality of life today: methodological aspects. *Oncology.* 1990; **4**: 29–38.

Chipas A. Do current educational programmes address critical thinking in nurse anaesthesia? *J Am Assoc Nurse Anesth.* 1995; **63**: 45–9.

Cooley C, Coventry G. Cancer and older people. *Nurs Older Person.* 2003; **15**: 22–6.

Department of Health. *Policy Framework for Commissioning Cancer Services: a Report to the Chief Medical Officers of England and Wales (Calman–Hine Report).* London: Department of Health; 1995.

Department of Health. *The NHS Cancer Plan.* London: The Stationery Office; 2000.

James ND, Guerrero D, Brada M. Who should follow up cancer patients? *Clin Oncol.* 1994; **6**: 283–7.

Jenkinson C. Measuring health and medical outcomes: an overview. In: Jenkinson C, editor. *Measuring Health and Medical Outcomes.* London: UCL Press; 1994. pp. 1–6.

Jenny MEM, Kane RL, Lurie N. Developing a measure of health outcomes in survivors of childhood cancer: a review of the issues. *Med Paediatr Oncol.* 1995; **24**: 145–53.

Johns C. *Becoming a Reflective Practitioner.* Oxford: Blackwell Science; 2000.

Langton H. *Cancer Nursing Education: literature review and documentary analysis. Research highlights.* London: English National Board; 1999.

Meadows AT, Black B, Nesbit ME *et al.* Long-term survival. Clinical care, research and education. *Cancer.* 1993; **71**: 3213–15.

Montazeri A, Gillis CR, McEwen J. Measuring quality of life in oncology: is it worthwhile? I. Meaning, purposes and controversies. *Eur J Cancer Care.* 1996; **5**: 159–67.

National Audit Office. *Tackling Cancer in England: saving more lives.* London: The Stationery Office; 2004.

Ottery F (2004) Issues of nutrition, weight and cancer: an overview for clinicians. Business briefing. In: *US Oncology Review;* www.toughbriefings.com (accessed 30 November 2004).

Peck B. Effects of childhood cancer on long-term survivors and their families. *BMJ.* 1979; **1:** 1327–9.

Pendersen-Bjergaard J. Long-term complications of cancer chemotherapy (editorial). *J Clin Oncol.* 1995; **13:** 1534–6.

Selby P. Measuring the quality of life in patients with cancer. In: Walker SR, Rosser R, editors. *Quality of Life Assessment: key issues in the 1990s.* Lancaster: Kluwer Academic Publishers; 1993. pp. 235–69.

Souhami R, Tobias J. *Cancer and its Management.* 2nd ed. Oxford: Blackwell Science; 1995.

Stark D, Kiely M, Smith A *et al.* Anxiety disorders in cancer patients: their nature, associations and relationship to quality of life. *J Clin Oncol.* 2002; **14:** 3137–48.

Tesauro GM, Rowland JH, Lustig C. Survivorship resources for post-treatment cancer survivors. *Cancer Pract.* 2002; **10:** 277–83.

Wen KY, Gustafson DH. Needs assessment for cancer patients and their families. *Health Qual Life Outcomes.* 2004; **2.** www.hqlo.com/content2/1/11 (accessed 27 September 2005).

World Health Organization. *WHO Constitution. Basic texts.* Geneva: World Health Organization; 2004.

Wykurz G, Kelly D. Developing the role of patients as teachers: literature review. *BMJ.* 2002; **325:** 818–21.

Further reading

- National Institute for Clinical Excellence. *Supportive and Palliative Care for the Adult with Cancer.* London: National Institute for Clinical Excellence; 2004.
- Gronwald SL, Hansen Frogge M *et al. Cancer Nursing: principles and practice.* 3rd ed. London: Jones & Bartlett; 1987.

Chapter 21

Health and social policy education: universally relevant, studiously avoided

Lorna Foyle

> *If we, as health workers, or teachers, or students, or civil servants, do not feel that we, and the groups or organisations we belong to, have some power to alter policy that affects our lives, or the lives around us, then why bother getting up in the morning?*
>
> Gill Walt (1994, p. 10)

Aim

This chapter aims to explore the pertinent issues and provide a range of teaching strategies for educationalists delivering cancer and palliative care education that is specifically related to health and social care policies.

Learning outcomes

- Identify teaching strategies to raise awareness of policy and organisational processes relevant to cancer and palliative care education.
- Explore the evolving landscape in which health policy education is delivered.
- Explore the motivating and constraining factors that inhibit students from fully engaging with health and social policy issues relating to cancer and palliative care.
- Identify the relevance of cancer and palliative care health and social policy education in healthcare professionals' portfolio of knowledge, skills and understanding.

Introduction

This author sat writing the outline of this chapter on General Election Day 2005 on a journey to Edinburgh. On leaving the house that morning the discussion was not about who would win the general election, but how many people would turn out to vote. In fact, the turnout for this election was up by 2% from 59.2% to 61.3% (BBC, 2005). Nevertheless, not a very high number when one considers the plight of citizens in oppressed countries where the opportunity to vote would be seized in order to make their contribution to the governing of their country.

It is accepted by most people living in democratic countries that they are entitled to vote at general elections. Paradoxically, in the UK, the very knowledge that the individual is entitled to vote appears to have generated the opposite effect, with people choosing not to cast their votes.

This attitude of indifference is often mirrored in healthcare policy education. So why has this incipient apathy crept into our society? Is it about individuals' beliefs that they are unable to influence, participate in or change public policy making? Or is it simply that these individuals, and some healthcare professionals in particular, do not know how to access, influence and participate in the processes involved in the formulation and delivery of healthcare policy? If this is the case, educationalists are failing to stimulate interest or provide the necessary knowledge and skills that would empower healthcare professionals to be proactive and engage in health policy development and implementation.

The health and social care policy processes in relation to cancer and palliative care are particularly relevant at the moment, and all healthcare professionals involved in the delivery of care in these specialties need to heighten their awareness of public policy processes so that they become more active in policy making and politics, whether at a clinical, organisational, national or global level.

This puts the responsibility for improving healthcare professionals' political sophistication and knowledge acquisition in these topics firmly on the education-alists' shoulders.

Health and social care policy no longer remains the concern of government officials. In the UK in the twenty-first century there are numerous opportunities for many individuals and more specifically healthcare professionals to influence the future delivery of healthcare.

The fundamental aspects of policy making, interpretation, implementation and evaluation should be within the grasp of every healthcare professional, regardless of the country, culture or prevailing politics.

The word 'politics' has now entered the equation. Throughout this book the authors have maintained that certain topics, such as spirituality and sexuality in cancer and palliative care (*see* Chapters 16 and 17), are rarely discussed or taught formally in educational programmes. The general response from students and the reluctance of some educationalists to link health and social policy with politics demonstrate how this topic is often perceived as being distasteful, slightly contro-versial, and likely to generate strong emotions.

The symbiotic relationship between policy and politics does not lead to a natural dichotomy, as both paradigms are linked inextricably. To separate one from the other is virtually impossible, and when educationalists attempt to do this, the inevitable impact on the subject matter means that the contents can often become tedious, muted and lacklustre.

However, it is possible to deconstruct the various facets that contribute to politics, policy and policy making so that the different aspects can be incorporated into educational programmes by either an integrated approach or a topic-specific session as part of an ongoing course. Before paring down to this micro-perspective, it is essential to look at the relationship of policy, policy making and politics to cancer and palliative healthcare provision at a macro-level.

A macro-perspective encompasses the concept of healthcare policy 'global-isation' – a term that is increasingly used to note that boundaries between individ-uals, organisations, societies and nations are vanishing (International Federation of

Trading and Development Organisations, 1998). This infers the notion of a global network where there are common forces shaping the lives of practically every person on earth (Clifford, 2000). The notion of a global village expressed by Clifford (2000) highlights several concepts that are applicable to healthcare delivery and healthcare professionals. These are exemplified by common values such as humanness, caring and commitment to healthcare improvements. The erosion of international borders between many countries enables healthcare professionals to deliver care in virtually any country in the world. Consequently, there is a need to educate healthcare professionals who can function within this global scenario and who are capable of developing reciprocity and partnerships in the provision of healthcare. These healthcare professionals need to be fully conversant with international healthcare policies and politics. It is incumbent on all healthcare professionals to become aware of the social environment, economy, employment, civil unrest or war, poverty, crime levels, education, political regime in ascendance and the use of power and control in any country if they are to recognise the influences that such factors have on the health status of the people who live there (Slevin, 2000). This is a challenging task for healthcare educationalists, as the world stage is changing on an hourly basis. Cancer and the more explicitly palliative healthcare professionals have disseminated its ethos globally. This philosophy has transcended many barriers across the world, and where possible resources and expertise have been shared. Worldwide, 52 million people die each year, and approximately 1 in 10 of these deaths are due to cancer. However, each day millions of people suffer from other life-threatening illnesses, such as AIDS (Help the Hospices, 2006). Several of the countries involved in palliative care provision are resource poor, despite the overwhelming need for this type of care. There are many barriers to the implementation of palliative care for the dying. Some of the obstacles that need to be overcome include the following:

- non-availability of essential medicines
- minimal opportunities for training and support
- lack of resources to develop services and to train healthcare workers
- a history of long-standing wars and natural disasters.

Despite these impediments to the planning and delivery of palliative care globally, the principles of hospice and palliative care are proliferating. It is now estimated that hospice/palliative care initiatives exist or are in the process of being initiated in approximately 100 countries. The Help the Hospices website (Help the Hospices, 2006) provides information on the international provision of palliative care. A similar, clear and research-based website is www.eolc-observatory.net, where information about hospice and palliative care in an international context can be accessed. Relevant public health and policy data relating to hospice and palliative care services in 61 countries from around the world are readily available. This information is supplemented with material drawn from analysis of end-of-life issues, including historical, ethical and cultural perspectives (International Observatory on End-of-Life Care, 2006).

   A teaching strategy that this author has used for this aspect of global palliative care, which has proved popular with students and has developed their knowledge and understanding, will now be outlined. It is designed for post-registration oncology and palliative care nurses, but would be transferable to most disciplines and grades of staff. The group size should be between 6 and 12 students. A sample student preparation sheet is shown in Box 21.1.

Box 21.1   Global Palliative Care Documentary Worksheet

In 2 weeks' time you are going to make a short (15- to 20-minute) video about global palliative care.

You are to work as a team to make this video as creative and informative as possible.

The video is to inform the British public about the provision of palliative care globally.

Although you are going to look at global perspectives to highlight your news articles, you are to examine three countries in particular and make them featured items in your video presentation.

These countries are Russia, India and Uganda. (You can select others. It is useful to select countries that vary widely in terms of palliative care provision.)

You are to include in as innovative a way as possible the following information where possible:

- the main life-threatening illnesses in each of these countries
- the mortality rates
- the models of palliative care service provision that are implemented in these countries
- the barriers to palliative care service provision in these countries.

Include any other information that will help to make your stories as human and interesting as possible.

There is a map of the world and the flags of these countries are available. Please place the flags of the above three countries on the map.

Each member of the group is to participate in front of the camera.

You will have 50 minutes of preparation time prior to recording.

Remember that this is a real opportunity to extend your knowledge of how palliative care is delivered across the globe, and what influences or hinders the process.

A programme title and cast list would add interest. Good luck, and have fun.

Students are presented with a short reading list, but are asked to provide further evidence for their commentaries with a reference list. This type of session can be described as an informed and evidence-based debate. Despite an initial reluctance to stand in front of a video camera, most students gave feedback which suggested that they found the experience enjoyable. This type of activity promotes teamworking and student cohesion. Watching the completed video is also useful, as the teacher can stop it at relevant points and check the students' knowledge, or provide further information and allow the students to debrief.

Palliative care education has overcome many barriers in order to deliver care to the far corners of the globe. Advocates of palliative care would readily acknowledge that there are still countries that do not have a system of healthcare provision that would support the development of palliative care services. These states or countries will continue to be a challenge.

Although a full exploration of policy analysis is beyond the scope of this chapter, it is essential to outline some of the concepts in order to clarify its relationship to healthcare professionals' education.

Walt (1994, p. 5) contends that health policy is best understood by looking at both processes and power, which means exploring the role of the state (both nationally and internationally), the actors within it, the external forces influencing it and the mechanisms within the political system for participation in policy making.

Countries and states are no longer insular – they are interdependent in many ways. Consequently, health policy decisions may be dependent on external influences and the inherent economic stability. This interdependence was illustrated at the 2005 G8 Summit held at Gleneagles in Scotland, where all of the nations that attended agreed to make poverty history in Africa. The UK led the way by proposing to eradicate the national debt of those African states that owed money to the Treasury. These international influences impact not only at a fiscal level but also at the point of policy making and healthcare provision, the above-mentioned proliferation of palliative care services being a prime example of this.

After scrutinising the international influences that affect policy making, it is important to explore national issues. Specifically, it is crucial to gain an understanding of the nature of the intrinsic political system and to gauge whether participation is tolerated or not. Identifying to what extent a country is a liberal democracy or an authoritarian state is pivotal to health policy analysis, as this will determine the degree to which the population can participate in the governing or decision-making processes within their country. This allows the analyst to explore the sources of power that will influence policy. The final component in the analysis equation is the exploration of the people involved and how they may be exerting an influence on policy (Walt, 1994).

This investigation should not just include politicians and government leaders, but should also focus on where individuals stand as members of groups, institutions, political parties or professions. In certain circumstances these groups can be as powerful in changing policy as heads of states and their colleagues within the government. The policy process does not have a life of its own, but is dependent on the inherent players to give it expression (Walt, 1994).

This policy analysis framework has been developed further by Walt (1994), who describes policy making as having four (not necessarily linear) stages.

1 *Identifying the problem.* What is put on and kept off the agenda for discussion?
2 *Formulating the policy.* What is the policy? Who decides this?
3 *Implementing policy.* What resources are available? Who is to be involved? How will it be enforced?
4 *Evaluating policy.* Does it meet the objectives? What are the unintended consequences?

This outline is a simplification of the issues involved in policy analysis. However, policy becomes more multifaceted as the finer points and intricate details of policy are introduced and processes activated. This framework for analysis can be utilised whatever the complexity of the prevailing issues or potential policy developments, and it is a useful educational tool. Healthcare professionals and educationalists should certainly be key players in the policy processes.

This is not meant to imply that there is only one essential underlying framework which provides coherence to the policy processes. On the contrary, there are other ways of analysing policy processes, and these should be utilised wherever appropriate. The value of this framework in relation to cancer and palliative health and social care is that it can be applied readily to all oncology and palliative care policy processes.

Equally, this framework can be applied to almost all countries and states worldwide. However, whilst acknowledging that an internationalist perspective is important to understand health policy processes at a macro-level, this chapter will now focus on politics, policy, processes, people and education in a UK context.

In the UK there has been a shift towards inter-professional education (IPE), which has been defined as occurring when two or more professions learn with, from and about one another in order to facilitate collaboration in practice (Barr, 2006, p. 3).

Core IPE content outlined by the World Health Organization (WHO) in 1988 included competencies for effective teamwork. Further elements have been added which incorporate ethics, conflict resolution, leadership, professional roles, healthcare systems, and healthcare and social policy (Barr, 2006). It is unclear how much health and social policy is included as IPE in the pre-qualification curricula, or how it is delivered. Students of nursing, medicine, allied health and social work are entering the workforce poorly prepared for the teamwork in which they will be required to engage (McNair, 2005). Furthermore, knowledge and understanding of health policy development, implementation and analysis, which they will undoubtedly encounter in the clinical setting post qualification, has universal relevance. The relevance may be universal, but its interpretation, significance and level of accountability for each profession may be entirely different. This provides the educationalist with a unique opportunity to examine the policy drivers, the national and local contexts and the value systems of each individual. The exploration of individual value systems provides the opportunity to identify whether these values are congruent with their chosen profession and those of students from other professions within their educational group. The content of this session can facilitate a greater understanding of the constraints and responsibilities of other professions and have a positive influence on attitudes towards other healthcare professionals (Horder, 1995). Medical, nursing and allied health students are found to enter their specific healthcare professional courses with preconceived and stereotyped ideas about their own and other disciplines (Horsburgh *et al.*, 2001; Tunstall-Pedoe *et al.*, 2003). Negative stereotyping of other disciplines can lead to professional arrogance and hamper future effective collaborative relationships (Carpenter, 1995). Exposure to the value systems of other professions and the encouragement of open debate on current health and social policy issues would go a long way towards eradicating preconceived negative attitudes and professional exclusivity.

Policy sessions could facilitate the discovery of profession-specific codes of conduct, a specific body of knowledge and skills and core sets of ethical principles.

The timing of these sessions in each professional curriculum is crucial, as are the chosen methods of teaching. The most commonly used method for teaching IPE groups of pre-qualification students is generally the lecture (the commonest teaching strategy in adult education) (Bligh, 1998). It is used extensively for the education of large groups of students, where the teacher:student ratio can often be as high as 1:150. The lecture is purported to be a useful vehicle for the transmission of knowledge to students (Ausubel *et al.*, 1978), and it has a place as a teaching strategy for delivering knowledge and understanding of health and social policy. However, Johnson (2000) contends that health and social policy in the nursing curriculum can mean nothing more than a description of the content of recent government publications, to which might be added the barest of analyses (Johnson, 2000). This assumption is probably based on the lecture as a teaching method that is deemed effective for conveying information, but less effective for promoting thinking skills and the changing of attitudes (Quinn, 2000). A similar supposition can be transposed to the lecture format in the delivery of health and social policy teaching to IPE students – it is useful if it is succeeded by mixed small group teaching strategies. The lecture should be short (student attention declines after 20 minutes) (Quinn, 2000), and should include policy analysis frameworks such as that of Walt (1994) (*see* above). This provides the opportunity to discuss other policy analysis frameworks and paradigms, enabling the teacher to cover the background information from disparate sources and clarify confusing or conflicting concepts (Billings and Halstead, 2005). In the past, students have complained that is the concept of disparate notions in health and social policy education that has caused them to become bewildered and lose interest.

Small group work should follow the keynote lecture, preferably with a suitable delay to allow adequate student preparation for the small group work. Students can then take part in three small discussion groups that examine current policy topics which can be presented in the case study format. Billings and Halstead (2005) suggest that well-devised case studies/scenarios can stimulate critical thinking, associate the practical with the theoretical, and allow problem solving in a safe environment without putting patients at risk or harassing them. They can also engender peer interaction and elicit values and attitudes in a potentially non-threatening atmosphere. This facet is entirely reliant on the skills of facilitators.

Each small group discussion could look at a scenario that is relevant to one of the current national framework initiatives prevalent in the UK. It is important to ensure that the content matter is relevant, topical and within the reach of non- specialist groups. Yesterday's hot policy topic is today's dinosaur and will be of little or no interest to the very students whom you are trying to stimulate.

The following scenario is both relevant to oncology and topical at the time of writing. It may be of use for another two to three years before it becomes outdated. Students should be asked to read around the subject prior to the small group tutorial, and to prepare by using a framework. To assist clarification in this chapter, the Walt framework will be used.

The National Institute for Clinical Excellence (which covers England and Wales) said in draft guidance that Herceptin should be prescribed for women with early-stage breast cancer who could benefit from it. Final guidance was published in July 2006.

You should prepare using the concepts from the Walt (1994) policy analysis framework.

This preparation could be done using the format of questions and a list of potential references, although students should be encouraged to extend the literature search. Questions based on this framework can include any or all of the following.

- What are the international issues? (The manufacturers of the drug have an international perspective.)
- What are the national perspectives?
- Who are the key players in this scenario? Who has held the power and exerted the most influence?
- Has new policy been developed or old policy been changed and, if so, in what ways?
- What are the implications of this policy for clinical practice in your chosen profession?

The facilitation of this type of session benefits from a team teaching approach where each student discipline represented in the small group has an accompanying facilitator. When it works well, team teaching can provide greater stimulation and variety than the ordinary lecture, because each teacher can respond to the perspective of the others, affirm similarities between disciplines, and highlight any differences which can be supported by evidence and professional expertise. Pre-registration house officers (PRHOs), student nurses and pre-registration pharmacists are the groups involved in IPE at this author's academic institution. This type of IPE group work has been utilised before in the teaching of communication skills. Participants in these small group sessions evaluated them positively, emphasising that as a result of attending they had developed an increased awareness of others' roles (Kilminster *et al.*, 2004).

This type of team teaching requires a high degree of understanding and collaboration between the educators in order to overcome the exclusivity of their discipline, which may have become embedded in the subconscious from pre-qualification training (McNair, 2005).

Health service provision involves a variety of professions, and IPE can play a crucial part in developing an understanding of the politics and policy relationship. Despite the limited provision of IPE, healthcare professions still require discipline-specific training and education. It is widely recognised in the health service literature that the nursing profession delivers 80% of direct care (Beardshaw and Robinson, 1990). Nurses represent the largest single occupational group in the NHS, and their views need to be taken into account if modernisation is to occur (Hicks, 2000). In the UK, nurses' contribution to the policy process is not adequately documented or understood (Hewison, 2003). Similarly, the exact number of nurses involved in policy development and the extent to which they are politically aware is not known.

This lack of input from nursing on issues of political importance for health is not a new concern. Historically, nursing has lacked influence in policy formulation (Robinson, 1991). Throughout the last 20 years, the importance of policy as an issue for nursing has been an emerging area of discussion and debate (see, for example, Wilkinson, 1995; Meerabeau, 1996; Antrobus, 1997; Antrobus and Brown, 1997; Cheek and Gibson, 1997; Antrobus and Kitson, 1999; Hewison, 1999). This followed the ground-breaking work of White (1988). There has also been a reluctance among nurses to engage in the public policy arena, and West and Scott (2000) contend that this stems from a perceived lack of knowledge in such areas as political science and economics. Therefore the problem for educators is how to engage nurses in the province of health and social policy, become more politically aware and find inspirational ways of filling the gap in nursing knowledge. To address some of the prevailing issues with regard to this subject, the rest of this chapter will focus on nursing in the UK and its relationship with health and social policy, and the ramifications that this has for educationalists.

In the introduction to this chapter it was proposed that an incipient apathy had evolved in relation to voting and politics in the UK, and that perspective has been mirrored by nurses in their response to their profession and public policy involvement (Des Jardin, 2001).

In a recent survey of post-registration nurses entering degree courses that was undertaken by this author in the academic year 2005–6, exactly 50% of respondents stated that their reason for non-involvement was apathy.

This may be because of a lack of understanding or a mistaken belief that public policy has nothing to do with nursing (Maslin-Prothero and Masterson, 1998). However, this perception may be changing.

When the nurses in the above-mentioned survey were asked whether they avoided health and social policy teaching sessions, most of the respondents said that they did not. One student summed this up as follows: '[I] have avoided [them] in the past, but have found throughout my nursing career, issues re. health and social policy are relevant to many areas.'

When asked what deterred them from becoming more involved in health and social public policy, a range of answers were given, but these were eloquently summarised by one respondent:

> health and social policy sounds as if it is at a high level academically and so may prevent people with excellent knowledge, skills and expertise from taking part in policy teaching sessions and developments. It also implies that it does not apply to staff working at grass roots.

Many aspects of nursing are now being included in health policy arenas such as those determined by clinical effectiveness, quality and clinical governance agendas (Scott and West, 2001). Consequently, all healthcare professionals must develop broad health policy analysis skills so that they can at least understand political, social, economic and environmental theory (Adams, 2001).

Traditionally, nurses have viewed political involvement and behaviour as incompatible with the caring ethic. These tensions apply equally to other professions working in health and social care. Consequently, there will always be the potential for conflict between personal beliefs, professional values, organisational priorities and political ideologies. To counteract these tensions, students need to understand the worth of health and social policy reformation in the provision of care, and the benefits of political and policy involvement. This can only be achieved by assimilating health policy analysis and raising socio-political awareness early in their healthcare educational experience, and by the continued nurturing of their health policy consciousness throughout their careers (Whitehead, 2003). The current philosophy of developing socio-political roles later in their nursing career is restrictive, and the early recognition of nurses who have the qualities necessary to influence the nursing contribution to public policy making is essential. The RCN Political Leadership Programme, established in 2000, has concentrated on building confidence and skills to enable nurses to become more proactive in a national political arena (Antrobus and Kitson, 1999), although this programme has only been accessible to a minority of nurses, usually in senior management positions.

Davies (2004) exhorts nurses to explain what they do and to explain further the potential of nursing in service provision. Nursing needs to get its messages across to politicians and the public alike. This can only be achieved by working with the media and responding to policy consultations. It should not just be the business of a small number of individuals, but should also be the concern of those who are in the thick of clinical practice. Promoting the concepts of political awareness and policy engagement should be a core and accepted component of nursing practice and education (Davies 2004). Nursing is evolving with regard to its political activities and spheres of policy influence. It therefore needs to select representatives who can work alongside health policy experts and become generic health policy entrepreneurs, as well as developing careers in specific policy areas (Lavis and Sullivan, 2000). The cultivation of those students who demonstrate enthusiasm, commitment and insight is dependent on an educational system that delivers a broad range of health policy education.

Consequently, the integration of active health policy analysis and processes into educational curricula is essential if nurses are to assume a meaningful role in determining client care delivery systems (Taylor, 1995; De Witt and Carnell, 1999; Gebbie *et al.*, 2000). It is uncertain at present what the exact theoretical, political health policy content is in the current nursing curricula in the UK. One of the priorities in nursing education is to review current delivery of health and social policy. Clarification is needed to distinguish between establishments that provide tailor-made course and programmes that contain explicit policy themes throughout. These establishments may also differ in the level of active encouragement of the students with regard to policy involvement. This is particularly relevant in palliative care, where courses are often delivered in hospices and are subject to different internal and external influences and constraints. Nurse education should avoid the current situation where programmes with a political component concentrate on the descriptive elements of reports (Johnson, 2000), rather than contextualising them to contemporary clinical practice and exploring the drivers that initiated them originally.

There is an absence of literature that explores who teaches health and social policy. There is a debate as to who should deliver this education – whether it should be educationalists, policy analysts, politicians or lead clinicians. Surely the answer is to utilise those people who have the knowledge, skills and expertise necessary to deliver to the students, whatever their capability, and meet the required learning outcomes. As this debate continues, strategies need to be put in place to ensure the development of political acumen and policy analysis skills of healthcare professionals. A range of diverse activities is crucial in the delivery of health policy teaching. When planning and undertaking a health policy session, there are some key factors that this author considers. As a simple tool, the mnemonic REPACKED has been found to be of use, and those sessions in which this mnemonic has been applied have generally been positively evaluated.

- Relevant. Is the content of this session relevant to this group's sphere of practice? How can I funnel the macro-policy down to existing practice?
- Engage. What strategies do I need to employ in order to make students engage with policy analysis and processes?
- Political awareness. How can I increase students' awareness in a stimulating way without imprinting my own political values?

- Activities. What educational activities will develop their knowledge and understanding and ensure their attention?
- Communicate. Who will be the best person to deliver the session? (Myself, another healthcare tutor, or an acknowledged expert in that field.)
- Knowledge and understanding. What is the level of the students' existing knowledge and understanding? What do they need to know in order to achieve the learning outcomes?
- Evaluation. Ensure that the groups have an opportunity to evaluate the session and provide feedback. Mediocre sessions have improved and been adapted in the light of evaluation. Students can generate some extremely useful ideas for improving the session.
- Discussion time. It is important that this is built into delivery time. Students are rarely encouraged to express political opinions, and this gives them an opportunity to do so in a safe, non-threatening environment.

Hostad (2004) outlines the qualities and skills of effective cancer and palliative care teachers. Passion is deemed to be a core quality for delivering this form of education. Likewise, a passion for health policy education is crucial. The lecturer's disinterest is readily transmitted to students, and the potential for apathy thus perpetuated. Sessions can be made relevant to the students' particular discipline, background or specialty. In cancer and palliative care there are many policy opportunities for utilising group work. For example, a group of registered oncology nurses can be asked to look at the safe administration and delivery of chemotherapy in a new outreach primary care centre. They can be asked to prepare for the discussion by looking at the following questions. Why was the policy written (inputs and drivers)? How will it be implemented (processes)? Who are the stakeholders? How will they be consulted? How will the service be implemented? How will this service initiative impact on their clinical practice (outcomes)? There are other examples of policy implementation in the oncology and palliative care setting, and a repertoire of case studies can be developed to match the needs of each individual group.

Key points

- Health policy decisions can impact globally as well as at a national and local level.
- Applying policy analysis frameworks can assist educationalists in enabling students to make sense of the policy arena.
- Nursing is slowly emerging from its former position of non-involvement to take its place alongside other professions in the construction of healthcare policy, but it still needs to extend its realms of influence further.
- The delivery of healthcare policy education in the UK urgently needs to be reviewed.
- There is a place for inter-professional teaching in the delivery of health and social policy education.
- Teachers of health policy need to enthuse and be passionate about the topic in order to engage the students' interest.
- Assessment of the students' level of knowledge and understanding is crucial in order to tailor the mode of education delivery to their needs.

Conclusion

Health policy activity is no longer the exclusive domain of medicine, and other healthcare professions need to be conversant with its attributes and processes. Public health professionals who understand the political dimensions of healthcare policy can influence future healthcare provision and better anticipate the opportunities and constraints that government initiatives may produce. To ensure that healthcare professionals have gained this policy wisdom and political sophistication, whether it is in oncology, palliative care or other healthcare specialties, educationalists need to develop programmes that engage students proactively in the policy arena. When this outcome has been achieved, it may be true to say that health policy education is universally relevant, and that it is no longer studiously avoided, but positively embraced.

Implications for the reader's own practice

1 What aspects of healthcare policy education do you currently deliver?
2 How do you relate your policy teaching to clinical practice?
3 What steps do you need to take to develop an inter-professional approach to health policy education?
4 Who is available in your area with specialist knowledge whom you could call upon to help to deliver healthcare policy education?
5 How could you use the Walt model of policy analysis and the Foyle mnemonic REPACKED to alter your teaching strategies?
6 What do you need to do to develop your political awareness?
7 How does your institution involve itself in global policy issues?

References

Adams L. The role of health authorities in the promotion of health. In: Scriven A, Orme J, editors. *Health Promotion: professional perspectives.* 2nd ed. Basingstoke: Palgrave; 2001. pp. 35–42.

Antrobus S. An analysis of nursing in context: the effects of current health policy. *J Adv Nurs.* 1997; **25:** 447–53.

Antrobus S, Brown S. The impact of the commissioning agenda upon nursing practice: a proactive approach to influencing health policy. *J Adv Nurs.* 1997; **25:** 309–15.

Antrobus S, Kitson S. Nursing leadership: influencing and shaping policy and nursing practice. *J Adv Nurs.* 1999; **29:** 746–53.

Ausubel D, Novak I, Hanesian H. *Educational Psychology: a cognitive view.* New York: Holt, Rinehart and Winston; 1978.

Barr H. *Interprofessional Education, 1997–2000: a review.* UK Centre for the Advancement of Interprofessional Education (CAIPE); www.caipe.org.uk (accessed 2 July 2006).

BBC News; www.bbcnews.co.uk (accessed 6 May 2005).

Beardshaw V, Robinson K. *New for Old? Prospects for Nursing in the 1990s. Research Report No. 8.* London: King's Fund Institute; 1990.

Billings DM, Halstead JA. *Teaching in Nursing. A guide for faculty.* 2nd ed. Philadelphia, PA: WB Saunders; 2005.

Bligh D. *What's the Use of Lectures?* 5th ed. Bristol: Intellect Books; 1998.

Carpenter J. Doctors and nurses: stereotypes and stereotype change in interprofessional education. *J Interprof Care*. 1995; **9**: 151–61.

Cheek J, Gibson T. Policy matters: critical policy analysis and nursing. *J Adv Nurs*. 1997; **25**: 668–72.

Clifford C. International politics and nursing education: power and control. *Nurse Educ Today*. 2000; **20**: 4–9.

Davies C. Political leadership and the politics of nursing. *J Nurs Manage*. 2004; **12**: 235–41.

Des Jardin K. Political involvement in nursing – politics, ethics and strategic action. *AORN J*. 2001; **74**: 613–30.

De Witt R, Carnell J. Public health nursing. In: Griffiths S, Hunter DJ, editors. *Perspectives in Public Health*. Oxford: Radcliffe Medical Press; 1999. pp. 235–49.

Gebbie KM, Wakefield M, Kerfoot K. Nursing and health policy. *J Nurs Scholarship*. 2000; **32**: 307–15.

Help the Hospices. www.helpthehospices.org.uk (accessed 16 June 2006).

Hewison A. The new public management and the new nursing: related by rhetoric? Some reflections on the policy process and nursing. *J Adv Nurs*. 1999; **29**: 1377–84.

Hewison A. Modernizing the British National Health Service (NHS) – some ideological and policy considerations: a commentary and application. *J Nurs Manage*. 2003; **11**: 91–7.

Hicks C. Of rites, research and reforms: a systems perspective on the maintenance of clinical nursing rituals. In: Hennessy D, Spurgeon P, editors. *Health Policy and Nursing: influence, development and impact*. Basingstoke: Macmillan Publishers Ltd; 2000. pp. 176–89.

Horder J. Interprofessional education for primary health and community care: present state and future needs. In: Soothill I, McKay I, editors. *Interprofessional Relations in Health Care*. London: Arnold; 1995.

Horsburgh M, Lamdin R, Williamson E. Multiprofessional learning: the attitudes of medical, nursing and pharmacy students to shared learning. *Med Educ*. 2001; **35**: 876–83.

Hostad J. An overview of hospice education. In: Foyle L, Hostad J, editors. *Delivering Cancer and Palliative Care Education*. Oxford: Radcliffe Publishing; 2004.

International Federation of Trading and Development Organisations (IFTDO). IFTDO and ISPI dialogue on the challenges of globalisation. *IFTDO News*. 1998; **2**: 2–4.

International Observatory on End-of-Life Care; 2006. www.eolc-observatory.net

Johnson M. International politics and nursing education: power and control – a response. *Nurse Educ Today*. 2000; **20**: 10–11.

Kilminster S, Hale C, Lascelles M *et al*. Learning for real life: patient-focused interprofessional workshops offer added value. *Med Educ*. 2004; **38**: 717–26.

Lavis JN, Sullivan TJ. The state as a setting. In: Poland BD, Green LW, Rootman I, editors. *Settings for Health Promotion: linking theory and practice*. London: Sage Publications; 2000. pp. 175–99.

Maslin-Prothero S, Masterson A. Continuing care: developing a policy analysis for nursing. *J Adv Nurs*. 1998; **28**(3): 548–53.

McNair R. The case for educating health care students in professionalism as the core content of interprofessional education. *Med Educ*. 2005; **39**: 456–66.

Meerabeau L. Managing policy research in nursing. *J Adv Nurs*. 1996; **24**: 633–9.

Quinn F. *Principles and Practice of Nurse Education*. 4th ed. Cheltenham: Stanley Thornes; 2000.

Robinson J. Introduction: beginning the study of nursing policy. In: Robinson J, Gray A, Elkan R, editors. *Policy Issues in Nursing*. Milton Keynes: Open University Press; 1991. pp. 1–8.

Scott C, West E. Nursing in the public sphere: health policy research in a changing world. *J Adv Nurs*. 2001; **33**: 387–95.

Slevin E. International politics and nursing education: power and control. A response to Clifford. *Nurse Educ Today*. 2000; **20**: 15–16.

Taylor G. Politics and nursing: an elective experience. *J Adv Nurs.* 1995; **21:** 1180–85.

Tunstall-Pedoe S, Rink E, Hilton S. Student attitudes to undergraduate interprofessional education. *J Interprof Care.* 2003; **17:** 161–72.

Walt G. *Health Policy: an introduction to process and power.* London: Zed Books; 1994.

West E, Scott C. Nursing in the public sphere: breaching the boundary between research and policy. *J Adv Nurs.* 2000; **32:** 817–24.

White R. The influence of nursing in the politics of health. In: White R, editor. *Political Issues in Nursing: past, present and future. Volume 3.* Chichester: John Wiley & Sons; 1988. pp. 15–31.

Whitehead D. The health-promoting nurse as a health policy career expert and entrepreneur. *Nurse Educ Today.* 2003; **23:** 585–92.

Wilkinson M. Love is not a marketable commodity: new public management in the British National Health Service. *J Adv Nurs.* 1995; **21:** 980–87.

World Health Organization (WHO). *Learning to Work Together for Health. Report of a WHO Study Group on Multiprofessional Education of Health Personnel: the team approach.* Technical Report No. 769. Geneva: World Health Organization; 1988.

Further reading

- Foyle L, Hostad J. *Delivering Cancer and Palliative Care Education.* Oxford: Radcliffe Publishing; 2004.
- Walt G. *Health Policy: an introduction to process and power.* London: Zed Books; 1994.

Useful websites

- BBC News; www.bbcnews.co.uk
- Centre for the Advancement of Inter-Professional Education (CAIPE); www.caipe.org.uk
- Department of Health; www.dh.gov.uk
- Help the Hospices; www.helpthehospices.org.uk
- International Observatory on End-of-Life Care; www.eolc-observatory.net
- National Association for Palliative Care Educators; www.pceig.org.uk
- National Council for Palliative Care; www.ncpc.org.uk
- National Institute for Clinical Excellence (NICE); www.nice.org.uk

Index

action learning 24
Agenda for Change (DoH 2004) 18–19
alternative therapies *see* complementary
    therapies
art and spiritual care 191
audits, as educational tool 89

benchmarking 77–8
bereavement
    and learning disability 154–5
    and young people 175–7
A Billion Seconds (video) 156, 159
black and ethnic minorities, information
    needs 115
Bland, Tony 101
BMT (bone-marrow transplantation)
    programmes 49
body image issues 204
Body Image (Price) 204
bone-marrow transplantation (BMT)
    programmes 49
breaking bad news
    ethical issues 99–100
    to learning-disabled patients 152–3
bulletin boards 92

Calman–Hine Report (1995) 38
Cancer Care Alliance 42
cancer care education
    global perspectives 262–4
    key teaching areas 128
    for paediatric care 137–43
    policy making and politics 260–71
    pre-registration 127–31
    see also individual disciplines; training and
        education
Cancer Networks, on chemotherapy
    education 42–3
cancer pain education 70–82
    background 70–1
    impact of national initiatives 80–1
    implications for practice 82
    importance and need 71–2
    international initiatives 80–1
    methods in clinical settings 75–8
    methods in educational settings 78–80
    multi-professional 74–5
    pre-registration 73

    post-registration 73–4
    for patients 78
    timing considerations 72–3
    use of benchmarking 77–8
    use of guidelines 76–7
    use of structured home visits 79–80
Cancer Pain Objective Structured Clinical
    Examination (OSCE) 78–9
Cancer Pain Relief (WHO 1986/1996)
    70–1
Cancer Research UK 241
Cancer Services Users Information Project
    (Spencer-Grey 2005) 110–12
Cancer Ward (Solzhenitsyn) 203
cancers
    incidence predictions 71
    survival rates 252
care homes *see* nursing homes and palliative
    care education
case-based teaching 25
    cancer pain management 80
    symptom management 91–2
CD-ROMs, cancer pain education 80
chemotherapeutic drugs
    administration risks 40
    settings for administration 40–1
chemotherapy care 37–46
    background and recent changes 37–9
    current training requirements 38–9
    education requirements 41–3
    guidelines and standards 38–9
    home nursing responsibilities 41
    implications for practice 46
    primary care training needs 41–2
    settings 40–1
Childhood Bereavement Network 175–6,
    177
The Children Act-2004 141
clinical decision support systems 88
clinical education *see* training and education
clinical guidelines *see* guidelines
clinical simulation centres 4–6
Cochrane Collaboration 222
collaborative models (education) 55
communication issues
    language barriers 115
    with learning-disabled patients 150,
        152–3

competencies
  background to educational use 14
  concepts and definitions 15–16
  domains 16–17
  for chemotherapy care 40, 42
  further developments 20–1
  implications for practice 21
  importance 14–15
  and models of clinical education 55
  and pay scales 18–19
  use in cancer care education 14, 17–21,
    42
  use in information development
    education 112
complementary therapies 220–32
  background trends 221
  definitions 221–2
  key issues and considerations 228–30
  models and approaches 222–4
  patient benefits 225–6, 228–9
  research evidence 226–7
  role of learning and investigations
    224–8, 229–31
  role of literature 235–6
  use of relaxation therapies 227–8
computer simulators see high-fidelity patient
    simulators
computer-based learning see e-learning
confidentiality issues, group work 201
consent issues, and ethics education 102–3
Core Competency Framework (Royal College of
    Nursing 2003) 14
Core Curriculum for Professional Education in
    Pain (IASP 1997) 71
Council of Europe 63–4, 68
The Counsellor's Workbook (McLeod) 180
crisis avoidance, training methods 8
critical analysis, of clinical evidence 116
cultural issues, information needs 115
cytotoxic agents see chemotherapeutic drugs

debriefing, group-mediated 4, 8
decision support systems see clinical decision
    support systems
descriptive models (educational) 54
developmental models (education) 55
Disability Distress Assessment Tool
    (DisDAT) 153–4
DISCERN 117
discussion groups 92
DisDAT see Disability Distress Assessment
    Tool

district nurses, role in chemotherapy
    care 41
Down's syndrome 150, 156
dyslexia, information needs 114

e-learning
  challenges 44
  and chemotherapy education 43–5
ecomaps 174
Edmonton Assessment Scale 88
education see training and education
educators, skills needed 270
English National Board (ENB)
  courses 138–42
  on sexual health education 202
ethical theories 98–100
ethics education 96–105
  aims and purpose 97–8
  content and subject matter 98
  implications for practice 105
  inter-professional learning 103–4
  and reflective learning strategies 103
  teacher profiles 104–5
  teaching legal issues 100–1
  teaching methods 102–3
  teaching theories 98–100
ethnic minorities, information needs 115
European Association of Palliative Care
    (EAPC)
  on nurse education 18, 131–3
  on pain management education 74–5
European Blood and Marrow
    Transplantation (EBMT) 49
European Oncology Nursing Society
    (EONS)
  curriculum guidance 129
  curriculum standards 139
euthanasia, legal and ethical
    considerations 100–1
evidence-based healthcare, evaluating
    skills 116
experiential learning 90
  key elements 178

facilitators, and problem-based
    learning 25–6
family care education 169–82
  approaches and systems theory 170–1
  background 169–70
  belief systems and organisation
    principles 171–2
  clinical assessments 172–6

genograms 172–6
implications for practice 182
methods of teaching 178–81
organisation of teaching 176–8
teaching evaluations 181–2
workshop planning 179–82
family trees 172–6
First Aid Kit (Sunderland and
Engleheart) 181
Fitness for Practice Report (UKCC for Nursing,
Midwifery and Health Visiting
1999) 125–6, 128
focus groups 78, 119
Foundation for the Accreditation of Cellular
Therapy (FACT) 48–9
A Framework for Adult Cancer Nursing
(RCN 2003) 54, 129

gay and lesbian relationships 207–9
genograms 172–6
global perspectives on palliative care 262–4
group work
debriefing sessions 4
ground rules 201–2
groups, and problem-based learning 26–7
*A Guide to the Development of Children's
Palliative Care Services* (ACT/RCPCH
2003) 143
guided imagery 227–8
guidelines
dissemination 76–7
evaluation 116
for pain management 76–7
for symptom management 88–9

haematological oncology 48–59
health and social policy education 260–71
background and global influences 260–3
current drivers for change 261–4
policy making and healthcare
education 264–70
strategies and techniques 269–70
high-fidelity patient simulators
background and history 1–3
benefits and drawbacks 3–4
for cancers 6–7
clinical centres 4–6
costs 4
educational value and effectiveness
8–10
future developments 10–11
implications for practice 11

multi-professional applications 7–8
paediatric uses 10
portable versions 11
holism 222–4
home care, chemotherapy
administration 41
home visits, education opportunities 79–80
homosexuality 207–9
hospices, development of training
packages 28–9
Hostad, J 177, 178, 198, 202–3, 270
human actors 3

*Improving Supportive Care for Adults with
Cancer* (NICE 2004) 176–7, 237
*Improving Supportive and Palliative Care for
Adults with Cancer* (DoH 2004)
148–9
individual performance reviews (IPRs),
and competencies 20
information development and delivery
education 66, 107–22
background 107–8
content of courses 110–12
identifying local needs 118
impact of policy initiatives 113–14
implications for practice 122
key teaching requirements 110–11
mandatory attendance 112–13
methods of educating staff 111–13
methods of evaluation 118–19
overview 120–1
patient characteristics and needs
114–15
principles of learning 109–10
quality issues 115–18
role of educator 113
teaching demographics and
epidemiology 114–15
terminology and language issues
114–15, 117
use with pain management 72
use of technologies 112
informed consent *see* consent issues
integration models (education) 54–5
inter-professional education (IPE) 265–7
see also multi-professional education
interactive process models (education) 55
International Council of Nurses (ICN), on
specialisation 137
International Society for Cellular Therapy
(ICST) 48–9

JACIE *see* Joint Accreditation Committee of
        ISCT and EBMT
Joint Accreditation Committee of ISCT and
        EBMT (JACIE) 48–9
    standards 49–50
journal-keeping, and spiritual
        education 191–2

Knowledge and Skills Framework (KSF)
        (DoH 2004) 52, 55, 59, 112

language use, information delivery
        considerations 114–15
Last Acts 131
learning disability and palliative care
        education 148–57
    background and importance 148–50
    characteristic needs 149–50
    communication issues 152–3
    controversial issues 156
    disease profiles 150
    evidence of good practice 155–6
    future developments 156
    implications for practice 157
    information needs 114
    loss and bereavement issues 154–5
    multi-professional applications 150–2
    particular issues and concerns 152–5
    symptom control issues 153–4
learning processes
    key principles 109–10
    post-registration 51–3
    role of experience 53
learning styles 56
lecture formats 43
legal issues, and ethics education 100–1
'Link trainers' 1
literacy 114, 117
literacy screening tools 117
literature and spiritual care 191
Liverpool Integrated Care Pathway
        (LCP) 88–9
Loss and Learning Disability (Blackman) 154

Macmillan Cancer Relief 163–4
Making a Difference (DoH 1999) 128–9
Manual of Cancer Services (DoH 2004) 38–9
Manual of Cancer Services Standards
        (DoH 2000) 38
Marie Curie Cancer Care
    on protocol and policy development 212
    on staff competencies 189

massage therapies 224–5
medication administration, chemotherapy
        agents 40
Mexborough Hospital 4–6
Mini Clinical Evaluation Exercise
        (Mini-CEX) 92
models of clinical education 53–6
Montagu Clinical Simulation Centre 4–10
'mourning' tasks (Worden) 155
multi-professional education
    definitions 63
    degree-level 63, 64
    importance and need 63–6
    and learning objectives 67
    use with ethics teaching 103–4
    use with radiotherapy education 64–8
    use in rehabilitation 243–4
    use with symptom management
        education 91–2
    see also inter-professional education (IPE)

National Audit Office 252
National Council for Hospices and Specialist
        Palliative Care Services 239, 248–9
National Institute for Clinical Excellence
        (NICE)
    on cancer care education 18, 64
    on children's cancer services 142
    on evaluating clinical evidence 116
    on rehabilitation 237
    on spiritual care 189
National Service Frameworks, for Children,
        Young People and Maternity Services
        (DoH 2005) 141–2
The NHS Cancer Plan (DoH 2000) 14, 64, 66,
        128, 130
NHS Toolkit 116
No – You Don't Know How We Feel!
        (video) 175–6
'novice to expert' (Benner) 15–16, 52–3
NSFs *see* National Service Frameworks
nurse education *see* training and education
nurse specialists, cancer care 42
The Nursing Contribution to Cancer Care
        (DoH 2000) 128–9
nursing homes and palliative care
        education 160–7
    background and policy directions 160–1
    benefits of education 162
    costs 162
    current provisions and
        recommendations 162–4

learning needs assessments 165
legislation issues 164
projects and initiatives 163
resource opportunities 165–6
staff turnover issues 164
teaching packages 164
tools and techniques 165–6
Nursing and Midwifery Council (NMC), on standards in nursing 142

OSCE *see* Cancer Pain Objective Structured Clinical Examination

paediatric oncology education 136–46
background and early developments 136–8
current state 138–41
future directions 143–6
key policy influences 141–3
masters programmes 145
in palliative care 143
Paediatric Oncology Nurse Educators (PONE) group 138–9, 145
paediatric oncology outreach nurses (POONs) 144
pain link groups 75–6
pain management
guidelines 70–1, 76–7
national and international initiatives 80–1
and patient education 78
use of benchmarking 77–8
use of clinical guidelines 76–7
see also cancer pain education
palliative care education
for children and young peoples care 143–5
global perspectives 262–4
policy making and politics 260–71
pre-registration 131–3
see also cancer care education; training and education
patient education, pain management 78
patient information leaflets 66
patient involvement 255–6
Picker Institute for Europe 119
PLISSIT assessment tool 209–11
policy analysis frameworks (Walt) 264–5
A Policy Framework for Commissioning Cancer Services (Calman and Hine 1995) 38, 66, 127

politics and policy making 261–5
frameworks for understanding 264–5
international perspectives 262–4
PONE group *see* Paediatric Oncology Nurse Educators (PONE) group
POONs *see* paediatric oncology outreach nurses
Positive Approaches to Palliative Care (Jones and Tuffrey-Wijne) 155
post-registration training
cf. pre-registration 51–3
family work courses 177
pre-registration training 125–34
background 125–6
cf. post-registration 51–3
in cancer care 127–31
in palliative care 131–3
Pretty, Dianne 101
problem-based learning (PBL) 24–35
concepts and definitions 24–7
criticisms 31
future developments 33–4
and palliative care 27–30
processes involved 27
strengths and effectiveness 30–3
for symptom management education 91–2
training packages 28–9
use of facilitators 25–6
use of group work 26–7
web-based technologies 33–4
Producing Patient Information (Duman 2003) 117
profiling service users 114
psychological support needs 176–7
psychoneuroimmunology (PNI) 228

Quality Education for Quality Care (RCN 2002) 125
quality issues
challenges 57
in patient information development 116–18
quality of life assessment tools 257
quality of life issues, and surviving cancer 252–3

race, and information needs 115
race impact assessments 116
radiographers, roles 65–6
radiotherapy education 62–8
multi-professional approaches 64–8

readability assessment tools 117
Recommendations for Nursing Practice in Pain Management (Pain Society 2002) 71
'reflecting upon experience' (Dewey) 53
reflection
    and family care education 178
    and learning needs (10 'Cs' – Johns) 256
    and problem-based learning 27–8
    and spiritual education 192
reflective practices 27–8, 53, 90–1
reflexology 224–5
rehabilitation 236–49
    with advanced illnesses 238–9
    aims and goals 238–9
    background and policies 236–7
    current approaches 237–9
    effectiveness evaluations 239–42
    essential components 237
    implications for practice 248–9
    integration of services 244–5
    multi-disciplinary education 243–4
    responding to uncertainties 246
    role of education 242–3
    survival rates 237–8
    teaching strategies 242–3
    see also surviving cancer
relationship issues 204–6
relaxation therapies 227–8
REPACKED mnemonic 269–70
resource management, training methods 8
role modelling 80, 165–6
role play, and family care education 180
Royal College of Nursing, on pre-registration cancer care education 127–8, 130
Royal Marsden NHS Trust, pain management benchmarking 77

St Michael's Hospice (Hereford) 28
Saunders, Dame Cicely 236
Schon, D 16–17, 53, 193
SCIM *see* Structured Clinical Instruction Module
The Scope of Professional Practice (UKCC for Nursing, Midwifery and Health Visiting 1992) 137–8
sculpting techniques, and family care education 180–1
self-help approaches 228–9
sexual health and sexuality 197–216
    attitudes and beliefs 198–9
    definitions 199–200

educational approaches 202–4
    group work ground rules 201–2
    implications for practice 216
    issues of body image 204
    love and relationships 204–6
    organisation policies and protocols 211–12
    sexual orientation issues 207–9
    supervision issues 212–15
    support needs assessments 209–11
sexual orientation issues 207–9
Sexualities in Health and Social Care (Wilton) 209
'Sim One' 2
simulation techniques *see* high-fidelity patient simulators; human actors
SMOG Formula (McLaughlin) 117
social work training, and family care education 176
Spencer-Grey, SA 108, 110, 112, 116–19, 121, 228
spirituality 185–95
    definitions 186–7
    identifying educators 193–4
    as a 'journey' 187–8
    literature and art-based approaches 191–3
    models 192
    professional caregiver roles 188–9
    role of education 188
    skills required 189–90
Standards of Proficiency for Pre-Registration Nursing Education (Nursing and Midwifery Council 2004) 126, 129
Structured Clinical Instruction Module (SCIM), cancer pain 79
suicide attempts 240
    legal and ethical considerations 100–1
supervision, and models of clinical education 55
surviving cancer 251–8
    epidemiological data 252
    implications for practice 258
    late effects 253–4
    quality of life issues 252–3
    teaching strategies 254–7
    see also rehabilitation
symptom management 85–94
    attitudes towards 86
    background 85–6
    challenges 86–7

methods of education 89–93
timing considerations 87–9

Tavistock Clinic 177
teacher–manager model (education) 56
teachers, skills needed 270
therapeutic radiographers 65–6
time constraints 57
TNA *see* training needs analysis (TNA)
total quality management (TQM) 49
touch therapies 224–5, 229
TQM *see* total quality management
training and education
    general goals 51
    in chemotherapy care 37–46
    in complementary therapies 220–32
    in family care 169–82
    in haematological oncology 49–59
    in information management 107–22
    in learning disability care 148–57
    in nursing home care 160–7
    in paediatric care 136–46
    in pain management 70–82
    in rehabilitation and survivor care
        236–58
    in sexual health care 197–216
    in spiritual care 185–95
    in symptom management 85–94
    international perspectives 262–4
    local small-scale initiatives 18
    models 53–6

pre- cf. post-registration differences
    51–3
problems and challenges 57
role of politics and policy making 260–71
skills needed for teaching 270
use of competencies 13–21, 42
use of high-fidelity simulation 6–11
use of problem-based learning
    techniques 24–35
web links 21
training needs analysis (TNA) 53
transactional analysis, and sexuality
    education 211
trigonal model of clinical education
    (Farmer and Farmer) 54
truth-telling 99–100

undergraduate education, 'cancer care'
    degrees 63
user involvement 255–6

Valuing People (DoH 2001) 149

When My Dad Died (West) 156
World Health Organization
    on pain management education 70–1,
        73–4
    on sexual health 199

You'll Always Remember Them (video)
    176